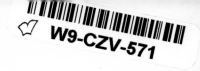

COMPREHENSIVE CARDIAC CARE

A text for nurses, physicians, and other health practitioners

COMPREHENSIVE CARDIAC CARE

A text for nurses, physicians, and other health practitioners

KATHLEEN G. ANDREOLI, R.N., B.S.N., M.S.N.

Associate Professor of Nursing, School of Nursing; Associate Professor of Medicine
in Nursing, Department of Medicine; Associate Professor, Department of Public
Health, University of Alabama Medical Center, Birmingham, Alabama

VIRGINIA HUNN FOWKES, R.N., B.S.N.

Lecturer, Departments of Surgery and Family, Preventive,
and Community Medicine; Director, Primary Care Associate Program,
Stanford University Medical Center,
Stanford, California

DOUGLAS P. ZIPES, M.D.

Professor of Medicine; Director of Cardiovascular Research,
and Senior Research Associate, Krannert Institute of Cardiology,
Indiana University School of Medicine,
Indianapolis, Indiana

ANDREW G. WALLACE, M.D.

Walter Kempner Professor of Medicine; Chief,
Division of Cardiology; and Assistant Professor of Physiology,
Duke University Medical Center,
Durham, North Carolina

FOURTH EDITION
with **699** illustrations

The C. V. Mosby Company

ST. LOUIS • TORONTO • LONDON   1979

FOURTH EDITION

Copyright © 1979 by The C. V. Mosby Company

All rights reserved. No part of this book may be reproduced in any manner without written permission of the publisher.

Previous editions copyrighted 1968, 1971, 1975

Printed in the United States of America

The C. V. Mosby Company
11830 Westline Industrial Drive, St. Louis, Missouri 63141

Library of Congress Cataloging in Publication Data

Main entry under title:

Comprehensive cardiac care.

Includes bibliographies and index.
1. Cardiovascular disease nursing. 2. Coronary care units. I. Andreoli, Kathleen G.
RC674.C65 1979   616.1'2'0024613   78-9905
ISBN 0-8016-0256-4

C/VH/VH 9 8 7 6 5 4 3 2 1   03/B/313

PREFACE

Advances in cardiac research and technology, coupled with new approaches in management, continually effect changes in patient care. The adequate reflection of this progress is the mission of the fourth edition of *Comprehensive Cardiac Care*. Accordingly, all chapters in this new edition have been revised and updated, and in some cases they have been expanded. As with previous editions, the goals of prevention and early rehabilitation of the patient are emphasized. Furthermore, the book continues to serve as a basic text for all health professionals participating in the care of patients with coronary artery disease.

The fundamental aspects of the anatomy and physiology of the heart remain the focus of Chapter 1. Chapter 2 presents the common clinical syndromes resulting from coronary artery disease, with considerable revision in the section on risk factors. The continued intent of Chapter 3 is to focus on the data collection process as it pertains to the patient's cardiovascular status. In order to bring a more comprehensive approach to this section, the content has been expanded in the sections on patient interview, physical examination, and common laboratory and physiological tests specifically for individuals with coronary artery disease. Additionally, twelve new figures appear in this chapter to reinforce the presentation. New content in Chapter 4 includes current approaches to the management of patients with myocardial infarction with new information about vasodilators. Because the existing format for Chapter 5 has served our readers well, the organization of this section remains essentially the same, with sequential development of the basic principles of electrocardiography preceding information on vector analysis and electrocardiographic diagnosis of common heart disorders. Chapter 6 reflects suggestions from our readers in that all electrocardiogram tracings have been enlarged to facilitate examination and study. The visual format continues to provide two examples of all arrhythmias discussed, with a self-test section on 12-lead electrocardiograms and arrhythmia tracings at the end of the chapter. Finally, data on the significance and therapy of the arrhythmias have been updated.

Chapter 7, concerning cardiac pacemakers, has had the benefit of review and update on current pacemaker therapy by Dr. John W. Fitzgerald, Assistant Professor of Medicine, Stanford University School of Medicine. Chapter 8 represents a significant revision by three contributing authors: Donna J. Rogers, R.N., M.S.N., Assistant Professor of Nursing; Martha E. Branyon, R.N., M.S.N., Associate Professor of Nursing; and Marguerite R. Kinney, R.N., D.N.Sc., Associate Professor of Nursing, all from the University of Alabama School of Nursing in Birmingham. This chapter has traditionally addressed the care of the patient with myocardial infarction in a sequential fashion, beginning with admission to the cardiac care unit and extending through the period of rehabilitation. Special attention has been given to problems that may be encountered in the acute, intermediate, and posthospitalization stages of illness, with practical approaches toward their resolution. In addition, the use of new technology in patient care is included.

Appendix A has been updated and expanded to include a section on investigational or experimental drugs, and Appendix B continues to focus on the differential diagnosis of chest pain.

To all who assisted in the preparation of this book we extend our thanks. We are especially grateful to the contributing authors, typists, and illustrators. A very special thanks to you, our readers, for your thoughtful suggestions and continued support, which have made this publication a pleasant experience over the past decade.

Kathleen G. Andreoli
Virginia Hunn Fowkes
Douglas P. Zipes
Andrew G. Wallace

CONTENTS

Donna J. Rogers, R.N., M.S.N.
Martha E. Branyon, R.N., M.S.N.
Marguerite R. Kinney, R.N., D.N.Sc.

COMPREHENSIVE CARDIAC CARE

A text for nurses, physicians, and other health practitioners

CHAPTER ONE

ANATOMY AND PHYSIOLOGY OF THE HEART

This chapter reviews very briefly the anatomy and physiology of the heart. It is not intended to be a detailed discussion, but merely to serve as a general background for the material to follow. More complete consideration of the subject can be found in textbooks of anatomy and physiology.

The major physiologic roles of the circulatory system are to deliver oxygen and other essential substrates to the tissues of the body and to remove carbon dioxide and other products of cellular metabolism. Many of the substances carried to and from the tissues are simply dissolved in plasma, and their transport depends solely on the volume of flow. In the case of oxygen and carbon dioxide, however, which are transported almost entirely by red blood cells, the characteristics of the hemoglobin association-dissociation curve are such that gas transport to and from the tissues is affected not only by flow, but also by the local rate of metabolism. Local rates of metabolism, for example, in an exercising muscle, are probably the most important determinant of local blood flow and thus the distribution of cardiac output.

To maintain the flow of blood to and from the tissues (cardiac output = volume of blood pumped by the heart per minute) the heart must generate an arterial pressure (approximately 120/80 mm Hg) that will ensure that all the organs and tissues are adequately perfused. Although developing this arterial pressure is essential to organ perfusion, it is equally essential that the heart maintain a low venous pressure (usually 5 to 10 mm Hg) that will not impede the return of blood to the heart. Competent one-way valves at the entrance and exit of the muscular pumping chambers (the ventricles) allow the heart to achieve these pressures while maintaining a continuous forward flow of the blood.

The heart may be viewed as a muscular pump that propels blood into the arterial (delivery) system and receives blood from the venous (return) system. As illustrated schematically in Fig. 1-1, the heart is divided into right and left sides, which are anatomically distinct. Each side consists of a receiving chamber (atrium) and a pumping chamber (ventricle). The right atrium, a thin-walled structure, receives unoxygenated venous blood from three sources: the inferior vena cava, which drains blood from the lower half of the

1

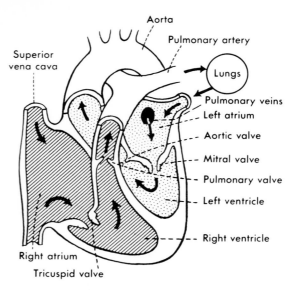

Fig. 1-1. Internal anatomy of the heart (Adapted from Guyton, A. C.: Function of the human body, ed. 3, Philadelphia, 1969, W. B. Saunders Co.)

body; the superior vena cava, which drains blood from the upper half of the body, and the coronary sinus, which drains venous blood from the heart muscle. The blood that collects in the right atrium passes through the tricuspid valve (three leaflets) into the right ventricle. The three leaflets of the tricuspid valve are attached to the papillary muscles, which lie in the floor of the ventricle, by chordae tendineae that run from the free margin of the valve leaflets. Contraction of the papillary muscles prevents the leaflets from everting into the right atrium during ventricular contraction (systole). During ventricular systole, blood is ejected by the right ventricle (through the pulmonary valve) into the pulmonary artery and then into the lungs. The blood returning from the lungs enters the left atrium through four pulmonary veins. It passes from the left atrium to the left ventricle through the mitral valve (two leaflets). Each leaflet of the mitral valve is attached to the wall of the left ventricle by chordae tendineae that insert at the free margin of the leaflets and connect to the papillary muscles. The left ventricle ejects blood through the aortic valve into the aorta, and the aorta distributes the cardiac output to peripheral tissues.

The right heart collects blood from the peripheral (systemic) circulation and distributes it to the pulmonary (lesser) circulation. The left heart collects blood from the lesser circulation and distributes it to the systemic circulation. As blood passes through the systemic capillary bed, which joins peripheral arteries and veins, the red blood cells surrender their oxygen to metabolizing tissues and accumulate carbon dioxide. Conversely, as blood passes through

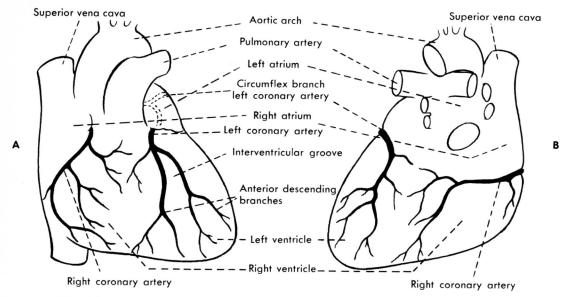

Fig. 1-2. A, Coronary arteries supplying the anterior aspect of the heart. **B,** Coronary arteries supplying the posterior aspect of the heart.

the pulmonary capillaries, red blood cells exchange carbon dioxide for oxygen in the inspired air within pulmonary alveoli in preparation for returning to the systemic circulation.

Coronary arteries

The function of the coronary artery system is to maintain an adequate blood supply to the heart muscle (myocardium). As subsequent chapters will indicate, impairment of the coronary circulation by atherosclerosis constitutes the most frequent cause of heart disease in modern clinical medicine.

There are two major coronary arteries, the left and the right, which arise from the aorta immediately behind their respective cusps of the aortic valve. The left coronary artery divides into two branches shortly after its origin (Fig. 1-2). One of these, the anterior descending branch (A), passes down the groove between the two ventricles on the anterior surface of the heart. The anterior descending artery gives off diagonal branches that supply the left ventricular wall and septal perforating branches that supply the anterior portion of the interventricular septum and the anterior papillary muscle of the left ventricle. The anterior descending artery usually supplies the entire apical portion of the interventricular septum before turning at the apex to terminate in anastomotic channels with the posterior descending coronary artery. The circumflex branch of the left coronary artery passes to the left and posteriorly in the groove between the left atrium and the left ventricle. It gives off several small and one or two large marginal branches that supply the lateral aspects of the left ventricle. Ordinarily, the circumflex artery terminates before it reaches the posterior interventricular groove. However, should the circumflex artery continue and supply the posterior interventricular groove, the coronary circulation is then referred to as a "dominant left" circulation.

More commonly, the right coronary artery passes around the right atrioventricular (A-V) groove, giving off branches to the right ventricle, and then turns at the crux of the heart to descend in the posterior interventricular groove. The posterior descending artery supplies the posterior aspect of the septum and the posterior left ventricular papillary muscle before terminating in anastomotic channels with the anterior descending branch of the left coronary artery. The right coronary artery gives off important branches that supply the sinoatrial (S-A) node and the A-V node in the majority of human hearts. When the right coronary artery turns at the crux and supplies the posterior aspect of the left ventricle and interventricular septum, the coronary circulation is said to be a "dominant right" circulation.

Conduction system

The normal cardiac impulse arises in the specialized pacemaker cells of the S-A node (Chapter 6), located about 1 mm beneath the right atrial epicardium at its junction with the superior vena cava (Fig. 1-3). The S-A node artery passes through the center of the S-A node, nourishing it and most of the

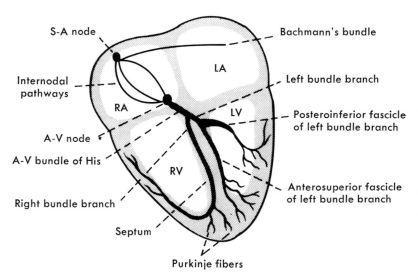

Fig. 1-3. Transmission of the cardiac impulse from the sinoatrial (S-A) node over atrial myocardium, Bachmann's bundle, and internodal pathways, then through the A-V node and bundle of His and down the left and right bundle branches, emerging into the Purkinje fibers, which distribute the impulse to all parts of the ventricle.

right atrium. In 60% of humans, this artery arises from the right coronary artery; in the remainder, it arises from the left circumflex artery.

The impulse spreads over the atrial myocardium from its origin at the sinus node, to the left atrium and region of the A-V node via atrial muscle, and over defined preferential routes or pathways, that is, Bachmann's bundle to the left atrium and the anterior, middle, and posterior internodal tracts connecting S-A and A-V nodes. When the impulse reaches both atria, they depolarize electrically, producing a P wave on the electrocardiogram, and they contract mechanically, producing the "a" wave of the atrial pressure pulse and propelling blood forward into the ventricles.

When the impulse reaches the A-V node, conduction slows markedly. The A-V node is located on the top of the interventricular septum anterior to the coronary sinus and receives its blood supply from a branch of whichever coronary artery crosses the crux of the heart (in 80% to 90% of humans, the right coronary). The term *"A-V junction"* includes the A-V node–His area.

After emerging from the A-V node, conduction resumes its rapid velocity through the His bundle and down the left and right bundle branches. The left bundle branch divides into anterosuperior middle and posteroinferior divisions. Left and right bundle branches supply the inner shell (endocardium) of their respective ventricles with a profusely branching terminal network called Purkinje fibers. These fibers allow almost simultaneous depolarization of both ventricles by distributing the impulse rapidly throughout the ventricular endocardium.

Conduction to the point just prior to an impulse's leaving the Purkinje fibers takes place within the time of the P-R interval. When the impulse emerges from the Purkinje fibers, ventricular depolarization occurs, producing the QRS complex on the electrocardiogram (ECG) and mechanical contraction of the ventricles that propels the blood forward into the pulmonary artery and aorta. It is of great interest, considering the many different parts in the specialized conduction system just detailed, that only atrial depolarization (P wave), ventricular depolarization (QRS complex), and ventricular repolarization (T wave) are apparent in the standard ECG recording.

Nervous control of the heart

Although the heart has an intrinsic control system and will continue to operate without nervous system influences, the autonomic nervous system plays an important role in the rate of impulse formation, the speed of conduction, and the strength of cardiac contraction. The autonomic nervous system regulates the heart through two different sets of nerves: the parasympathetic (chiefly the right and left vagus nerves) and the sympathetic (Fig. 1-4). Vagal nerve fibers are found primarily in the S-A node, atrial muscle fibers, and A-V node; they supply the ventricular myocardium, but the density of innervation is less than that of atrial chambers and the physiologic consequences of vagal innervation to the ventricles has been a subject of

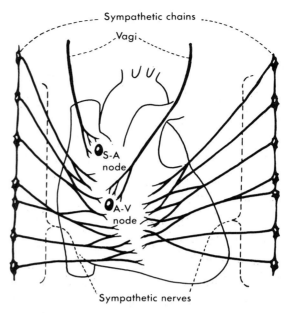

Fig. 1-4. Connections of parasympathetic nerves (vagi) and sympathetic nerves with the heart. (Adapted from Guyton, A. C.: Function of the human body, ed. 3, Philadelphia, 1969, W. B. Saunders Co.)

conjecture. However, recent data suggest that vagal innervation may affect ventricular electrophysiology more than previously considered. The sympathetic nerve fibers supply all areas of the atria and ventricles. The influence of the autonomic nerves on the heart is mediated by neurotransmitters, acetylcholine in the case of the vagus nerve and norepinephrine in the case of sympathetic nerves. These neurotransmitters are contained within the postganglionic nerve fibers, are released by electrical impulses traveling down the nerve fibers, and exert their effects by binding to specific receptors on the surface membrane of myocardial cells.

Stimulation of the vagus nerve causes the following effects on the heart: (1) decreased rate of firing of the S-A node, (2) decreased force of contraction of atrial (and probably ventricular) muscle, and (3) decreased speed of conduction of impulses through the A-V node, which lengthens the delay period between atrial and ventricular contractions (P-R interval). Vagal stimulation speeds conduction through the atrial muscle and shortens the atrial refractory period. Stimulation of the sympathetic nerves has essentially the opposite effects on the heart. These include (1) increased heart rate, (2) increased speed of conduction through the A-V node, and (3) increased vigor of cardiac contraction.

The activity of the autonomic nerves can be modulated by the central nervous system (such as in fear or pain) or by reflex changes caused by stimulation of sensors that detect changes in pressure (pressoreceptors). These receptors are located in the aortic arch and carotid arteries. Sensory fibers extend from the aortic arch pressoreceptors by way of the vagus nerve to the vasomotor center in the medulla. Impulses from the carotid sinus pressoreceptors reach the vasomotor center over the glossopharyngeal nerve. From the vasomotor center, efferent impulses are transmitted to the heart by the cardiac branches of the vagus nerve and by sympathetic nerves. The frequency of nerve impulses is modulated by the vasomotor center, and in general there is a reciprocal relation between vagal and sympathetic activity.

Consequently, sudden elevation of blood pressure within the aorta or the carotid sinus, for example, by a hypertensive drug or by carotid sinus massage, stimulates the pressoreceptors in these vessels. This stimulates the cardioinhibitory center, which in turn inhibits the accelerator center. Conversely, a sudden drop in blood pressure within the aorta or carotid sinus stimulates pressoreceptors less intensely. The cardioinhibitory center is stimulated less, producing less depression of the accelerator center and consequently reflex acceleration of the heart. This phenomenon becomes apparent during hypotension.

Although pressoreflexes constitute the dominant control mechanism of heart rate, there are other influential factors, including the levels of oxygen and carbon dioxide in the blood, drugs, electrolytes, and the degree of alkalinity or acidity.

REFERENCES

Abboud, F. M., Heistad, D. D., Mark, A. L., and Schmid, P. G.: Reflex control of the peripheral circulation, Prog. Cardiovasc. Dis. **18**:371, 1976.

Guyton, A. C.: Textbook of medical physiology, ed. 5, Philadelphia, 1976, W. B. Saunders Co.

Heymans, C., and Neil, E.: Reflexogenic areas of the cardiovascular system, London, 1968, Churchill Livingstone.

Hirsch, E. F.: The innervation of the human heart, Arch. Pathol. **75**:378, 1963.

James, T. N.: Anatomy of the coronary arteries in health and disease, Circulation **32**:1020, 1965.

Katz, A. M.: Physiology of the heart, New York, 1977, Raven Press.

Rushmer, R. F.: Structure and function of the cardiovascular system, ed. 2, Philadelphia, 1976, W. B. Saunders Co.

Wellens, H. J. J., Lie, K. I., and Janse, M. J.: The conduction system of the heart, Leiden, 1976, H. E. Stenfert Kroese B. V.

CHAPTER TWO

CORONARY ARTERY DISEASE

Coronary artery disease and its complications are presently the leading cause of death in Western civilizations. The terms "coronary artery disease" (CAD) and "arteriosclerotic heart disease" (ASHD) are essentially synonyms. What is the nature of arteriosclerosis?

The term "arteriosclerosis" means "a chronic disease of the arteries characterized by abnormal thickening and hardening of the vessel walls resulting in loss of elasticity." This process, however, may have divergent etiologies, and its manifestations differ according to the type of vessel involved and the site of the disease within the vessel. Accordingly, it is convenient to categorize the disease into the following types:

Type I: Intimal atherosclerosis. This form of arteriosclerosis affects the internal membranes (intima) of arteries and consists of irregular thickening and "plaque" formation. Plaques consist of lipid, proliferating smooth muscle cells, and variable amounts of collagen. The process affects primarily the large vessels, begins at a very young age, and is almost universally present in people over the age of 20 years.

Type II: Medial sclerosis. This process consists of calcification and hypertrophy of the muscular portion of the artery (media). The process involves medium-sized blood vessels such as the brachial and femoral arteries, which become thickened, rigid, and tortuous. This process can be detected frequently at the wrist as hard pipestem arteries. However, it is not necessarily associated with any reduction in the caliber of the involved vessel.

Type III: Arteriolar sclerosis. This type of involvement of small blood vessels is characterized by hypertrophy of the muscular media and thickening of the intima and is usually seen in patients with long-standing hypertension. It often affects the small vessels in the fundus of the eye and in the kidneys.

It should be recognized that although these processes may exist separately, there is in fact considerable overlap. Type I, or intimal atherosclerosis, is the cause of most coronary artery disease but may be enhanced or accelerated by coexisting hypertension.

As noted previously, atherosclerosis starts in the intima, or the innermost layer of the artery, which is bounded on the inside by the endothelium and on the outside by the internal elastic lamella. The earliest evidence of atherosclerosis is a fatty streak consisting of lipid accumulation in the intima. This lipid may be extracellular or contained within macrophages or small smooth muscle cells, and it usually cholesterol-rich β-lipoprotein. The accumulation of lipid within the intima appears to result from some form of initial injury to the endothelium that increases its permeability to molecules such as low-density lipoproteins (LDLs). These molecules, perhaps together with components released by platelets that aggregate over the injured area, cause smooth muscle cells to migrate from the media to the intima and to proliferate. As they proliferate, these muscle cells also produce increased amounts of collagen, and together lipid, muscle cells, and collagen form a plaque. Small blood vessels grow into the fibrous plaque and may, from time to time, rupture, producing small hemorrhages. Such subintimal hemorrhage increases the size of the plaque and is frequently followed by scarring and fibrosis, which further enlarge the lesion. Rupture of blood vessels within the plaque may cause sudden major obstruction of the lumen of the vessel. Enlargement of a plaque, however, is usually slow and gradual, with the additional deposition of fat and scar tissue. The intima covering a plaque may break, and as a result a small clot may form on the surface. This clot may then obstruct the lumen of the vessel. The clot or plaque may embolize and occlude the vessel farther downstream. In addition to compromising blood supply by obstruction, the atherosclerotic process may also cause weakening of the arterial wall and aneurysm formation. In coronary arteriograms, we not infrequently see coronary arteries where there is obstruction and aneurysm formation in the same artery.

Pathology

The atherosclerotic process affects large- and medium-sized arteries, and lesions dominate at branch points and forks in the arterial tree. In the carotid arteries, the disease is worst at the bifurcation, and in the aorta, atherosclerosis is worse distally at its bifurcation and in the iliac arteries. Coronary arteries are particularly susceptible to atherosclerosis. Although it is rare to have peripheral disease without coronary artery involvement, coronary disease without involvement of the peripheral arteries is not rare. In the coronary circulation, it is interesting that the atherosclerotic process is confined to the portions of the vessels that lie on the epicardial surface. The intramural arteries are spared from the atherosclerotic process. This pattern of distribution and sparing of the disease has suggested to some that turbulence of flow at branch points and rhythmic torsion on untethered vessels may contribute to the genesis of the lesion.

In patients with symptoms of coronary artery disease, involvement is most frequent in the left anterior descending artery, next in the right coronary artery, and least frequent (although not rare) in the circumflex artery. Compromise of the lumen of the coronary artery by 75% or more is required to produce any significant reduction of coronary blood flow. In fatal coronary artery disease, the coronary arteries are diffusely involved by atherosclerosis, all portions of the extramural coronary tree are involved, and usually at least two of the major coronary arteries are narrowed by more than 75%. The most severe narrowing tends to be in the proximal 2 to 3 cm of each artery, but distal involvement, particularly of the right coronary artery, is not uncommon. Myocardial infarction takes place only rarely in the absence of significant disease involving at least two coronary arteries. The coronary artery responsible for perfusing an area of infarction is not necessarily the most severely diseased but is rarely less than 75% obstructed. Thus significant disease of the right coronary artery can be expected in inferior myocardial infarction and disease of the left anterior descending artery in anterior infarction. Insidious in onset, coronary atherosclerosis may be without signs or symptoms for many years until the disease process produces a degree of obstruction that interferes with the arterial blood supply to the myocardium. If the obstructive process is gradual, over a period of years, intercoronary collateral circulation may develop, and clinical evidence of disease may be long deferred or never occur. In this instance, although there is marked obstructive disease, the myocardial cells may receive adequate oxygen regardless of demand.

In contrast, when an artery is partially obstructed and sufficient collateral circulation has not yet developed, the obstruction may impair blood flow during conditions of increased demand. Consequently, symptoms of intermittent vascular insufficiency may occur. Thus the patient with arterial insufficiency in the legs may complain of cramps on walking (intermittent claudication); patients with intestinal arterial insufficiency may feel abdominal pain (abdominal angina) following meals; and finally, patients with partial obstruction of the coronary vessels may have angina pectoris when the myocardial demands exceed the blood supply, such as during exertion. Transient ischemic attacks in patients with carotid artery disease are most often thought to represent embolic episodes, arising from the discharge of platelets and other debris from the ulcerated plaque.

Incidence and predisposition

Overt coronary artery disease affects about 5% of the men between ages 45 and 64 years and 11% of the men over the age of 65 years. It causes about 1.25 million heart attacks and nearly 600,000 deaths per year in the United States alone. About one third of these deaths are sudden, about one third result from acute myocardial infarction, and about one third occur as a consequence of heart failure secondary to ischemic heart disease. Regardless of the immediate cause of death, fatal coronary artery disease is nearly always associated with diffuse and significant atherosclerosis of the coronary arteries, as noted previously. In recent years, large-scale epidemiologic studies have identified so-called "risk factors" that help to define the risk of developing coronary artery disease and presumably contribute to the cause of atherosclerosis. Because several apparently unrelated risk factors exist, it seems most likely that coronary atherosclerosis is a multifactorial disease, and it also seems highly probable that the disease develops when more than one factor exists over a relatively long period of time. In this context, then, risk is viewed as a probability of developing coronary heart disease, and that probability is determined by the number of risk factors in any given individual, by the level of each factor, that is, blood pressure, cholesterol, and so on, and by time, that is, age.

It is important to distinguish between primary and secondary risk factors. Primary factors are those that are thought to contribute to the development of coronary atherosclerosis, and secondary factors are those that are thought to enhance the risk of any specific manifestation of the disease, that is, sudden death, arrhythmias, myocardial infarction, and so forth, in those who already have coronary atherosclerosis. The likelihood or probability of developing coronary heart disease is influenced by and can be predicted from several primary risk factors.

Age, sex, and race. Atherosclerosis is more prevalent in older people than in young ones. In the United States the death rate is nearly six times higher in white men than in white women between 35 and 55 years of age. After menopause, however, the incidence of the disease in women rapidly approaches that in men. It is generally held that atherosclerosis develops more rapidly in white people than in blacks.

Blood pressure. In the Coronary Heart Disease Study in Framingham, Massachusetts, middle-aged men with arterial pressures in excess of 160/95 showed a fivefold increase in the incidence of ischemic heart disease compared with that in subjects having blood pressures of 140/90 or less. Both systolic and diastolic pressure elevations correlate positively with ischemic heart disease; the diastolic pressure may be more important as a high-risk factor in younger people and systolic pressure more important in older age groups.

Hyperlipidemia and diet. The lipids in the plasma that are of general importance are cholesterol, triglycerides, and free fatty acids. Cholesterol has been measured more extensively than the other lipids and when elevated is associated with an increased incidence of coronary heart disease. Cholesterol and triglycerides are insoluble in plasma and are transported by lipoproteins that are soluble. These lipoproteins can be separated and quantitated. In the fasting state, very low-density lipoproteins (VLDLs) carry mostly triglycerides and lesser amounts of cholesterol. LDLs are derived from the metabolism of VLDLs and carry most of the cholesterol in plasma. High-density lipoproteins (HDLs) are mostly protein and carry about 35% cholesterol. Recent epidemiologic studies have shown that the relation between total serum cholesterol level and risk of coronary atherosclerosis is even stronger if LDL cholesterol is related to risk. Conversely, there is an inverse relation between HDLs and coronary risk, suggesting that HDLs or a high ratio of HDL to LDL conveys protection against vascular disease. The significance of these associations is heightened by pathophysiologic studies that have shown that high levels of LDL cholesterol damage the endothelial lining of vessels and promote proliferation of smooth muscle cells and other components of the atherosclerotic lesion. Among patients with premature atherosclerosis the two most common patterns of hyperlipidemia are type IV (elevated triglyceride levels with a normal or only slightly elevated cholesterol level), caused by elevated VLDL levels, and type II (elevated cholesterol levels with a normal or only slightly elevated triglyceride level), caused by elevated LDL levels. Dietary and pharmacologic methods are moderately effective in lowering serum cholesterol and triglyceride levels, and only recently have the effects of treatment on HDLs and LDLs been explored in detail. Population studies have shown a relation between the fat content of the diet and serum lipid levels, and animal studies have shown that reduction of elevated serum lipid levels protects against atherosclerosis. At the present time, studies are under way to assess whether lowering serum lipid levels in man prevents or causes regression of atherosclerosis, but conclusive results are not yet available.

Smoking. The relation of cigarette smoking and the development of coronary heart disease has been established. Statistical evidence supports a mean increase of about 70% in the death rate from coronary artery disease in middle-aged men who smoke one pack of cigarettes per day as compared with nonsmokers. This percentage decreases with advancing age, and the relation is less firm in women. Pipe and cigar smokers do not have an increased risk, probably because they do not inhale. The mechanism for the relation between smoking and increased heart disease is not clear. The chief effects of nicotine on the cardiovascular system are cardiac stimulation and peripheral vasoconstriction. The former results in an increase in heart rate, stroke volume, cardiac output, and cardiac work. The peripheral vasoconstriction caused by nicotine is not greater in patients with vascular disease than in normal persons, but the resultant decrease in blood flow is more conspicuous in the patient with circulatory impairment and enhances the ischemia already present.

Glucose intolerance. Coronary heart disease is more prevalent in patients with diabetes mellitus. It is proposed that insulin may act to modify either lipid metabolism or the response of the artery to its environment. Furthermore, diabetics have an increased tendency to degeneration of connective tissue, which may increase the tendency to atheroma formation.

Physical activity. Many studies in the past have suggested that physical inactivity is associated with an increased risk of coronary heart disease. However, the strength of the relation was low, and after correcting for other inequalities between active and inactive subjects, physical inactivity was generally regarded as a minor risk factor. One problem with most of these studies was the lack of a precise method to "quantitate" activity. More recently, a careful study of California longshoremen has demonstrated a strong inverse relation between energy expenditure at work (excess caloric expenditure) and the incidence of fatal and nonfatal heart attacks. The reduced risk was evident in all age groups, but most striking in the young, and it was still evident after correcting for excess weight, smoking patterns, and serum cholesterol level. The most significant finding of this study of over 3000 men was that the habitual expenditure of about 1800 calories per day above basal consumption through physically demanding work reduced by nearly 50% the incidence of fatal heart attacks as compared to the incidence in those who expended less than 1000 calories per day above basal consumption.

Personality factors. For many years it has been suspected that coronary heart disease was more prominent among individuals subject to chronic anxiety or stress. Subsequently, a personality type, so-called type A, was identified that was related to coronary heart disease. The characteristics of this behavioral pattern included enhanced aggressiveness, ambitiousness, competitive drive, and chronic sense of time urgency. The report of the Western Collaborative Study showed that the incidence of coronary heart disease was twice as high in type A individuals than in type B (absence of these traits) individuals even after correcting for other risk factors. These observations are of considerable interest, but a firm link between the type A personality and the pathophysiology of coronary atherosclerosis remains to be defined. Furthermore, it remains to be shown that modification of behavioral patterns will be feasible or effective in altering risk.

It is vitally important to recognize that risk is multifactorial, that the influence of two or more factors may be additive or synergistic, and that the risk with any given factor is influenced by the degree of abnormality—not just its presence or absence.

REFERENCES

Friedman, M., et al.: The relationship of behavior pattern A to the state of the coronary vasculature, Am. J. Med. 44:525-537, 1968.

Goldstein, J. L., and Brown, M. S.: The low-density lipoprotein pathway and its relation to atherosclerosis, Annu. Rev. Biochem. 46:897, 1977.

Gordon, T., et al: High density lipoprotein as a protective factor against coronary heart disease, Am. J. Med. 62:707, 1977.

Kannel, W. B.: Coronary risk factors: The Framingham study, J. Occup. Med. 9:611, 1967.

'Kannel, W. B., Castelli, W. P., Gordon, T., and McNamara, P. M.: Serum cholesterol, lipoproteins and the risk of coronary heart disease: The Framingham study, Ann. Intern. Med. 74:1, 1971.

McGill, H. C.: The geographic pathology of atherosclerosis, Lab. Invest. 18:463-653, 1968.

Paffenbarger, R. S.: Physical activity and fatal heart attack: Protection or selection? In Amsterdam, E., et al., editors: Exercise in cardiovascular health and disease, Chapter 3, New York, 1977, Yorke Medical Books.

Roberts, W. C.: Coronary arteries in fatal acute myocardial infarction, Circulation 45:215-230, 1972.

Stamler, J.: Epidemiology of coronary heart disease, Med. Clin. North Am. 57:1, 1973.

Wolinsky, H.: A new look at atherosclerosis, Cardiovasc. Med. 1:41, 1976.

CHAPTER THREE

ASSESSMENT OF PATIENTS WITH CORONARY ARTERY DISEASE

Patients with coronary artery disease enter the health care system at varying stages of disease progression. Thus in order to determine the individual goals of care and complementary management plans, a clinical data base must be generated. This information can be systematically procured through an interview with the patient and through a complete physical examination, plus pertinent laboratory and physiologic tests. Here begins the process of identifying and solving patient problems, a process that continues throughout the therapeutic relationship. As plans are developed and implemented toward the resolution of each problem, subjective and objective data are collected concomitantly to evaluate the success of the plan and determine the necessity of management revision.

The intent of this chapter is to focus on the data collection process as it pertains to the patient's cardiovascular status. It is important to remember, however, that other body systems may affect, or be affected by, cardiac disease, and other systems may be involved in disease processes that secondarily affect the heart. Consequently, any patient who develops a new problem should have a complete evaluation.

The discussion that follows includes the patient interview, physical examination, and common laboratory and physiologic tests specific to the individual with coronary artery disease. This process of data gathering can be used to explore a patient's problem in an outpatient clinic, to develop a patient care plan in the coronary care unit, or to acquire further information about a new or acute problem.

Patient interview

The patient interview is the first step in the data collection process. Its purpose is to gather pertinent information about the patient's present complaint or problem, past health history, and family and social history. The accuracy and completeness of the subjective data gathered during this interaction depend on the examiner's ability to establish effective communication and rapport with the patient. A gentle, confident approach will help the anxious patient describe his illness. Structure can be provided by the interviewer through simple, open-ended questions, and the patient's facial expression and attitude should be observed to make sure the patient understands the questions. Listening to the patient is essential for learning about the disease as well as for learning about the patient as a person.

THE PATIENT'S PRESENT COMPLAINT OR PROBLEM

The patient's chief problem, whether it be chest pain, shortness of breath, or palpitations, among others, precipitated his contact with the health care system. It is his chief concern and therefore the first subject of the interview. As the patient expresses his perceived physical and/or mental changes, the interviewer should reorganize the patient's words into a clinical format to help identify the bodily or mental processes underlying each symptom. This reorganization is accomplished by employing seven basic characteristics or descriptors that differentiate a symptom of one disease from that of another.

Descriptors

Bodily location. Where did the symptom originate? Did it radiate? To what site? It is helpful if the patient indicates the location of the symptom and the radiation pattern with his hand.

Quality. How did the symptom feel to the patient? It may be described as being "like" something else. For example, the chest pain of myocardial infarction is often compared to "being squeezed in a vise." Other qualifiers include "choking," "burning," and "constricting."

Quantity. How intense is the symptom? Is it mild, moderate, severe, or unbearable?

Chronology. When did the symptom first occur? Was its onset sudden or gradual? How long did it last in terms of minutes, hours, or days? Over time, has the symptom stayed the same or become better or worse?

Setting. Describe the circumstances when the symptom first occurred. Look for associations between the symptom and the patient's physical activity, emotional status, and personal interactions.

Aggravating and alleviating factors. Are the symptoms influenced by certain activities or physiologic processes? What produces relief—resting, avoiding food, medication? What aggravates the problem—exertion, eating, body position, coughing?

Associated symptoms. Rarely is a disease process present with only one symptom. Therefore the presence or absence of symptoms commonly associated with cardiovascular conditions should be noted. The patient should be asked specifically about each of these and affirmative responses should be characterized and described as stated in the six previous steps. Questions for eliciting this information should explore whether or not the patient is experiencing: (1) chest pain or discomfort, (2) unexplained weakness or fatigue, (3) weight loss or gain, (4) swelling of ankles *(edema)*, (5) shortness of breath on exertion *(dyspnea)*, (6) shortness of breath while sleeping that wakens the patient *(paroxysmal nocturnal dyspnea)*, (7) a need to sleep on more than one pillow to breathe comfortably *(orthopnea)*, (8) dizzy or fainting spells *(syncope)*, (9) coughing at night, (10) coughing up blood *(hemoptysis,* (11) rapid heart beat or palpitations, (12) a need to get up several times during the night to urinate, and (13) pain or cramps in the legs while walking that is relieved by rest *(intermittent claudication).* Finally, asking the patient generally about his daily activities, and any self-imposed restrictions on these, can provide clues as to the severity of the existing problem.

THE PATIENT'S PAST HEALTH HISTORY

The patient's past health history may contribute to defining the problem and planning interventions. He should be asked if he has ever had a problem related to his heart, such as a heart murmur, an enlarged heart, heart failure, or a heart attack. Does he have or has he had rheumatic fever, hypertension, elevated cholesterol or triglyceride levels, or diabetes? What medications is he taking? Has he been under the care of other physicians? Further information should include previous diseases, emotional or mental problems, hospitalizations, surgical procedures, injuries, and allergies, including drug, contact, or food.

THE PATIENT'S FAMILY AND SOCIAL HISTORY

The patient's family background and social profile may also contribute significant information to the assessment. The age, sex, and health of parents, siblings, children, and spouse and the age and cause of death of deceased members are relevant. In addition, certain familial diseases that grandparents and close relatives may have had are pertinent. These include hypertension, coronary artery disease, rheumatic fever, stroke, kidney disease, and diabetes.

Knowledge concerning certain aspects of the patient's current life situation leads to an understanding of the patient as a person and, accordingly, gives more relevance to the therapeutic program. These include place of birth; habits, including sleep, exercise, diet, use of alcoholic beverages, tobacco, and medications; armed service affiliation; religion; level of education; occupation; marital relationship; reaction to stress; and home environment. It is helpful to ask the patient to select a typical day and describe his activities and what foods and drugs he consumes in the course of that day. Asking the patient what upsets him may identify issues that contribute causally to the problem and may be considerations in planning management. For example, family stress may have contributed to the onset of a patient's myocardial infarction.

Other aspects of the patient's social situation may be pertinent to the plan of care and rehabilitation. A veteran may be entitled to hospitalization in a Veterans Administration hospital, an important resource for some people. A patient's religion may influence management significantly. Blood transfusions may not be acceptable to the Jehovah's Witness and last rites may be an important consideration to the critically ill Roman Catholic.

Physical examination

The cardiovascular physical examination is performed to collect objective data about the patient's complaint, symptoms, or illness. The information that has been obtained from the patient interview is then correlated with the physical findings as the next step in the evaluation process. Often an adequately and accurately obtained history establishes the nature of the problem prior to the physical examination.

The examiner evaluates the cardiovascular system in an orderly fashion using the techniques of inspection, palpation, percussion, and auscultation, as appropriate.

inspection visual examination of the parts of the system. It includes whatever the examiner can see, such as pulsations, deformities, color, manner of breathing, and so forth.

palpation employs the examiner's sense of touch. He feels or presses with the fingers or hands to locate possible vibrations, thrills (blood flowing past an obstruction), impulses, grating sensations, and so on.

percussion tapping the patient's body surface to determine, through touch and hearing, the relative amount of air or solid material underneath the skin.

auscultation act of listening with or without the stethoscope to internally produced sounds. Such sounds include breath sounds, heart sounds, bruit (murmur over a peripheral vessel), friction rubs, and heart murmurs.

The physical examination actually begins when the patient meets the examiner. At this time the examiner makes general observations about the patient regarding apparent age versus stated age, grooming, speech, posture, gait, nutritional state, attitude, color, and degree of distress, if any. The collection of objective data begins with the recording of the patient's vital signs, including temperature, pulse, respiration, and blood pressure.

TEMPERATURE

A temperature elevation above the normal value of 98.6° F or 37° C is common during the first few days following acute myocardial infarction. The elevation is usually to less than 101° F and is associated with necrosis of cardiac muscle. Prolonged, high, or late development of fever suggests other complications. Although fever may indicate the onset of infectious processes, it may also be the first sign of thrombophlebitis, pulmonary embolism, pericarditis, or atelectasis. Moreover, prolonged temperature elevation in the patient with a myocardial infarction may be harmful, since it causes a rise in the metabolic rate of body tissues and, therefore, a demand for increased circulation and oxygenation. This, in turn, increases the myocardial oxygen demands, a threatening situation in the face of infarction.

Temperature assessment is therefore a part of routine examination and daily monitoring activities for critically ill patients. The temperature is taken orally, rectally, or in the axilla for a period of 3 minutes. Rectal temperatures are most accurate. In the past the taking of rectal temperatures was avoided in patients with myocardial infarctions as a precaution against undue vagal stimulation. However, recent studies suggest that taking rectal temperatures is quite safe.

Temperature is measured on a Fahrenheit or centigrade scale. The formula for converting centigrade measurement to Fahrenheit and vice versa follows:

$$\text{Fahrenheit} = 1.8\,(°C) + 32$$
$$\text{Centigrade} = \frac{°F - 32}{1.8}$$

PULSE

Arterial pulse. The arterial pulse is a propagated wave of arterial pressure resulting from left ventricular contraction. The pulse wave begins in the aorta with the opening of the aortic valve and the ejection of blood from the left ventricle (Fig. 3-1). The pressure in the aorta rises sharply, since blood enters the vessel more rapidly than it runs off to the peripheral vessels. A notch may appear during the sharp rise in the central arterial pressure curve. This is called the *anacrotic notch* and is generally absent from peripheral pulse recordings but may be prominent in valvular aortic stenosis. After peak pressure has been reached, aortic pressure decreases, ventricular ejection slows, and blood continues to flow to peripheral vessels. As the ventricles relax, there is a brief reversal of flow (from the central arteries back toward the ventricle) and the aortic valve closes. This produces the *dicrotic notch* on the peripheral pressure pulse tracing, corresponding to the *incisura* recorded centrally. Following this, aortic pressure increases slightly and then decreases as diastole continues and blood flows to the periphery, a result of energy imparted to the elastic tissue in the great vessels during systole. In the graphic recording of aortic pressure in Fig. 3-1 the peak of the pulse wave represents systolic pressure and the lowest point on the wave represents diastolic pressure.

The pulse wave changes in shape as it travels to the periphery. The height, or amplitude, of the wave (the systolic reading) increases as it moves from the aortic root to the peripheral arteries, with a slight decrease in the diastolic pressure. The ascending part of the wave becomes steeper and the peak becomes sharper.

Examination. The arterial pulses are palpated to evaluate patency, heart rate and rhythm, and character of the pulse. This examination covers the carotid, brachial, radial, femoral, popliteal, dorsalis pedis, and posterior tibial pulses. These pulses can best be evaluated with the patient in a reclining position and the trunk of the body elevated about 30 degrees. If diffuse atherosclerosis in an elderly patient has resulted in absence of the dorsalis pedis or posterior tibial pulse, this observation should be noted on initial examination, so that the hospital staff do not interpret this finding as a new catastrophic event, such as arterial embolus, at a later time during the patient's hospitalization.

Although the radial pulse is commonly used in determining heart rate, the carotid pulse best correlates with central aortic pressure and reflects cardiac function more accurately than peripheral vessels. Furthermore, if the patient develops marked vasoconstriction, the radial pulse may be difficult to palpate. However, caution must be exercised in palpating the carotid pulse to avoid pressure on the carotid sinus, since palpating at that site may result in severe bradycardia.

The pulse is examined for rate and rhythm, equality of corresponding pulses, contour, and amplitude. To obtain information about cardiac rate and rhythm, the pulse should be palpated for 30 seconds in the presence of a regular rhythm and for 1 to 2 minutes in the face of an irregular rhythm. If an irregularity exists, an apical pulse should be recorded. The term *"peripheral pulse deficit"* indicates that the heart rate counted at the apex by auscultation exceeds the heart rate counted by palpation of the radial pulse. A deficit

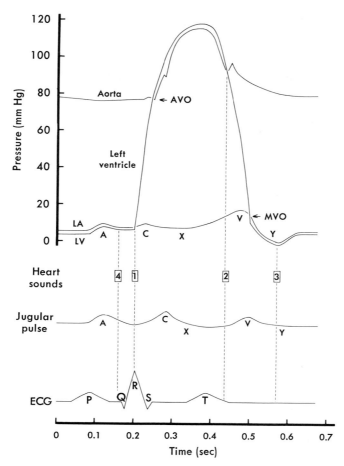

Fig. 3-1. Simultaneous ECG, pressures obtained from the left atrium, left ventricle, and aorta, and the jugular pulse during one cardiac cycle. For simplification, right heart pressures have been omitted. Normal right atrial pressure closely parallels that of the left atrium, and right ventricular and pulmonary artery pressures time closely with their corresponding left heart counterparts, only being reduced in magnitude. The normal mitral and aortic valve closure precedes tricuspid and pulmonic closure, respectively, whereas valve opening reverses this order. The jugular venous pulse lags behind the right atrial pressure.

During the course of one cardiac cycle, note that the electrical events *(ECG)* initiate and therefore precede the mechanical *(pressure)* events, and that the latter precede the auscultatory events *(heart sounds)* they themselves produce. Shortly after the P wave, the atria contract to produce the A wave; a fourth heart sound may succeed the latter. The QRS complex initiates ventricular systole, followed shortly by left ventricular contraction and the rapid buildup of left ventricular *(LV)* pressure. Almost immediately LV pressure exceeds left atrial *(LA)* pressure to close the mitral valve and produce the first heart sound. When LV pressure exceeds aortic pressure, the aortic valve opens *(AVO)*, and when aortic pressure is once again greater than LV pressure, the aortic valve closes to produce the second heart sound and terminate ventricular ejection. The decreasing LV pressure drops below LA pressure to open the mitral valve *(MVO)* and a period of rapid ventricular filling commences. During this time a third heart sound may be heard. The jugular pulse is explained under the discussion of the venous pulse. (Modified with permission from Hurst, J. W., et al.: The heart arteries and veins, ed. 3, New York, 1974 McGraw-Hill Book Co.)

means that not every cardiac systole is forceful enough to produce a palpable radial pulse and may occur in the presence of premature extrasystoles or atrial tachyarrhythmias, such as atrial fibrillation. Bilateral, simultaneous palpation of the radial and pedal pulses is helpful in determining whether the pulses arrive without delay and provides information about the peripheral arterial blood supply.

The character of the arterial wall, which normally feels soft and pliable, is noted by palpation. With significant atherosclerotic disease the vessel may be resistant to compression and feel much like a rope.

The pulse contour may be assessed by extending the patient's arm and palpating the radial or brachial pulse or the carotid pulse in the neck. The artery should be compressed lightly with a finger while the examiner ascertains the contour of the pulse wave. Variations in the contour of the arterial pulse are depicted in Fig. 3-2.

The *normal arterial pulse* (Fig. 3-2, *A*) has a pulse pressure of about 30 to 40 mm Hg; the systolic pressure measures the peaks of the waves, the diastolic pressure measures the troughs. One can feel a sharp upstroke and a more gradual downstroke (the dicrotic notch of the descending slope of the wave is too weak to be palpable). The contour of the normal pulse is smooth and rounded.

With *large bounding pulses* (Fig. 3-2, *B*), the pulse pressure is increased and one feels a rapid upstroke, a brief peak, and a fast downstroke. This type of pulse wave is encountered most often in conditions termed "hyperkinetic circulatory states." These states include exercise, anxiety, fear, hyperthyroidism, anemia, patent ductus arteriosus, aortic regurgitation, and complete heart block with bradycardia and hypertension. It is also found as a result of generalized arteriosclerosis and rigidity of the arterial system in aging people.

Small weak pulses (Fig. 3-2, *C*) are characterized by diminished pulse pressure and pulse contour that is felt as a slow gradual upstroke, a delayed systolic peak, and a prolonged downstroke. This pulse is found in severe cases of left ventricular failure as a result of decreased stroke volume and in moderate or severe cases of aortic stenosis as a result of slow ejection of blood through the narrowed orifice.

Pulses alternans (Fig. 3-2, *D*) refers to a pulse pattern in which the heart beats with a *regular* rhythm, but the pulses alternate in size and intensity. When this alternation is present in lesser degrees, the difference may not be palpable, but it can be readily detected by measuring blood pressure by auscultation.

As the sphygmomanometric cuff (see p. 22) is slowly deflated from a pressure above the systolic level, the sounds from the alternate beats are heard first. Then one hears the alternating loud and soft sounds or a sudden doubling of the rate as the cuff pressure declines. Pulsus alternans often accompanies left ventricular failure and can masquerade as a bigeminal pulse.

The *bigeminal pulse* (Fig. 3-2, *E*) is usually produced by premature ven-

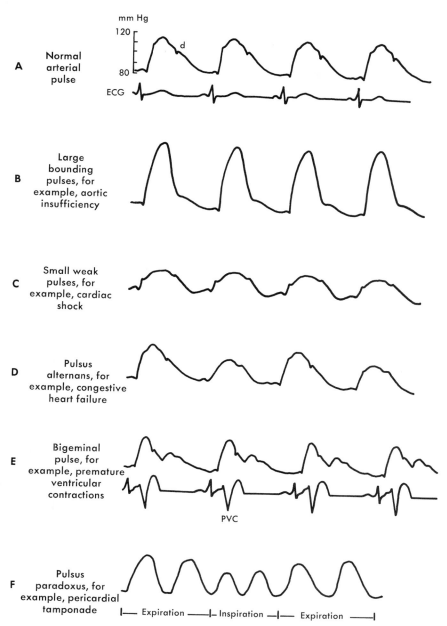

Fig. 3-2. Variations in contour of the arterial pulse with correlated ECGs for the normal arterial pulses (A) and bigeminal pulse (E). See text for description.

tricular extrasystole that occurs regularly following a normally conducted beat. The stroke volume of the premature beat is less than that of the normal beat, since contraction occurs before complete ventricular filling. The rhythm is *irregular*, since the time between the normal beat and the premature beat is shorter than the time between the pairs. The irregularity may be consistent. Simultaneous arterial palpation and cardiac auscultation assist in diagnosing this cardiac irregularity.

Pulsus paradoxus (Fig 3-2, *F*) refers to the phenomenon in which the pulse diminishes perceptibly in amplitude during normal inspiration. Although the differences in pulse volume can be palpated, they can be more precisely demonstrated with sphygmomanometry. Under normal conditions of rest the systolic blood pressure ordinarily decreases by 3 to 10 mm Hg. The procedure for detecting pulsus paradoxus is as follows:

1. Have the patient breath *normally*.
2. Pump up the sphygmomanometer, then lower the pressure until the first sound (systolic) is heard.
3. Observe the patient's respirations. The systolic sound may disappear during normal inspiration.
4. Slowly deflate the cuff until all systolic sounds are heard, regardless of the respiratory cycle. The change (in millimeters of mercury) from the point at which systolic sounds were first heard to the point where they are heard during the entire respiratory cycle represents the millimeters of paradox observed. A paradox greater than 10 mm Hg is usually abnormal.

To be significant, a paradoxical pulse must occur during normal cardiac rhythm and with respirations of normal rhythm and depth. In short, it is an exaggeration of a normal response during respiration. Pulsus paradoxus is found in cases of pericardial tamponade, adhesive pericarditis, severe lung disease, advanced heart failure, and other conditions.

Ascultation of arteries. Arteries are normally silent when auscultated with the bell or diaphragm of the stethoscope, which is placed lightly over them. Occlusive arterial disease, such as arteriosclerosis, will interfere with normal blood flow through the artery, resulting in a blowing sound called a *bruit*. Auscultation of the carotid arteries should be done with the patient holding his breath so that the bruits can be distinguished from the sounds of respiration. Often these abnormal arterial vibrations can be *felt* as *thrills*. Auscultation is also done over the abdominal aorta and femoral arteries to detect the presence of bruits.

Venous pulse. Examination of the neck veins provides diagnostic information about the dynamics of the right side of the heart. For this clinical evaluation, one must study the waveform of the venous pulsations, correlate them with the cardiac rhythm, and determine the venous pressure.

The character of the venous pulse is determined by (1) the rate at which blood is returned from the peripheral tissues to the venous system; (2) the amount of resistance to flow presented by the right atrium and ventricle dur-

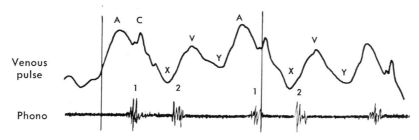

Fig. 3-3. Relationship of the jugular venous pulse to right atrial activity.

ing different phases of the cardiac cycle; (3) the pressure-volume properties of the segment of the vein; and (4), in part, the nature of the tissues overlying the veins at the focus of observation.

Examination. The examination begins with observation of the external and internal jugular veins on both sides of the neck as well as of the venous pulsations that may be present in the supraclavicular fossae or in the suprasternal notch. For accurate evaluation of the venous waveform the *right internal jugular vein* is usually selected, although one of the other veins may be preferable and just as revealing. If the venous pressure is relatively normal, the patient can assume a comfortable recumbent position with the head and trunk elevated to about a 30 degree angle without flexing the neck. If the venous pressure is greatly elevated, the pulses can be examined better with the patient in a completely upright position so that the pulsations appear at the jugular level.

The patient's head should be gently rotated away from the examiner. A light shined tangentially across the area being examined may help detect a slightly distended vein. A series of undulant waves that are better seen than felt characterize the venous pulse, a graphic recording of which is shown in Fig. 3-3. These pulsations are evaluated in relation to the cardiac cycle and therefore the carotid pulse or heart sounds can be used for timing them.

A WAVE. The A wave is produced by right atrial contraction and the retrograde transmission of the pressure pulse to the jugular veins. It occurs at the time of the fourth heart sound, preceding the first heart sound. The A wave can be easily identified by placing the index finger on the carotid pulse opposite the side being inspected. Because of the compliance of the great veins and the low pressures in the right heart, the A wave will be seen to start just slightly before the carotid pulse is palpated in the neck. The A wave is absent during atrial fibrillation. Giant A waves reflect an elevated right atrial pressure and may be seen in such conditions as pulmonary hypertension and pulmonic and tricuspid stenosis. *Cannon A waves* are an exaggerated form of the giant A wave. In this situation the right atrium contracts during ventricular systole, when the tricuspid valve is closed, and the blood regurgitates into the neck veins. *Regular* cannon waves may occur during A-V junctional (nodal) rhythm when the atria and ventricles contract almost simultaneously. *Irregular* cannon waves may occur during A-V dissociation of any cause and during ectopic beating.

C WAVE. The C wave begins shortly after the first heart sound and may result from impact of the carotid artery on the adjacent jugular vein or from retrograde transmission of a positive wave in the right atrium, generated by the bulging tricuspid valve during right ventricular systole. The C wave is often difficult to visualize by inspecting the neck veins.

V WAVE. Continued atrial filling during ventricular systole produces the V wave, which peaks just after the second heart sound, when the tricuspid valve opens. Tricuspid insufficiency causes a very large V wave.

X DESCENT. The X descent is the downslope of the A and C waves and results from right atrial diastole, plus the effects of the tricuspid valve being pulled downward during ventricular systole. Tricuspid insufficiency blunts or eliminates the X descent, whereas elevated right ventricular output and constrictive pericarditis may enhance it.

Y DESCENT. The Y descent represents the fall in the right atrial pressure from the peak of the V wave following tricuspid valve opening and occurs during the period of rapid atrial emptying in early diastole. Impedance to right atrial emptying, caused by tricuspid stenosis or atresia or by right atrial myxoma, dampens the Y descent. Constrictive pericarditis produces a speedy Y descent and prominent trough, followed by a rapid Y ascent as the ventricular, atrial, and venous pressures promptly rise when the nondistensible right ventricle becomes filled with blood.

* * *

Respiration alters the venous pulse. Deep inspiration lowers the level of the venous pressure pulsation (actual amplitude of the pulse waves may be increased) by a decrease in intrathoracic pressure. This increases venous return, reduces central venous pressure, and increases right heart filling to lower the level of the venous pulse in the neck and collapse the neck veins. Expiration produces reversed effects. The *Valsalva maneuver,* that is, forced expiratory straining against a closed glottis, elevates the venous pressure by obstructing flow into the chest.

KUSSMAUL'S SIGN is a paradoxical rise in venous pressure and neck vein distention during inspiration and is seen in the patient with severe right heart failure or pericardial constriction. The limited capacity of the right ventricle to receive the increased volume of venous return generated by inspiration results in a backing up of blood into the superior vena cava and distention of the neck veins.

HEPATOJUGULAR REFLUX is a sustained rise in the level of venous pressure during abdominal compression when the patient is breathing normally. As the liver or splanchnic vessels are compressed, the volume of venous blood returning to the right heart is thought to increase. The normal heart accepts this extra load easily. During right heart failure, constrictive pericarditis, or hypervolemia the venous pressure rises because the right ventricle is unable to accommodate the increased blood volume. The prominent V wave of tricuspid insufficiency may be exposed by this maneuver. Manual abdominal compression may cause discomfort resulting in muscular guarding. This muscle tension may increase intra-abdominal pressure (Valsalva maneuver) and give a falsely positive hepatojugular reflux.

RESPIRATION

The rate and character of the patient's respirations should be carefully observed. Under normal conditions the adult should breathe comfortably about 16 to 20 times per minute. Variations in the normal rate and character of respirations include the following:

tachypnea rapid shallow breathing that may indicate pain, cardiac insufficiency, anemia, fever, or pulmonary problems.

bradypnea slow breathing as a result of opiates, coma, excessive alcohol, and increased intracranial pressure.

hyperventilation simultaneous rapid, deep breathing found in extreme anxiety states, in diabetic acidosis, and after vigorous exercise.

Cheyne-Stokes respiration periodic breathing with *hyperpnea* (increased depth of breathing) alternating with *apnea* (cessation of breathing), encountered in cardiac failure and central nervous system disease.

sighing respiration normal respiratory rhythm interrupted by a deep inspiration, followed by a prolonged expiration accompanied by an audible sigh. This variation is often associated with emotional depression.

dyspnea conscious difficulty or effort in breathing. When the patient assumes an elevated position of the trunk at rest to breathe more comfortably, this is called *orthopnea*. Dyspnea is a cardinal sign of left ventricular failure and may also occur in certain lung disorders.

obstructive breathing (air trapping) In obstructive pulmonary diseases such as emphysema and asthma, it is easier for air to enter the lungs than for it to leave. During rapid respiration, sufficient time for full expiration is not available and air becomes trapped in the lungs. The patient's chest overexpands and his breathing becomes more shallow. Expiratory wheezes may be present. Further examination of lung function is discussed later in this chapter.

BLOOD PRESSURE

Arterial blood pressure. Cardiac contraction maintains blood pressure in both arteries and veins. The arterial blood pressure is an overall reflection of the function of the ventricles as pumps. Blood pressure in the arterial system is represented by the peak systolic and diastolic levels of the pressure pulse and is modified by cardiac output, peripheral arteriolar resistance, distensibility of the arteries, amount of blood in the system, and viscosity of the blood. Accordingly, changes in blood pressure reflect changes in these measurements. For example, the decrease in vessel distensibility in the elderly lowers diastolic pressure and increases systolic pressure to produce systolic hypertension. Increments in blood volume may raise both systolic and diastolic components.

Normal blood pressure in the aorta and large arteries, such as the brachial artery, varies between 100 and 140 mm Hg systolic and between 60 and 90 mm Hg diastolic. Pressure in the smaller arteries is somewhat less, and in the arterioles, where the blood enters the capillaries, it is about 35 mm Hg. However, wide variation of normal blood pressure exists, and a value may fall outside the normal range in healthy adults. The normal range also varies with age, sex, and race. A pressure reading of 100/60 may be normal for one person but hypotensive for another.

Observing changes in blood pressure and in pulse pressure (the difference between systolic and diastolic pressures and normally 30 to 50 mm Hg) is important in the care of a patient with an acute myocardial infarction. A reduction in blood pressure from a prior level of 150/100 mm Hg to 115/70 after myocardial infarction may indicate impending cardiovascular decompensation, such as congestive heart failure or shock. Tachycardia and pericardial tamponade also may reduce arterial pressure and narrow pulse pressure.

Measurement. Arterial blood pressure can be measured directly or indirectly. The *indirect* method is performed with a sphygmomanometer. It is a simple procedure and accurate enough for most determinations. With this method, systolic pressures may be slightly below and diastolic pressures slightly above directly obtained values. Rather than measuring one complete beat, the indirect method measures the systolic pressure of some beats and the diastolic pressure of other beats; it does not measure a mean pressure.

For routine indirect blood pressure measurements the patient may be either sitting or reclining. In some cases blood pressure may change with body position, and in this situation the pressure should be recorded with the patient in reclining, sitting, and standing positions. In order to obtain a realistic measurement the patient should have had the opportunity to relax for awhile.

The collapsed cuff should be affixed snugly and smoothly to the patient's arm, with the distal margin of the cuff at least 3 cm above the antecubital fossa. The arm should be rested on a table or a bed and the examiner should palpate for the location of the brachial artery pulse. Pressure in the cuff is then rapidly increased to a level about 30 mm Hg above the point at which the palpable pulse disappears. As the cuff is deflated, observations may be made by either palpation or auscultation. The point at which the pulse can be felt is recorded from the manometer as the palpatory systolic pressure. The auscultatory method is usually preferred; with this method, vibrations from the artery under pressure, called "*Korotkoff sounds*", are used as indicators.

For auscultatory blood pressure measurement the bell or diaphragm of the stethoscope is pressed lightly over the brachial artery while the cuff is slowly deflated, and pressure readings begin at the time the sounds first become audible. As the cuff is deflated further, the sounds become louder for a brief period; then they become muffled and finally disappear. The systolic blood pressure is the point at which sounds become audible, and the diastolic blood pressure is the point at which the sounds cease to be heard. If sounds continue to zero pressure, as they may at times in aortic regurgitation and thyrotoxicosis, three values may be recorded: the first value is the point of audibility of sounds; the second value is when sounds become muffled; and the third value is zero, when sounds disappear. The second value should be accepted as the diastolic pressure, since a diastolic pressure of zero is impossible.

Although the sounds may disappear at a certain reading on the manometer, one should continue to listen at zero pressure to detect the possible presence of the *auscultatory gap.* In this situation the examiner may first detect systolic sounds at a high level, only to have them suddenly disappear and then reappear at a lower level. For example, sounds may be heard first at 180 mm Hg, disappear at 160 mm Hg, and then reappear at 120 mm Hg. This phenomenon is depicted in Fig. 3-4. One can appreciate the problem only by inflating the cuff to 150 mm Hg. In this instance a patient might be considered normotensive when actually he is hypertensive.

The patient's blood pressure should be checked in both arms and any difference noted. A difference of 5 mm Hg may exist. If the patient has hypertension or reduced pulses in the lower extremities, the blood pressure readings are also taken in the legs. In this situation the cuff is placed around the lower third of the thigh and the stethoscope is applied to the popliteal artery. In the event that the thigh is too thick for cuff placement the examiner may place the cuff around the calf and palpate the dorsalis pedis or posterior tibial pulse.

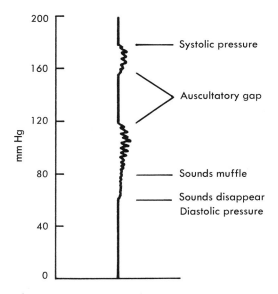

Fig. 3-4. Detection of auscultatory gap in blood pressure measurement. The systolic sounds are first heard at 180 mm Hg. They disappear at 160 mm Hg and reappear at 120 mm Hg; the silent interval is called the auscultatory gap. The Korotkoff sounds muffle at 80 mm Hg and disappear at 60 mm Hg. The blood pressure is recorded as 180/60, noting the presence of the auscultatory gap.

The blood pressure in the leg should be equal to or slightly greater than that in the brachial artery. If the patient has hypertension, is taking medication that may affect blood pressure, or is just beginning to ambulate following a period of bed rest, it is also important to check the blood pressure in the standing, sitting, and supine positions.

Direct measurement of arterial pressure may be indicated for the patient in shock whose blood pressure is too low to be determined accurately by the cuff method. It also may be useful in managing patients who have a low blood volume or who are being treated with hypertensive or hypotensive drugs. An arterial catheter, in addition to directly measuring blood pressure, provides continuous recording without disturbing the patient and allows frequent blood sampling to determine blood gas levels and arterial pH during the management of patients with cardiogenic shock or respiratory insufficiency and those using mechanical ventilators.

For direct measurement of arterial blood pressure, a needle or catheter is inserted into the brachial, radial, or femoral artery. A catheter may be advanced centrally into the aorta or even into the left ventricle. A catheter in the central aorta permits accurate assessment of the diastolic and mean aortic pressures and is very important for the patient who has a myocardial infarction, because these pressures may significantly affect coronary blood flow. Catheters should not remain in the left ventricle or ascending arch of the aorta proximal to the origin of the cephalic arteries because of the risk of embolization. They may be maintained safely in the subclavian artery or descending thoracic aorta for several hours or even several days with proper attention.

A plastic tube filled with heparinized saline solution connects the catheter to a pressure-sensitive device or a strain-gauge transducer. This device converts the mechanical energy that the blood exerts on the recording membrane into changes in electrical voltage or current that can be calibrated in millimeters of mercury. The electrical signal can then be transmitted to an electronic recorder and an oscilloscope, which continually record and display the pressure waves. The transducer and oscilloscope method is more accurate than the sphygmomanometer method and yields an electrically integrated mean pressure.

On the oscilloscopes, the arterial pressure wave forms for the brachial and radial arteries appear identical. The more distal the catheter is from the aorta, the higher the systolic pressure, resulting from the amplification effect in the arterial system during systole. The normal arterial waveform should be clearly discernible, reflecting a rapid upstroke to the peak of systolic pressure, followed by a more gradual downslope. Approximately at the end of ventricular systole, a secondary smaller upstroke, termed the "dicrotic notch" and caused by a rebound against the closing aortic valve, occurs (see Fig. 3-2, A). The accuracy of intra-arterial pressure readings depends on accurate catheter placement, solid connections between the parts of the system, and arterial line patency. The daily care of this system is discussed in Chapter 8.

Venous blood pressure. In addition to evaluating the contour of the jugular venous pulse, one can obtain further information about the right side of the heart by determining the level of venous pressure. Venous pressure refers to the pressure exerted within the venous system by the blood. It is highest in the venule of the extremities and lowest at the point where the vena cava enters the heart. Venous blood flow is continuous rather than pulsatory. In the arm, venous pressure normally ranges from 5 to 14 cm H_2O and in the inferior vena cava, from 6 to 8 cm H_2O. Blood volume, tone of the vessel wall, patency of veins, competence of venous valves, function of the right heart, respiratory function, and force of gravity all influence venous pressure. The veins most commonly used in this estimation are the hand and arm veins, the internal jugular veins, and the external jugular veins.

Measurement. When the examiner is using the veins on the dorsum of the hand to determine venous pressure, the patient should be sitting with his hand held sufficiently below the level of the heart to permit venous distention. As the arm is slowly raised, one can observe the level at which venous collapse occurs. Normally this occurs when the dorsum of the hand reaches a point just above the sternal notch. In cases of elevated venous pressure, the vertical distance above the sternal notch at which the veins collapse provides a rough estimate of the venous pressure.

The *external jugular vein* is commonly used because of its easy accessibility. It is considered less reliable in determining venous pressure than the internal jugular veins, since it is smaller and takes a less direct route to the superior vena cava. To evaluate the pressure in the external jugular vein, the examiner should have the patient recline with the trunk elevated at an angle of 30 to 60 degrees and the head rotated slightly away from the vein being examined. Semielevation is important because the external jugular veins are normally collapsed above the level of the suprasternal notch when the person is upright. The examiner gradually elevates the head of the bed or table until venous distention is visible. The examiner then occludes the external jugular vein by pressing the neck just above and parallel to the clavicle. After waiting approximately 20 seconds for the vein to fill, the examiner quickly withdraws the finger and observes the height of the distended fluid column within the vein. If visible at all, the level will normally be less than 3 to 5 cm above the sternal angle of Louis (Fig. 3-5).

As previously mentioned, the *internal jugular vein* is the most reliable indicator of indirect venous pressure as well as venous pulse waveform. The patient's trunk should be elevated to the optimum angle for the observation of venous pulse. The highest point of visible pulsation of the internal jugular vein is determined and the vertical distance between this level and the level of the sternal angle of Louis is recorded. The angle of elevation of the patient should also be recorded.

It is important to note that the sternal angle is used as a bedside reference point for the sake of convenience. The ideal reference level for venous pressure measurement is the midpoint of the right atrium. This level is established by running an imaginary anteroposterior line from the fourth interspace half-

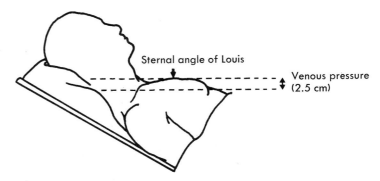

Fig. 3-5. Sternal angle of Louis as a reference point for measuring venous pressure. The height of the distended fluid column in the external jugular vein is less than 3 cm above the sternal angle.

way to the back. A horizontal plane through this point is the zero level for the measurement of venous pressure. The vertical distance from this plane to the head of the blood column, or the meniscus, approximates the venous pressure (Fig. 3-6). Elevations of pressure above 10 cm H_2O are considered abnormal. mal.

Central venous pressure. The direct measurement of central venous pressure (CVP) becomes important if there is a doubt about the value obtained by indirect measurement, or when monitoring a critically ill patient, a situation in which CVP is considered an important sign to follow (Chapter 4).

The CVP indicates right atrial pressure, which primarily reflects alterations in right ventricular pressure and only secondarily reflects changes in the pulmonary venous pressure or the pressure in the left side of the heart. The CVP provides valuable information with regard to blood volume and adequacy of central venous return.

The CVP can be obtained by inserting a polyethylene catheter into the external jugular, antecubital, or femoral vein and threading it into the vena cava. The medial antecubital veins are used more commonly than the others. The catheter offers a method for CVP measurement as well as an intravenous route for drawing blood samples, administering fluid or medications, performing phlebotomy, and possibly inserting a pacing catheter.

The procedure for setting up the CVP system is as follows:

1. Using a three-way stopcock, attach the catheter to a water manometer and an intravenous infusion line. When the venous pressure is not being read, the stopcock is adjusted so that the intravenous fluid will run through the catheter and keep it patent.

2. Mount the manometer on a pole by placing the zero marking at the level of the right atrium. The level of the right atrium can be determined by placing the patient flat and measuring 5 cm down from the top of the

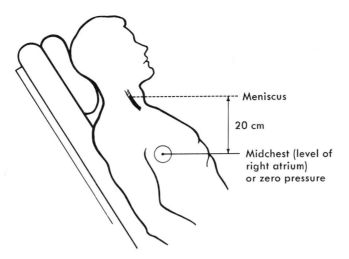

Fig. 3-6. Estimation of venous pressure accomplished by elevating the head until the meniscus is visualized. The venous pressure is measured as the vertical distance between the meniscus and midchest, or right atrial level, in this case, 20 cm and elevated above normal.

chest at the fourth interspace. Run a yardstick from the patient's chest to the baseline of the manometer.

3. Flush the line as necessary to maintain patency.

4. To prevent infection, place an antibiotic ointment and a 2 × 2 inch dressing over the catheter insertion site.

The procedure for measuring CVP is as follows:

1. Place the patient flat in bed and be certain that the zero point of the manometer is at the level of the right atrium.

2. Determine patency of the catheter by opening the intravenous infusion line briefly to a rapid flow rate.

3. Turn the stopcock to allow the intravenous solution to run into the manometer to a level 10 to 20 cm above the expected pressure reading.

4. Turn the stopcock to allow the intravenous solution to flow from the manometer into the catheter. The fluid level in the manometer falls rapidly and fluctuates during respiration, decreasing with inspiration and increasing with expiration. Ventilatory assistance should be stopped during the measurement.

5. When the fluid level is constant, read the CVP. Some fluctuation will occur during respiration.

6. After the reading has been obtained, return the stopcock to the intravenous infusion position.

The normal CVP range is 4 to 10 cm H_2O. The CVP may be measured either in centimeters of water or in millimeters of mercury. The value in centimeters of water may be converted to millimeters of mercury by dividing the former by 1.36, since 1 mm Hg = 1.36 cm H_2O.

Abnormal CVPs must be interpreted according to the clinical situation and other considerations—urine output, skin turgor, temperature, systemic blood pressure, heart rate, and so on. An elevated CVP (above 10 cm H_2O) may indicate right ventricular failure secondary to left heart failure, pulmonary disease such as pulmonary hypertension or embolism, or cardiac tamponade. A low CVP (below 4 cm H_2O) may indicate hypovolemia or peripheral blood pooling, as in septic shock. Taking a single CVP value is less useful than noting repeated measurements, particularly after administering a challenge volume load. Further discussion of this measurement appears in Chapter 4, and the daily care of the CVP system is discussed in Chapter 8.

INSPECTION AND PALPATION OF THE HEART

The anterior part of the chest is inspected with the patient in a supine position and the trunk elevated to about a 30-degree angle. The approach should be made from the patient's right side. Certain landmarks on the anterior chest wall are useful as points of reference in describing the location of the heart. The heart rests on the diaphragm and is located beneath and to the left of the sternum. The base of the heart is situated approximately at the level of the third rib; the apex of the heart lies approximately at the level of the fifth rib in the midclavicular line. The anterior surface of the heart proceeding from the examiner's left to right, facing the patient, is composed of the right atrium, right ventricle, and left ventricle (Fig. 3-7). The anterior surface of the chest closest to the heart and aorta is called the *precordium*.

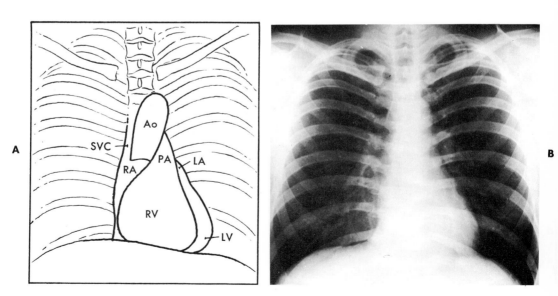

Fig. 3-7. A, Schematic illustration of the parts of the heart whose outlines can be detected in **B.** *Ao,* Aorta; *SVC,* superior vena cava; *RA,* right atrium; *PA,* pulmonary artery; *LA,* left atrium; *RV,* right ventricle; *LV,* left ventricle. **B,** Frontal projection x-ray film of the normal cardiac silhouette.

Inspection begins by observing the precordium for abnormal pulsations. Tangential lighting may be helpful in detecting these pulsations. Any visible impulse medial to the apex and in the third, fourth, or fifth interspace generally originates in the right ventricle and is usually abnormal. In pronounced right ventricular enlargement, one can usually see the lower sternum heave with the heartbeat. It is important to determine when the movements occur by correlating them with the heart sounds or carotid artery pulsations.

Following inspection, palpation of the precordium is performed to confirm the findings of inspection and to locate further *impulses* and *thrills*. The palmar bases of the fingers are used, since this area is most sensitive to feeling vibrations. First palpate the areas where pulsations are visible, then feel specific areas of the precordium systematically (Fig. 3-8).

Aortic area. The second interspace to the right of the sternum is felt for a pulsation, thrill, or vibration of aortic valve closure. Abnormal pulsations may be produced by dilation of the ascending aorta. A vibratory thrill is associated with aortic stenosis, and an accentuated aortic valve closure is felt in patients with arterial hypertension. Thrills at the base can best be palpated with the patient sitting up and leaning forward.

Pulmonic area. The second and third left interspaces are evaluated for abnormalities in the pulmonary artery or valve. A relatively slow, sustained, and forceful pulsation of the pulmonary artery may be felt in mitral stenosis and primary pulmonary hypertension. A palpable sustained pulse and a thrill are associated with pulmonary stenosis.

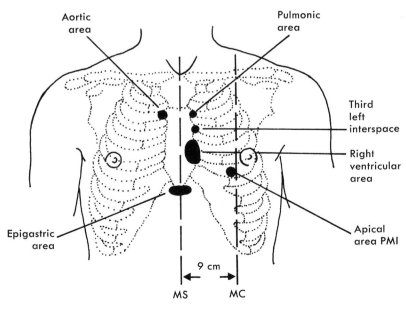

Fig. 3-8. Palpation areas on the precordium for detecting normal and abnormal cardiac pulsations. See text for description.

Right ventricular area. The lower left sternal border, incorporating the third, fourth, and fifth intercostal spaces, is palpated. Abnormal pulsations here are most commonly found in conditions associated with right ventricular enlargement. When the sternum can be felt to move anteriorly during systole, this movement is termed a *"substernal heave"* or *"lift."* Furthermore, a thrill in this area may be palpated in patients who have a ventricular septal defect.

Apical area. The fifth intercostal space at or just medial to the left midclavicular line is palpated for the *point of maximum pulse* (PMI) and the thrills of mitral valve disease. The PMI is evaluated for its location, diameter, amplitude, and duration. In normal adults the PMI is located at or within the left midclavicular line in the fifth intercostal space (Fig. 3-8). The impulse is normally less than 2 cm in diameter and often is smaller. It is felt as a light tap, beginning approximately at the time of the first heart sound, and is sustained during the first one third and one half of systole.

When the PMI is displaced lateral to the midclavicular line, it indicates left ventricular enlargement. A weak PMI may be palpated and may indicate inadequate stroke volume or reduced left ventricular contraction. This finding is difficult to detect in a muscular or obese chest or in patients with emphysema. A sustained or forceful apical impulse usually indicates left ventricular enlargement, such as that associated with aortic stenosis or arterial hypertension. A diffuse systolic thrill may be found in patients with mitral regurgitation, whereas a localized diastolic thrill generally is associated with mitral stenosis. Thrills at the apex are best felt with the patient in the left lateral decubitus position. This maneuver helps one find the impulse, but since this position displaces the PMI, no assessment can be made about location.

Epigastric area. The upper central region of the abdomen can have visible or palpable pulsations in some normal individuals. Abnormally large pulsations of the aorta may be produced by an aneurysm of the abdominal aorta or by aortic valvular regurgitation. In right ventricular hypertrophy right ventricular pulsations may also be detected in this area, which may be the best location to palpate the apical impulse in a patient with a distended chest, as in emphysema. In order to distinguish aortic from right ventricular pulsations, the palm of the hand should be placed on the epigastric area, sliding the fingers up under the rib cage. The palmar surface feels the aorta pulsating as the fingertips feel the impulses of the right ventricle.

AUSCULTATION OF THE HEART

Listening over the precordium with a stethoscope remains the most useful physical examination technique for providing information about heart function. Since the examiner depends on the stethoscope to register normal and abnormal sounds for interpretation, attention must be given to selection of the proper instrument. The stethoscope should have properly fitting earpieces, double tubes that are approximately 12 inches in length and 1/8 inch in internal diameter, a bell, and a diaphragm. The bell accentuates the lower frequency sounds, such as diastolic gallops and the rumbling murmur of mitral stenosis, and filters out high-pitched notes. It should be placed very lightly on the skin, with just enough pressure to seal the edge of the unit. More pressure on the bell will cause the skin itself to act as a diaphragm, accentuating high-frequency sounds. Since the diaphragm brings out high-pitched sounds, it should be pressed very firmly against the skin. This will make high-frequency murmurs, such as the murmurs of aortic or mitral insufficiency, audible.

The environment and the patient's position also play important parts in the auscultation procedure. The room should be quiet and the patient should be on a table or bed that will accommodate him comfortably when he is instructed to lie flat, sit up, or roll to one side.

Finally, auscultation of the heart should not be performed as an isolated event. The findings should be correlated with the other results of the physical examination, such as the arterial pulse contour, venous pulse waves, and precordial movements, in order to understand the altered cardiac physiology and anatomy.

Auscultation of the heart requires selective listening for each component of the cardiac cycle while "inching" the stethoscope over the five main topographic areas for cardiac auscultation (Fig. 3-9). Note that these auscultatory areas do not correspond to the anatomic locations of the valves, but rather to the sites at which the particular valve sounds are best heard. Accordingly, one listens with the stethoscope over the following areas:

1. *Aortic area* at the base of the heart in the second intercostal space close to the sternum

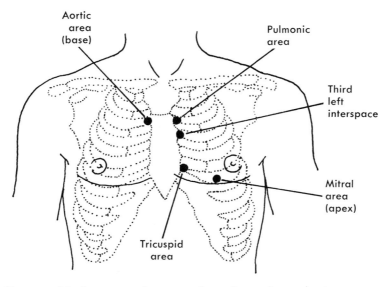

Fig. 3-9. Topographical areas on the precordium for cardiac auscultation. The auscultatory areas do not correspond to the anatomic locations of the valves but rather to the sites at which the particular valves are heard best. See text for description.

2. *Pulmonic area* at the second left intercostal space close to the sternum
3. *Third left intercostal space* where murmurs of both aortic and pulmonic origin may be heard
4. *Tricuspid area* at the lower left sternal border
5. *Mitral area* at the apex of the heart in the fifth left intercostal space just medial to the midclavicular line.

Auscultation is conducted in a systematic fashion. By beginning the process at the aortic area, one can determine the cardiac cycle time by identifying the first and second heart sounds. This will serve as a frame of reference as the

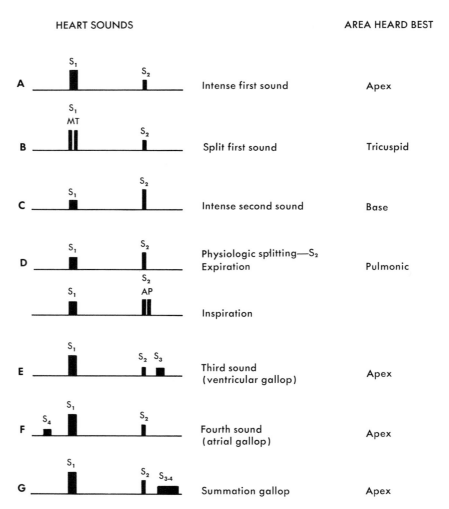

HEART SOUNDS   AREA HEARD BEST

A — Intense first sound — Apex

B — Split first sound — Tricuspid

C — Intense second sound — Base

D — Physiologic splitting—S_2 Expiration / Inspiration — Pulmonic

E — Third sound (ventricular gallop) — Apex

F — Fourth sound (atrial gallop) — Apex

G — Summation gallop — Apex

Fig. 3-10. The intensity and splitting of the first and second heart sounds, their relationship to the third and fourth heart sounds, and the auscultatory areas where these sounds are heard best.

examiner moves to other auscultatory areas of the precordium. At each site the procedure is as follows:

1. Listen to the first heart sound, noting its intensity and splitting.
2. Listen to the second heart sound, noting its intensity and splitting.
3. Note extra sounds in systole, identifying their timing, intensity, and pitch.
4. Note extra sounds in diastole, identifying their timing, intensity, and pitch.
5. Listen for systolic and diastolic murmurs, noting their timing, intensity, quality, pitch, location, and radiation.
6. Listen for extracardiac sounds, such as a pericardial friction rub.

Changes in the intensity of heart sounds may be clinically significant. The intensity of valve sounds is probably related to the speed and force of the valve closure, the excursion of leaflets during closure, and the physical condition of the cusps. Intensity is modified by the proximity of the valve to the chest wall and by the nature of the tissues interposed between valve and stethoscope. Accordingly, the first sound heard at the mitral area (apex) may not only become softer at the aortic area (base), but may also seem shorter and have a different quality which is caused by the dampening effect of the interposed soft tissues. Similarly, the second sound loses intensity as the stethoscope is moved toward the apex. The diagrams in Fig. 3-10 indicate the intensity and splitting of the first and second heart sounds, their relationship to the third and fourth heart sounds, and the auscultatory areas where these sounds can be heard best.

First heart sound (S_1). S_1 is associated with the closure of the mitral and tricuspid valves. It is synchronous with the apical impulse and corresponds to the onset of ventricular systole (Fig. 3-11). It is louder, longer, and lower pitched than the second sound at the apex (Fig. 3-10, *A*). As the ventricles begin to contract and pressure rises within, the tricuspid and mitral valves close. Valvular sounds of the left side slightly precede those of the right and are of higher intensity; the mitral valve closes from 0.02 to 0.03 second before the tricuspid valve. *Splitting* of the first sound may therefore be heard, particularly in the tricuspid area (Fig. 3-10, *B*). Tricuspid closure is normally inaudible to the examiner's ear. The intensity of S_1 relates to the relative position of atrial contraction with respect to ventricular contraction, that is, P-R interval. When the P-R interval is prolonged, the intensity of the first heart sound is decreased, and when the P-R interval shortens up to a point, the S_1 is increased. During A-V dissociation (Chapter 6), the intensity of the first sound varies as the P-R interval varies.

As the pressure within the ventricles continues to rise and exceeds the pressure within the pulmonary artery and aorta, the pulmonic and aortic valves open. Usually opening of these valves is inaudible. If opening of the aortic valve is heard, this is called an aortic ejection sound or click. The same is true for the pulmonic valve. *Early systolic ejection clicks* occur shortly after S_1, as depicted in Fig. 3-11. Aortic ejection clicks are associated with aortic stenosis,

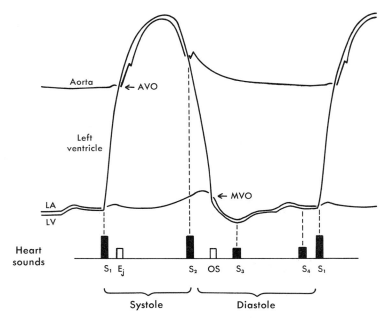

Fig. 3-11. Normal and abnormal heart sounds during one complete cardiac cycle as correlated with left heart pressure waves. Right heart pressures have been omitted for simplification. At the onset of ventricular systole, left ventricular *(LV)* pressure exceeds left atrial *(LA)* pressure to close the mitral valve, producing S_1 (in association with tricuspid valve closure). When LV pressure exceeds aortic pressure, the aortic valve opens *(AVO)*. With valvular disease and hypertension, aortic valve opening may be audible and heard as an early ejection click *(Ej)*. When aortic pressure exceeds LV pressure, the aortic valve closes to produce S_2 in association with pulmonic valve closure. When LV pressure drops below LA pressure, the mitral valve opens *(MVO)*. With thickening of the mitral valve as a result of rheumatic heart disease an opening snap *(OS)* is produced in early diastole. During rapid ventricular filling an S_3, or ventricular gallop, is produced in patients with myocardial failure. Late in diastole an S_4, or atrial gallop, is produced in association with atrial contraction, owing to increased resistance to ventricular filling.

dilation of the aorta, and hypertension and are heard at both the base and the apex. Pulmonary ejection clicks are associated with pulmonary stenosis, dilation of the pulmonary artery, and pulmonary hypertension and are heard in the pulmonic area. A common syndrome is the single or multiple midsystolic click that initiates a late systolic murmur of mitral insufficiency, caused by prolapse of the mitral valve. The click in this instance is a nonejection click.

Second heart sound (S_2). S_2 is associated with the closure of the aortic and pulmonic valves. With the completion of ventricular contraction the pressure within the ventricles and great vessels decreases. The ventricular pressure decreases more rapidly than the pressures within the aorta and pulmonary arteries, causing the aortic and pulmonic valves to close. This is followed by the start of ventricular diastole. At the aortic area, or base, the second sound is almost always louder than the first sound (Fig. 3-10, C).

The aortic component is widely transmitted to the neck and over the precordium. It is, as a rule, entirely responsible for the second sound at the apex. The pulmonary component is softer than the aortic and is normally heard only at and around the second left interspace (pulmonic area). Splitting of the second sound is therefore usually heard best in this region.

Again, events of the left side of the heart occur before those on the right and aortic valve closure slightly precedes that of the pulmonic valve. Transient *splitting* of the second sound may be demonstrated in most normal people during inspiration. Closure of the aortic and pulmonary valves during expiration is synchronous or nearly so because right and left ventricular systoles are approximately equal in duration. With inspiration, venous blood rushes into the thorax from the large systemic venous reservoirs. This action increases venous return and prolongs right ventricular systole by temporarily increasing right ventricular stroke volume, which delays pulmonary valve closure. At the same time, venous return to the left heart diminishes because of the increased pulmonary capacity during inspiration, which decreases left ventricular stroke volume and shortens left ventricular systole. Thus the aortic valve tends to close earlier. These two factors combine to produce transient "physiologic splitting" of the second sound (Fig. 3-10, D).

As the pressure in the ventricles decreases below the pressure in the atria, the atrioventricular valves open. The opening of these valves is characteristically silent. However, when either the mitral or the tricuspid valve is thickened or otherwise altered, as by rheumatic heart disease, it produces an *opening snap* in early diastole (Fig. 3-11). The opening snap of the mitral valve is differentiated from a third heart sound at the apex because it occurs earlier, is sharper and higher-pitched, and radiates more widely.

Third heart sound (S_3). S_3 occurs early in diastole during the phase of rapid ventricular filling, about 0.12 to 0.16 second after S_2 (Fig. 3-11). It is a low-pitched sound, heard best with the bell of the stethoscope pressed lightly over the apex and the patient in the left lateral decubitus position (Fig. 3-10, E). When S_3 is heard in healthy children and young adults, it is called a *physiologic third heart sound* and usually disappears with age. When an S_3 is heard in an older person with heart disease, it usually indicates myocardial failure and is called a *ventricular gallop*. In patients with cardiac disease, one should search carefully for the presence of a ventricular gallop, since it is a key diagnostic sign for the presence of congestive heart failure from any cause.

Fourth heart sound (S_4). S_4 occurs late in diastole, prior to S_1, and is related to atrial contraction (Fig. 3-11). It is a low-pitched sound heard best at the apex with the bell (Fig. 3-10, F). It is uncommon to hear this sound in normal individuals. S_4, or *atrial gallop*, is associated with increased resistance to ventricular filling and is frequently heard in hypertensive cardiovascular disease, coronary artery disease, myocardiopathy, and aortic stenosis. It is a common finding in patients who have had a myocardial infarction. An S_4 may also be heard in patients with A-V block where there is a delayed conduction between the atria and the ventricles.

Summation gallop. In adults with severe myocardial disease and tachycardia, summation of S_3 and S_4 may occur, producing the so-called summation gallop (Fig. 3-10, *G*).

Murmurs

Although the physical principles governing the production of murmurs are complex, from a practical point of view murmurs are related to three main factors, which are as follows:

1. High rates of flow, either through normal or abnormal valves
2. Forward flow through a constricted or deformed valve or into a dilated vessel or chamber
3. Backward flow through a regurgitant valve

The identification of murmurs may contribute important information to the recognition and diagnosis of heart disease. Accordingly, murmurs should be carefully evaluated and described in a manner that provides maximum information. Murmurs are usually characterized in relation to the following criteria:

1. *Timing.* Does the murmur occur during systole, during diastole, or continuously through both? A murmur may be easily differentiated as systolic or diastolic by palpating the pulse. If the murmur occurs simultaneously with the pulse, it is systolic; if it does not, it is diastolic. If a murmur occupies all the time period measured, it is described as holosystolic (pansystolic) or holodiastolic (pandiastolic).
2. *Intensity.* How loud is the murmur? A graded point system is generally accepted to describe the intensity of murmurs, as follows:

   Grade 1: Softest audible murmur
   Grade 2: Murmur of medium intensity
   Grade 3: Loud murmur unaccompanied by thrill
   Grade 4: Murmur with thrill
   Grade 5: Loudest murmur that cannot be heard with the stethoscope off the chest
   Grade 6: Murmur audible with the stethoscope off the chest

3. *Quality.* What is the tonal characteristic of the murmur? Is it harsh? Musical? Blowing? Rumbling? The configuration or shape of a murmur further defines its quality. It may be a crescendo (increasing intensity), decrescendo (decreasing intensity), or crescendo-decrescendo (diamond-shaped) type. Fig. 3-12 depicts these configurations.
4. *Pitch.* What is the sound frequency of the murmur? Is it high? Medium? Low?
5 *Location.* Over what area on the precordium is the murmur heard best? The aortic area? The pulmonic area? The triscuspid area? The mitral area?

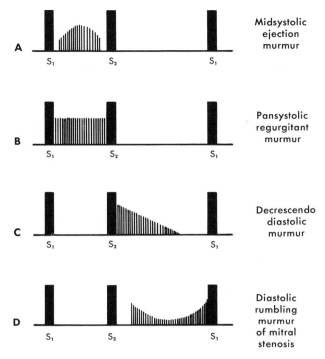

Fig. 3-12. Configuration of murmurs. **A,** Aortic and pulmonic stenosis produce systolic ejection murmurs that begin after the S_1, swell to a crescendo in midsystole, then decrease in intensity (decrescendo), and terminate before the S_2. **B,** Tricuspid and mitral regurgitation and ventricular septal defects produce pansystolic (holosystolic) murmurs that last throughout ventricular systole; usually no interval can be heard between S_1 and S_2 **C,** Aortic and pulmonic regurgitation produce murmurs that begin early in diastole immediately after the S_2 and then diminish an intensity (decrescendo). **D,** Mitral and tricuspid stenosis produce murmurs that begin during early diastole, have a rumbling or rolling quality, and terminate in late diastole with a crescendo effect.

6. *Radiation.* Is there transmission of the murmur elsewhere in the body? Does it radiate across the chest? Into the axilla? Into the neck? Down the left sternal border?

In addition, each of these characteristics is further evaluated as it is influenced by the patient's position and respiration. Certain other maneuvers may be used to further define murmurs, including Valsalva's maneuver, which decreases cardiac output and stroke volume during the strain and increases flow after release. Also, amyl nitrite can be administered, with resultant peripheral vasodilation and increased cardiac output. Changes in the intensity and character of murmurs with these maneuvers aid in determining the type of lesion involved. For instance, with the administration of amyl nitrite, murmurs associated with stenotic lesions usually become louder, whereas regurgitant murmurs decrease in intensity.

Systolic murmurs. Systolic murmurs are the most common murmurs and generally are either ejection or regurgitant murmurs. *Functional* or innocent systolic murmurs are commonly heard in young people and should be differentiated from those murmurs that represent valvular heart disease. Functional murmurs occur during ejection, are short, (less than two thirds of systole), are grade 2 or less in intensity (may become inaudible if the patient raises from a supine to a sitting position), and are heard best over the pulmonary outflow tract. It is important to remember that functional murmurs are intensified by fever, anxiety, anemia, and pregnancy. Therefore the patient should be reexamined under normal conditions.

Midsystolic (ejection) murmurs. *Aortic stenosis* and *pulmonic stenosis* produce systolic ejection murmurs that begin after the first sound, swell to a crescendo in midsystole, then decrease in intensity, and terminate before S_2, generated by closure of the appropriate valve (Fig. 3-12, *A*). The murmur may be harsh or musical and is usually high pitched because of the high velocity of blood flow. Aortic valve murmurs frequently radiate from the second right interspace to the cardiac apex and the carotid arteries. A systolic thrill may be present. Characteristically, pulmonic stenosis murmur is heard better at the second left interspace. Atrial septal defects increase pulmonary flow to produce a pulmonary ejection murmur.

Holosystolic (regurgitant) murmurs. Holosystolic murmurs last throughout ventricular systole (Fig. 3-12, *B*) and no interval can be heard between S_1 and S_2. *Tricuspid* and *mitral regurgitation* and *ventricular septal defects* produce holosystolic murmurs owing to the backflow of blood from the ventricle (high pressure) to the atrium (low pressure) through an incompetent tricuspid or mitral valve or from a high-pressure ventricle (left) to a low-pressure ventricle (right). Unlike the production of ejection murmurs, when a holosystolic murmur is produced one chamber maintains a greater pressure than the other throughout *all* of systole, causing regurgitant blood flow (and the murmur) to last through the entire systolic period. Murmurs caused by ventricular septal defects may seem louder during early systole and those of mitral regurgitation louder during late systole. The murmurs may be blowing, musical, or harsh and are often high pitched. The tricuspid regurgitation murmur is best heard along the lower left sternal border and the intensity commonly increases during inspiration. Mitral regurgitation is best heard at the apex with the patient lying on his left side and often radiates to the left axilla or back. Some forms of mitral regurgitation do not produce holosystolic murmurs. Ventricular septal defects are loudest at the third and fourth left interspaces along the sternal border; often a systolic thrill accompanies the murmur in that area.

During the acute phase of myocardial infarction the *interventricular septum* may *rupture*. Although uncommon, the resulting ventricular septal defect produces a loud systolic murmur, as described previously. The onset of this murmur is sudden and it may be accompanied by a thrill and the features of left and right heart failure.

Myocardial infarction may also produce *papillary muscle rupture*, with subsequent mitral insufficiency and predominantly left heart failure. The onset of the murmur is abrupt and may be difficult to differentiate from that of the perforated interventricular septum, since the features of both catastrophes overlap. Mitral valve dysfunction, without actual rupture of the papillary muscle or chordae tendineae, may establish less severe mitral insufficiency. Abnormalities of the chordae tendineae may produce clicking sounds that occur in the middle of ventricular systole and are referred to as *midsystolic clicks*. These may occur with or without a late systolic murmur. *Ventricular aneurysms* secondary to myocardial infarction may produce muffled heart sounds, gallop rhythms, and both systolic and diastolic murmurs; often a prominent systolic impulse may be palpated over the left precordium.

Diastolic murmurs. Diastolic murmurs generally can be classified into two types: the high-pitched decrescendo murmurs of aortic and pulmonic regurgitation and the lower pitched murmurs of mitral and tricuspid stenosis.

Murmurs of aortic and pulmonic regurgitation begin early in diastole, immediately after the S_2, and then diminish in intensity (decrescendo), as shown in Fig. 3-12, *C*. They are high pitched and blowing and may vary in intensity roughly according to the size of the leak. The murmur of aortic regurgitation may be heard best at the second right or third left interspace along the left sternal border with the patient holding his breath in expiration while leaning forward. The murmur of pulmonic regurgitation is heard at the upper left border of the sternum and cannot be distinguished from its aortic counterpart by auscultation alone. The pitch, timing, quality, and location of these murmurs are similar, although the murmur of pulmonic regurgitation tends to be more localized in the pulmonic area.

Mitral stenosis characteristically produces a low-pitched, localized apical, diastolic rumble, which may be accentuated in late diastole (Fig. 3-12, *D*) when atrial systole causes increased flow across the narrowed mitral valve. A sharp mitral "opening snap" frequently initiates the murmur in early diastole. In addition, a loud, sharp S_1 and accentuation of the S_2 often accompany mitral stenosis. The murmur of mitral stenosis is usually confined to the apex and may be enhanced by mild exercise or by the patient's lying on his left side. The *tricuspid stenosis* murmur is heard near the tricuspid area and is often accentuated along the left sternal border by inspiration.

Continuous murmurs. Murmurs audible in both systole and diastole are usually caused by connections between the arterial and venous or systemic and pulmonary circulations. A patent ductus arteriosus produces such a murmur. Table 3-1 summarizes the characteristics of the most common heart murmurs.

A benign sound heard at the lower border of the sternocleidomastoid muscle in some normal adults in the sitting position is called a *venous hum*. Although continuous, the venous hum is loudest in diastole and radiates to the first and second interspaces, with a soft to moderate intensity. It has a roaring quality, is low pitched, and can be obliterated by pressure on the jugular veins.

Table 3-1. Characteristics of types of valvular heart disease

Condition	Causes	Description of murmurs				Radiation or transmission	Other signs
		Time	Quality	Pitch (frequency)	Location of maximum intensity		
Aortic stenosis (narrowing of valve)	Rheumatic Calcification Congenital	Systolic (ejection)	Crescendo-decrescendo (diamond shaped) Harsh Rough	Variable pitch	Second interspace (aortic area)	Radiates to carotid arteries and apex	Slow rising "anacrotic" pulse Sustained pulse Left ventricular lift Systolic thrill Ejection "click" Diminished aortic closing sound
Aortic regurgitation (blood flows back from aorta into left ventricle)	Rheumatic Syphilitic Calcification Cystic medial necrosis	Diastolic	Blowing loudest just after S_2—diminishes during diastole decrescendo	High pitched	Second right interspace; third left interspace or along left sternal border with patient leaning forward and holding breath		Wide pulse pressure Left ventricular lift Brisk, quick pulses (water hammer) Tambour aortic closing sound
Mitral stenosis (narrowing of valve; blood flows through valve during diastole)	Rheumatic Congenital Tumor (myxoma)	Diastolic	Rumble presystolic accentuation in sinus rhythm	Low pitched	Well localized to apex, best heard in left lateral decubitus position		Atrial fibrillation often develops Loud S_1 Opening snap
Mitral regurgitation ("leaky" valve—blood reenters left atrium from left ventricle during systole)	Rheumatic Congenital Papillary muscle dysfunction/rupture Chordae tendineae dysfunction/rupture Heart failure associated with left ventricular dilation from any cause	Holosystolic	Blowing	High pitched	Apex, best heard in left lateral decubitus position	Axilla and back	S_3 common

Pericardial friction rub. An extracardiac sound that may be detected during the auscultation procedure is the pericardial friction rub. It is a sign of pericardial inflammation and, present in its complete form, exhibits three components. One is associated with ventricular systole, the second with the phase of rapid ventricular filling early in diastole, and the third with atrial systole. If only the systolic component of the rub is present, it may be misinterpreted as a scratchy murmur. The pericardial friction rub is best heard with the patient lying flat on his back in the third or fourth interspace to the left of the sternum, although the location may be variable. There is little radiation, and the quality of the sound is a leathery, high-pitched, multiphasic, scratchy rub that resembles the sound of two pieces of sandpaper being rubbed together.

EXAMINATION OF THE LUNGS

Disorders of the lungs may alter or be altered by cardiac conditions. Consequently, in assessing the cardiovascular status of a patient, one must also evaluate lung function. Examination of the anterior, lateral, and posterior chest is best accomplished with the patient in the sitting position. This may be done immediately following or just prior to the cardiac examination, before the patient assumes the supine position.

Understanding the anatomy of the lungs is essential to conducting a proper examination, since each bronchopulmonary lobe must be evaluated. The schematic illustrations of the lung lobes in anterior, posterior, and right and left lateral views in Fig. 3-13 may be helpful.

The lungs rest in the thorax, with the apex of each lung rising about 2 to 4 cm above the inner one third of the clavicles. The inferior border of the lungs runs from approximately the sixth rib at the midclavicular line to the eighth rib at the midaxillary line anteriorly and along the level of the tenth thoracic spinous process posteriorly. The lungs are divided by fissures into lobes, the left lung into two lobes, the right lung into three lobes. The locations of the fissures are identified by corresponding surface sites. On the anterior chest wall the horizontal fissure of the right lung runs from the fifth rib at the midaxillary line to the level of the fourth rib. On the lateral chest wall the spinous process of the third thoracic vertebra and the sixth rib at the midclavicular line denote the direction of the right and left oblique fissures. When the patient holds up his arms, the oblique fissures are close to the vertebral borders of the scapulae on the posterior chest wall.

The following discussion briefly covers the physical findings gathered during inspection, palpation, percussion, and auscultation of the chest with reference to the lungs.

Inspection and palpation. As discussed earlier in the chapter, the examiner observes the rate and pattern of respiration, the expansion of the chest with breathing, and the symmetry of the thorax. Normally the entire rib cage uniformly moves laterally and upward with respiration. Palpation refines the assessment of the degree and symmetry of expansion in respiration, detects any

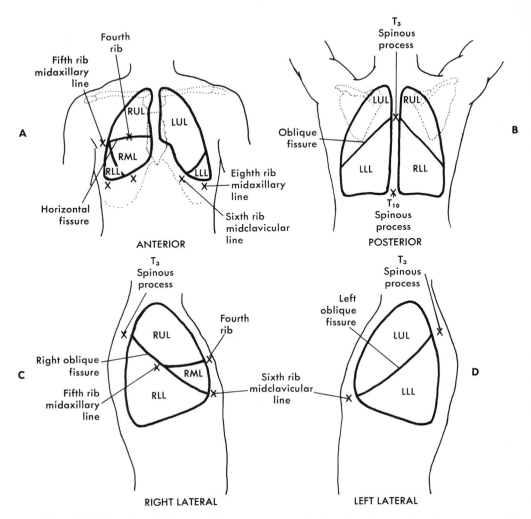

Fig. 3-13. The lung lobes and their anatomic landmarks in anterior, **A,** posterior, **B,** and right and left lateral **C** and **D,** views. See text for description.

areas of tenderness, and permits the examiner to feel *fremitus* (sound vibrations) when the patient speaks. Fremitus is most prominent over areas where the bronchi are relatively close to the chest wall and can be elicited by asking the patient to repeat words such as "one-one-one" or "ninety-nine." Fremitus increases as the intensity of the voice increases and its pitch drops; conversely, it decreases as the intensity of the voice decreases and the pitch rises. Fremitus may also decrease or be absent with an obstructed bronchus, pneumothorax, or pleural effusion. If the chest wall is markedly thickened, as in obesity, fremitus may be diminished. Increased fremitus is produced by consolidation of the lung in the presence of an intact airway.

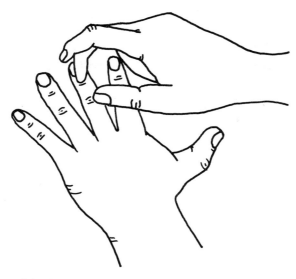

Fig. 3-14. Position of the hands in percussion. The distal two phalanges of the middle finger of the left hand for a right-handed examiner are placed firmly against the patient's chest in the intercostal space parallel to the ribs. The palm and other fingers of the left hand do not touch the chest wall. Then, as shown here, the examiner *quickly* strikes the distal phalanx of the stationary finger with the tip of the middle finger of the right hand.

Percussion. Percussion is performed to determine the relative amount of air or solid material in the underlying lung and to delineate the boundaries of organs or the portions of the lung that differ in structural density. The procedure of percussion involves placing the distal two phalanges of the middle finger of the left hand (for right-handed examiners) firmly against the patient's chest in the intercostal space parallel to the ribs. The palm and other fingers of the left hand should not touch the chest wall. Then with the tip of the middle finger of the right hand, *quickly* strike the distal phalanx of the stationary finger, as shown in Fig. 3-14. One or two rapid strikes in succession with a loose wrist action produces the desired percussion note. (To initially learn the technique of percussion, it may be helpful to percuss a wall in a room and note the difference in sound over the beams when compared with that over the hollows.)

The anterior and lateral chest walls are percussed in a top-to-bottom, side-to-side fashion while comparing the symmetry of sound and feeling. Similarly, the posterior lung fields are percussed, working down to the level of the diaphragm and comparing percussion notes.

The sounds produced by percussion should be evaluated with respect to four qualities:

1. *Resonance.* Resonance is the percussion note elicited over the normal lung. Although it may vary with the thickness of the chest wall, resonance projects a clear, low-pitched, and well-sustained note. A hyper-

resonant note, in general, is associated with hyperaeration of the lungs, as in pneumothorax or obstructive emphysema.

2. *Tympany.* The tympanic note is normally heard in the left upper quadrant of the abdomen over the air-filled stomach or over any hollow viscus. The note is loud, musical, and well-sustained, with a high-pitched, clear, hollow, and drumlike quality.

3. *Dullness.* Dullness is produced when the air content of the underlying tissue is decreased and its solidity increased, as in pneumonia or pleural effusion. The dull sound is soft, short, and high-pitched, with a thudding quality. It lacks the vibratory quality of the resonant note. A dull note is elicited normally over the heart or over bone. Of particular importance is the phenomenon of shifting dullness, that is, a change in the site of abdominal percussion dullness with a change in posture, since it suggests free fluid in the pleural cavity.

4. *Flatness.* Flatness is produced when no air is present in the underlying tissue. It is absolute dullness. The flat note is short, high pitched, and feeble. Normally the flat sound is percussed over the muscles of the arm and thigh and over the liver.

Diaphragmatic excursion can be measured by determining the distance between the levels of dullness on full expiration and full inspiration, normally about 5 cm. High levels of dullness over the posterior chest are associated with pleural effusion, atelectasis, or an elevated diaphragm.

Auscultation. Auscultation of the lung fields permits the examiner to make determinations about the state of bronchial patency of various lung divisions, to assess the quality and intensity of breath sounds, and to note any abnormal sounds. The patient should be asked to breathe somewhat deeper than usual, with the mouth open. Auscultation is then accomplished in a sequence similar to that of percussion, beginning with the upper lung fields, listening to one side, then the other, and then comparing both down to the level of the diaphragm. All portions of the lung fields—posterior, anterior, and lateral—must be systematically auscultated.

Normal breath sounds. Normal breath sounds can be categorized as vesicular, bronchial, and bronchovesicular. *Vesicular* breath sounds occur over most of the lungs and have a prominent inspiratory component and a brief expiratory phase. *Bronchial* breath sounds, also called tracheal breath sounds, are normally heard over the trachea and main bronchi. These sounds are hollow, tubular, and harsh and are heard best during expiration. *Bronchovesicular* breath sounds are heard over the main stem of the bronchi and represent an intermediate stage between bronchial and vesicular breathing.

Abnormal breath sounds. Normal breath sounds in one area may be pathologic when heard somewhere else. For example, bronchial and bronchovesicular breath sounds are heard over a consolidated, compressed, or fibrosed lung. Furthermore, diminished breath sounds occur with local or diffuse bronchial obstruction and with pleural disease associated with the presence of fluid, air, or scar tissue. With airways narrowed, the breath sounds are characteristically wheezing and whistling in nature, with a prolonged expiratory and a short inspiratory phase, as heard in patients with asthma.

Rales are abnormal sounds that occur when air passes through bronchi that contain fluid of any kind. They are subdivided into interrupted crackling sounds, termed *moist rales,* and continuous coarse sounds, called *rhonchi.* Rhonchi suggest a pathologic condition in the trachea or larger bronchi, whereas moist medium and fine rales imply bronchiolar and alveolar disease. *Fine rales* are short and high-pitched and can be simulated by rubbing a strand of hair between the thumb and forefinger next to the ear. *Medium rales* are louder and lower pitched.

In left ventricular failure the presence of rales is one of the earliest physical findings. Rales occur as a result of the transudation of edema fluid into the pulmonary alveoli. At first the alveolar fluid is dependent in location, and rales are present at the base of the lungs. As the failure becomes increasingly severe, the rales become more generalized. The rales of left ventricular failure are typically fine and crepitant, but as failure progresses, they may become moist and coarse. The findings may be difficult to differentiate from those caused by pulmonary infiltrations of an inflammatory nature. Rales from left ventricular failure often develop first at the right lung base but are frequently bibasilar.

Pleural friction rub. Inflammation of the visceral and parietal pleurae may result in loss of lubricating fluid so that apposing pleural surfaces rub together, producing a low-pitched, coarse, grating sound with respiration. When the patient holds his breath the rub disappears.

Finally, one should be wary of the adventitious sounds produced when a stethoscope is not held firmly against the chest. Body hair can rub across the instrument during respiration and produce an annoying crackling sound.

Laboratory studies

Certain laboratory studies may be useful in collecting objective data regarding the clinical status of the patient with coronary artery disease. Results from the laboratory studies are correlated with findings from the patient interview and the physical examination. From this complete data base, decisions are made regarding the nature of the problem and the plan of management. The laboratory tests frequently ordered under these circumstances that will be briefly described include chest x-ray films; electrocardiograms; exercise testing; tests of blood levels of cholesterol, triglycerides, and serum enzymes; phonocardiograms; echocardiograms; radionuclide studies; cardiac catheterization; and coronary arteriograms.

CHEST X-RAY FILMS

The posteroanterior (PA) chest film is routinely taken as part of the initial evaluation or may be ordered later if the patient develops new signs or symptoms (Fig. 3-7). A lateral film may be taken as well to aid in evaluating the findings of the PA film. The chest x-ray film provides information regarding overall heart size and individual cardiac chamber enlargement; the position of the heart in the chest; the size and configuration of the great vessels; the presence of calcification in the heart muscle, valves, aorta, or coronary arteries; and changes in the lungs or other thoracic structures secondary to heart disease.

ELECTROCARDIOGRAMS (ECGs)

The ECG provides valuable information regarding cardiac rhythm, conduction, and pathologic conditions that affect the heart. It is a routine part of assessing the patient's cardiac status and will be discussed in detail in subsequent chapters.

EXERCISE TESTING

Exercise testing, or stress testing, is a means of evaluating the patient's cardiovascular function and detecting abnormalities of coronary circulation. This procedure may be used to confirm a diagnosis of coronary artery disease in a patient with suspected angina or coronary insufficiency, to evaluate the functional capacity of a person with known disease for purposes of regulating activity or treatment, or to assess the effects of surgery in a patient postoperatively. Inasmuch as the majority of patients with exertional angina and no prior myocardial infarction will demonstrate a normal resting ECG, the progressively graded exercise test has become a valuable noninvasive aid in the clinical diagnosis of coronary heart disease.

Stress testing is designed to systematically and progressively increase myocardial oxygen demand. Accordingly, the exercise program may involve walking up and down steps (Master's test), exercising on a stationary bicycle, or walking on a variable speed and grade treadmill. The patient may be exercised to a predetermined heart rate, often 80% to 85% of the predicted maximum heart rate (submaximal testing), or the exercise may be continued until limiting symptoms develop, such as chest pain or fatigue (maximal or near maximal testing). The patient's ECG and blood pressure are monitored throughout and after the procedure. Indications that an exercise test should be terminated short of a target heart rate or work load include ventricular tachycardia (three or more consecutive premature ventricular systoles), falling blood pressure or heart rate in the face of progressive work loads, vertigo, visual disturbances, frequent premature ventricular extrasystoles or multiformed ventricular extrasystoles, S-T depression greater than 4 mm, intolerable chest pain, and severe anxiety.

The diagnostic criterion for coronary artery disease elicited by stress testing is a depression of 1.0 mm or more of the S-T segment, as depicted in Fig. 3-15. This positive S-T segment response may occur in patients with coronary artery disease during exercise and/or immediately afterward. The more extensive the coronary arterial involvement, the greater the S-T depression. The S-T segment depression is transient, lasting only a matter of minutes, and is observed more commonly in the lateral precordial leads V_4 to

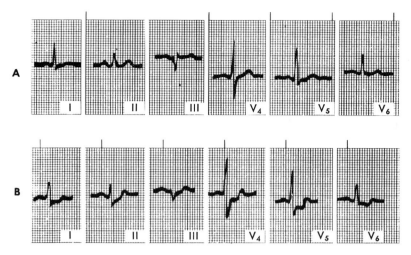

Fig. 3-15. A, Standard limb leads and lateral precordial leads at rest present a normal electrocardiogram. **B,** Immediately after exercise, the patient's ECG shows ischemic S-T segment depression in all the leads.

V_6. Arrhythmias occur often; S-T elevation results, rarely. Positive exercise tests may be followed by further evaluations such as coronary arteriography, which is discussed later in this chapter.

BLOOD LEVELS OF CHOLESTEROL, TRIGLYCERIDES, AND SERUM ENZYMES

Cholesterol and triglycerides. Cholesterol and triglycerides are the lipids of major clinical importance to the patient with coronary artery disease. Since hyperlipidemia is considered a risk factor contributing to coronary artery disease (Chapter 2), the search for this disorder is a routine laboratory test in cardiac patients; the concentration of cholesterol and triglycerides in serum or plasma can be detected clinically. Blood samples for lipid analysis should be obtained after a 14- to 16-hour fast and under the following conditions relative to the patient: (1) no acute illness or stress; (2) no alcoholic beverages for 48 hours prior to the test; and (3) no lipid-influencing drugs, with the exception of insulin in patients with diabetes mellitus. In adults less than 55 years of age, a cholesterol concentration greater than 250 mg/100 ml or a triglyceride level greater than 200 mg/100 ml clearly indicates hyperlipidemia. Elevated cholesterol levels are associated with the ingestion of cholesterol and saturated fats as well as hereditary influences. Triglyceride level elevation is frequently induced by carbohydrate ingestion and commonly accompanies diabetes mellitus.

Both cholesterol and triglycerides are transported in the blood in moieties called lipoproteins. These can be characterized by ultracentrifugation or electrophoresis. Five kinds of abnormalities of blood lipoproteins are described subsequently. Each type is classified according to the abnormal accumulation in the plasma of one or more lipoprotein species, and each may be caused by a primary, or congenital, condition or be secondary to a disease process.

Although it has not been proved that dietary modification and the use of drugs to reduce cholesteremia measurably decrease the progression of atherosclerosis in humans, some clinical trails have demonstrated that a fall in cholesterol produced by dietary management has a favorable effect on the overall incidence of complications of coronary artery disease. Accordingly, conservative measures are used to treat each of the following types of abnormalities.

Type I: Severe elevation in the concentration of chylomicrons. It is usually familial and detected in childhood. Clinical manifestations may include abdominal pains associated with the ingestion of fats. Reduction of fat content in the diet contributes to the resolution of this problem.

Type II: Associated with increased concentration of low-density lipoproteins (LDL). It is usually familial, occurs at all ages, and increases the likelihood of early atherosclerotic cardiovascular disease. Tendon xanthomas are the most common clinical signs. Dietary therapy includes reduction in the intake of cholesterol and saturated fats and increased consumption of polyunsaturated fats. Additionally, medications such as cholestyramine, D-thyroxine, and nicotinic acid may be effective.

Type III: Result of an unusual defect in the metabolism of lipoproteins and causes approximately equal elevations in both cholesterol and triglyceride levels in the plasma. It is present only in adults and produces palmar xanthomas and peripheral vascular disease. Clinical management includes reduction to ideal body weight, use of polyunsaturated fats, and administration of medications such as clofibrate or nicotinic acid.

Type IV: Common pattern secondary to many diseases. It is defined as an increase in plasma very low density lipoprotein (VLDL) content. This type is associated with weight gain and glucose intolerance and may be related to alcohol ingestion. Although external manifestations are not usually present, it probably increases the risk of early coronary artery disease. This abnormality is treated by maintaining the patient's ideal body weight and possibly with medication such as clofibrate.

Type V: Excess plasma levels of chylomicrons and VLDL and may be secondary to such disorders as diabetes, acidosis, alcoholism, and nephrosis. Clinical manifestations may be abdominal pain, glucose intolerance, or hyperinsulinism. Diet therapy includes reduction of caloric, fat, and carbohydrate intake and restricted use of alcohol. In addition, nicotinic acid may be used.

Serum enzymes. If a patient is suspected to have an acute myocardial infarction, evaluation of specific serum enzyme levels in an essential test that contributes to the diagnosis. With the occurrence of myocardial necrosis, intracellular cardiac enzymes leak into the circulation and can be measured in serum. Because the rate of liberation of these enzymes differs following infarction, the time-related pattern of enzyme release is of diagnostic importance. The serum glutamic-oxaloacetic transaminase (SGOT) and creatinine phosphokinase (CPK) levels rise and fall rapidly, whereas the lactic dehydrogenase (LDH) level rises later and remains elevated longer. Table 3-2 presents a summary of the standard enzymes and their activity in myocardial infarction.

Since these enzymes are present in a number of body tissues, there are

Table 3-2. Enzymes evaluated in myocardial infarction

Enzyme	Normal value (units per milliliter)*	Elevated value	
		In myocardial infarction	In other conditions
Serum glutamic-oxaloacetic transaminase SGOT	8-40	Occurs about 6 hours after infarction; in 24-48 hours reaches peak 2-15 times normal value; usually returns to normal after 3-4 days	Occurs in right ventricular failure with hepatic congestion; infarction of kidney, spleen, or intestine; acute pancreatitis; extensive central nervous system damage; primary muscle disease; toxemia of pregnancy; crushing injuries or burns; administration of salicylates, opiates, or coumarin-type anticoagulants; hypothyroidism
Serum lactic dehydrogenase LDH	150-300	Occurs 6-12 hours after infarction; in 3-4 days reaches a peak 2-8 times normal; usually returns to normal in 14 days	Occurs in a variety of muscle, renal, neoplastic, hepatic, and hemolytic diseases as well as in pulmonary conditions simulating myocardial infarction
Creatine phosphokinase CPK	0-4	Occurs within 2-5 hours after acute myocardial infarction; within 24 hours reaches a peak 5-15 times normal; usually returns to normal in 2 or 3 days	Occurs in skeletal muscle disease, stroke, hypothyroidism, myopathy associated with chronic alcoholism, clofibrate therapy, electrocardioversion, cardiac catheterization

*May vary with different laboratory determinations.

many conditions other than myocardial infarction that may produce elevations. For example, liver disease can elevate the SGOT level. If chest pain occurs in the context of a liver disorder, an elevated SGOT level may be mistaken as diagnostic of myocardial infarction. Furthermore, if a patient with chest pain of noncardiac origin has been given an intramuscular injection, for example, of a narcotic, the elevated CPK level that follows this injection may lead to an erroneous diagnosis of myocardial infarction.

In order to eliminate false positive elevated values resulting from causes other than myocardial necrosis, isoenzymes that are myocardial specific have been identified. Of the five LDH isoenzymes, LDH_1 is a more sensitive indicator of myocardial infarction than total LDH. The CPK isoenzyme designated MB is found only in myocardium, a characteristic that increases the accuracy of this enzymatic diagnosis of acute myocardial infarction.

PHONOCARDIOGRAMS

The phonocardiogram is a graphic recording of the audible vibrations produced by the heart and great vessels. It is used for timing cardiac sounds and murmurs and for documenting questionable physical findings. For example, it can provide a visible delineation of such cardiac events as the variation in the splitting of S_2 during respiration or the differentiation of separate systolic and diastolic murmurs from a continuous murmur that continues throughout late systole and early diastole. The phonocardiogram may be used to record preejection or ejection periods that relate to cardiac function, to assess the presence and timing of murmurs or pathologic heart sounds, or to noninvasively follow changes in cardiac function.

The phonocardiogram is obtained by placing microphones over the base and apex of the heart. Simultaneous recording from these two separate sites helps identify and differentiate heart sounds and murmurs. To provide a reference signal the ECG is recorded simultaneously with the phonocardiogram. Other noninvasive measurements that are helpful in timing auscultatory events are the carotid pulse wave (Fig. 3-2, A), the venous pulse (Fig. 3-4), and the apex cardiogram, and these may be recorded simultaneously with the heart sounds.

ECHOCARDIOGRAMS

Echocardiography is a noninvasive procedure that uses pulses of reflected ultrasound to evaluate the functioning heart. Since the anatomic components of the heart can be identified and their distances from a transducer measured, sizes of various chambers (left and right ventricles, left atrium) and vessels (aorta and pulmonary artery) can be estimated with accuracy.

To obtain an echocardiogram a special transducer that emits pulsed ultrasound waves and receives echoes is placed on the chest. If recording a left ventricular echocardiogram, the transducer is placed in the third to fifth intercostal space near the left sternal border. The transducer is tilted at various angles so that echo beams scan the segments of the left ventricle, and the tracings are recorded on a strip chart recorder. Recording the echos involves a time-motion presentation that plots distance from the chest wall against elapsed time and displays moving structures as undulating lines (Fig. 3-16). The ECG and time-distance markers are usually displayed on the oscilloscope and are used as reference signals on the recorded tracing as well.

Currently there is interest in cross-sectional echocardiography, which presents a two-dimensional planar image instead of the unidimensional time-motion display. The cross-sectional technique portrays regional anatomy and therefore provides diagnostic insight that supplements time-motion studies. Although two-dimensional scanning is relatively new, it has received favorable attention, since it provides information that cannot be obtained using conventional echocardiography.

Echocardiography has played an increasingly significant role in the evaluation of patients with certain cardiac conditions, such as valvular heart disease, congenital heart disease, cardiomyopathy, pericardial disease, and coronary artery disease. Valuable data can be obtained relative to left ventricular performance, including the dimensions of the ventricular cavity; thickness of

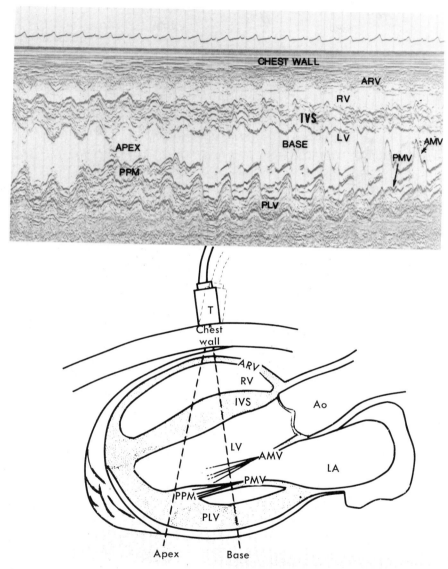

Fig. 3-16. Normal echocardiographic sector scan of the left ventricle and schematic presentation of the cardiac structures traversed by two echo beams. During ejection the left septal and posterior left ventricular wall echoes move toward the center of the left ventricular cavity. *AMV*, Anterior mitral valve leaflet; *AO*, aorta; *ARV*, anterior right ventricular wall; *IVS*, interventricular septum; *LA*, left atrium; *LV*, left ventricle; *PLV*, posterior left ventricular wall; *PMV*, posterior mitral valve leaflet; *RV*, right ventricle; *PPM*, posterior papillary muscle; *T*, transducer. (Reproduced with permission from Corya, B. C.: Applications of echocardiography in acute myocardial infarction, Cardiovasc. Clin. **2:**113, 1975.)

the left posterior ventricular wall and interventricular septum; estimates of diastolic, systolic, and stroke volumes; and motions of individual segments of the left ventricular wall in both systole and diastole. In short, the echocardiogram rapidly gives a comprehensive, noninvasive assessment of left ventricular function.

Finally, in addition to diagnostic information, serial echocardiograms may be obtained clinically to monitor and detect hemodynamic changes in cardiovascular patients. The uses of echocardiography are still being investigated and substantiated, and the ultimate role of this procedure has yet to be defined, but to date it has made a major contribution to the elevation of the cardiac patient.

RADIONUCLIDE STUDIES

Radionuclide studies of the cardiovascular system are accomplished through the external detection of photons emitted from the body after the administration of radioactive pharmaceuticals. Generally, these noninvasive studies are achieved in one of two ways: (1) radionuclide angiography and (2) "myocardial imaging." Radionuclide angiography involves the intravenous injection of a small bolus of a gamma emitter, such as pertechnetate Tc 99m, which allows rapid, sequential visualization of the heart, great vessels, and pulmonary vasculature via a high-speed scintillation camera. This technique is analogous to contrast angiography and is useful for detecting abnormalities in left ventricular wall motion in patients with coronary artery disease. Furthermore, it gives estimates of left ventricular volumes and ejection fraction.

Myocardial imaging selectively identifies normal or abnormal tissues with diffusible radiopharmaceuticals. For example, such isotopes as ^{43}K (potassium) or ^{201}Tl (thallium) concentrate in normal myocardium but not in areas of the myocardium that are unperfused. Therefore after intravenous injection of such radioactive tracers in patients with transient myocardial ischemia or a recent or previous myocardial infarction, "cold" defects (that do not take up the radionuclide) may be detected during isotope scanning. There is evidence to suggest that myocardial perfusion imaging at rest and during exercise may be more sensitive than electrocardiography during exercise in identifying patients with coronary artery disease. Other isotopes, such as pyrophosphate 99m, selectively accumulate in regions of recent myocardial

---

Fig. 3-17. Left coronary arteriogram, lateral projection. **A,** Occlusion of the left anterior descending artery (between left upper arrows). The distal segment *(LAD)* is almost totally opacified by collateral channels over the left ventricular free wall originating from diagonal *(D)* and marginal *(LM)* branches. A stenosis is present in the circumflex artery *(arrow on right)*. *S,* septal branches of left anterior descending artery. **B,** Diagrammatic representation of **A.** (Reproduced with permission from Soto, B., Russell, R. O., Jr., and Moraski, R. E.: Radiographic anatomy of the coronary arteries, Mount Kisco, N. Y., 1976, Futura Publishing Company, Inc. p. 151.)

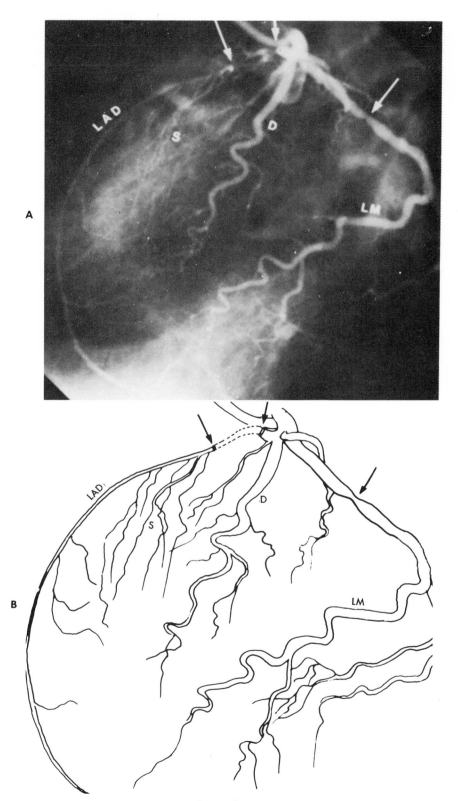

Fig. 3-17. For legend see opposite page.

necrosis, observed as "hot" areas. Radioactive tracers are therefore being advocated for the diagnosis of acute myocardial infarction. The ability to radiolabel infarcted myocardium in a living patient gives radionuclide studies considerable appeal, and their ultimate value will be determined by the results of future investigations.

CARDIAC CATHETERIZATION

Cardiac catheterization involves the introduction of catheters into various cardiac chambers, generally for diagnostic purposes. Cardiac catheterization and angiograms may be indicated as diagnostic studies in patients with valvular dysfunction, congenital heart disease, chest pain of uncertain cause, pulmonary hypertension, and other myocardial diseases for which surgical correction may be contemplated or wherein the diagnosis is in doubt. This procedure is a necessary part of preoperative evaluation and may also be done postoperatively to assess the effects of cardiac surgery.

With the patient under local anesthesia and the examiner using fluoroscopic control, catheters are inserted into the arterial and venous systems and passed into the great vessels and cardiac chambers. Blood samples are taken and evaluated, and pressures within the great vessels and chambers are measured with a catheter transducer system. Waveforms are studied and cardiac output is measured to assess valvular competency and myocardial function. Contrast angiography is usually done concurrently. Special catheters are also available to record intracardiac ECGs and phonocardiograms. The intracardiac phonocardiogram further characterizes murmurs and heart sounds. Recording electrical potentials from the right atrium, the bundle of His, and the ventricles may be useful in evaluating arrhythmias and heart block.

CORONARY ARTERIOGRAMS

Angiograms are intracardiac x-ray studies during which radiopaque contrast medium is injected into the cardiac chambers and vessels and its passage followed and filmed as the heart beats spontaneously. When moving pictures are taken, this process is called *cineangiography*. Similar studies of the arterial system are referred to as *arteriograms* and those of the venous system, *venograms*.

A *coronary arteriogram* is a radiographic study of the coronary vessels. With the patient under local anesthesia a catheter is inserted and advanced using fluoroscopic control to the base of the aorta and selectively placed in the ostium of each coronary artery. Contrast medium is injected and rapid serial x-ray films or cineangiograms are taken. Coronary arteriograms may be used to aid in the evaluation of patients who have atypical chest pain of uncertain etiology. In such instances, coronary arteriograms can establish the presence or absence of anatomic disease of the coronary arteries (Fig. 3-17). Coronary arteriograms are also helpful in evaluating patients who have known coronary disease for whom surgery may be comtemplated because of incapacitating angina or complicated acute myocardial infarction. Coronary arteriograms are often obtained as a part of preoperative evaluation for valvular surgery. In addition, they may be used postoperatively to assess the effects of coronary surgery, particularly with patients whose symptoms persist following coronary artery bypass surgery.

REFERENCES

Bailey, I. K., et al.; Thallium-201 myocardial perfusion imaging at rest and during exercise: Comparative sensitivity to electrocardiography in coronary artery disease, Circulation **55**:79-87, 1977.

Bates, B.: A guide to physical evaluation, Philadelphia, 1974, J. B. Lippincott Co.

Bilheimer, D. W.: Needed: New therapy for hypercholesterolemia, N. Engl. J. Med. **296**:508-509, 1977.

Bruce, R. A.: Methods of exercise testing: Step test, bicycle, treadmill, isometrics, Am. J. Cardiol. **33**:715-720, 1974.

Bruce, R. A.: Exercise testing for evaluation of ventricular function, N. Engl. J. Med. **296**:671-675, 1977.

Castelli, W. P. et al.: HDL cholesterol and other lipids in coronary heart disease: The cooperative phenotyping study, Circulation **55**:767-772, 1977.

Conti, R.: Coronary arteriography, Circulation **55**:227-237, 1977.

Coronary Drug Project Research Group: Clofibrate and niacin in coronary heart disease, J.A.M.A. **231**:360-381, 1975.

Corya, B. C.: Applications of echocardiography in acute myocardial infarction, Cardiovasc. Clin. **2**:113-127, 1975.

DeGowin, E. L., and DeGowin, R. L.: Bedside diagnostic examination, ed. 3, New York, 1976, Macmillan Publishing Co., Inc.

Feigenbaum, H.: Echocardiography, ed. 2, Philadelphia, 1976, Lea & Febiger.

Fisher, W. R., and Truitt, D. H.: The common hyperliproproteinemias: An understanding of disease mechanisms and their control, Ann. Intern. Med. **85**:497-508, 1976.

Fowkes, W. C., and Hunn, V. K.: Clinical assessment for the nurse practitioner, St. Louis, 1973, The C. V. Mosby Co.

Fowler, N. O.: Inspection and palpation of venous and arterial pulses. Examination of the heart. Part 2, New York, 1972, American Heart Association.

Friedewald, V. E.: Maximal-stress, multiple-lead exercise testing: The significance of ST-segment changes in the detection of coronary arterial occlusive disease, Heart Lung **5**:91-96, 1976.

Harris, A., Sutton, G., and Towers, M., editors: Physiological and clinical aspects of cardiac auscultation, Philadelphia, 1976, J. B. Lippincott Co.

Hobson, L. B.: Examination of the patient, New York, 1975, McGraw-Hill Book Co.

Hurst, J. W., et al., editors: The heart, ed. 4, New York, 1978, McGraw-Hill Book Co.

Hurst, J. W., and Schlant, R. C.: Inspection and palpation of the anterior chest. Examination of the heart. Part 3, New York, 1972, American Heart Association.

Judge, R. D., and Zuidema, G. D., editors: Methods of clinical examination: A physiologic approach, ed. 3, Boston, 1974, Little, Brown & Co.

Kelly, A. E., and Gensini, G. G.: Coronary arteriography and left-heart studies, Heart Lung **4**:85-98, 1975.

Leatham, A.: Auscultation of the heart and phonocardiography, ed. 2, London, 1975, Churchill Livingstone.

Leonard, J. J., and Croetz, F. W.: Auscultation. Examination of the heart. Part 4, New York, 1967, American Heart Association.

Lesser, L. M., and Wenger, N. K.: Carotid sinus syncope, Heart Lung **5**:453-456, 1976.

Levy, R. I.: Drug therapy of hyperlipoproteinemia, J.A.M.A. **235**:2334-2336, 1976.

Mann, G. V.: Diet—heart: End of an era, N. Engl. J. Med. **297**:644-650, 1977.

McHenry, P. L.: The actual prevalence of false positive ST–segment response to exercise in clinically normal subjects remains undefined, Circulation **55**:683-685, 1977.

Parisi, A. F., et al.: Noninvasive cardiac diagnosis. Part 1, N. Engl. J. Med. **296**:316-320, 1977.

Parisi, A. F., et al.: Noninvasive cardiac diagnosis. Part 2, N. Engl. J. Med. **296**:368-374, 1977.

Parisi, A. F., et al.: Noninvasive cardiac diagnosis. Part 3, N. Engl. J. Med. **296**:427-432, 1977.

Popp, R. L.: Echocardiographic evaluation of left ventricular function, N. Engl. J. Med. **296**:856-858, 1977.

Rasmussen, S., and Corya, B. C.: The diagnostic attributes of echocardiography in the patient with chest pain or pulmonary edema, Heart Lung **6:**660-670, 1977.

Ravin, A., et al.: Auscultation of the heart, ed. 3, Chicago, 1977, Year Book Medical Publishers, Inc.

Robb, C. P., and Seltzer, F.: Appraisal of the double two step exercise test, J.A.M.A. **234:**722-727, 1975.

Schroeder, J. P., and Daily, E. K.: Techniques in bedside hemodynamic monitoring, St. Louis, 1976, The C. V. Mosby Co.

Sheffield, L. T., et al.: The exercise test in perspective, Circulation **55:**681-682, 1977.

Silverman, M. E.: The clinical history. Examination of the Heart. Part 1, New York, 1975, American Heart Association.

Smith, L. K., et al.: Management of type IV hyper-liproproteinemia: Evaluation of practical clinical approaches, Ann. Intern. Med. **85:**22-28, 1976.

Soto, B., Russell, R. O., Jr., and Moraski, R. E.: Radiographic anatomy of the coronary arteries, Mount Kisco, N. Y., 1976, Futura Publishing Co., Inc.

Thorn, G. W., et al., editors: Harrison's principles of internal medicine, ed. 8, New York, 1977, McGraw-Hill Book Co.

Walker, H. K.: The problem−oriented medical system, J.A.M.A. **236:**2397-2398, 1976.

Weed, L.: Medical records that guide and teach, N. Engl. J. Med. **278:**593-600, 1968.

Winslow, E. H.: Visual inspection of the patient with cardiopulmonary disease, Heart Lung **4:**421-429, 1975.

Yeshurum, D., and Gotto, A. M., Jr.: Drug treatment of hyperlipidemia, Am. J. Med. **60:**379-396, 1976.

CHAPTER FOUR

COMPLICATIONS OF CORONARY ARTERY DISEASE

The function of the heart is to pump blood to all organs and tissues of the body. To accomplish this task the heart muscle requires a substantial flow of blood, called coronary perfusion, that can be increased appropriately when the demands on the heart increase with physical or emotional activity. Disturbances in the function of heart muscle develop when the supply of coronary blood flow is compromised by coronary artery disease. Coronary artery disease includes a spectrum of alterations of function in which the pathophysiology of the functional disturbance can be viewed as a complication of disease in the coronary arteries.

To understand the complications of coronary artery disease it is essential to understand the coronary circulation during normal conditions. The heart needs energy to contract and this energy is supplied by the metabolism of fuels (substrates) that yield high-energy phosphates; oxygen is necessary for this process to occur normally. Thus the function of the heart rests entirely on its ability to supply oxygen and substrates to meet the myocardial demand.

A remarkable feature of the coronary circulation is that even during normal activity, the heart extracts approximately 75% of the arterial oxygen supply. (Usual extraction of oxygen by other organs is approximately 25%). This demonstrates the limited oxygen reserve available to the heart when it is stressed. Under these circumstances an increase in coronary blood flow is the only means by which increased myocardial needs are satisfied. If the coronary blood flow fails to meet the myocardial need for oxygen, ischemia results.

The rate of blood flow in most arteries throughout the body is determined by the mean arterial blood pressure and the resistance to flow offered by smaller arteries and arterioles to the distribution of blood by the artery in which flow is measured. Coronary blood flow, in contrast to the flow in most other systemic arteries, is determined mainly by the diastolic arterial blood pressure. The reason for this is that during ventricular systole, the stress within the myocardial wall is high and the transmural coronary blood vessels are constricted by the heart muscle, increasing their resistance and effectively impeding coronary flow. In diastole, wall stress drops precipitously and coronary flow reaches its maximal velocity. The resistance of the coronary vessels in diastole is influenced by local factors: residual wall stress, tension

61

of oxygen and carbon dioxide, and by/products of cellular metabolism such as adenosine. Therefore under any given conditions, normal coronary blood flow is determined by a complex interaction between hydraulic factors—wall stress, arterial pressure, and heart rate—and local metabolic factors. Both of these in turn are modulated by the activity of the autonomic nervous system.

When these controls operate normally, the supply of coronary blood is closely matched to the metabolic requirements of heart muscle. When a hydraulically significant obstruction develops within a coronary artery, flow and the distribution of flow are compromised and ischemia develops. Obstructive coronary artery disease is generally insidious in its progression and produces ischemia only after approximately 75% of the arterial lumen is occluded. The functional significance of any given coronary artery stenosis depends in part on the demands placed on the myocardium and also on the extent of collateral vessels, which provide an alternative source of perfusion to the muscle in the distribution area supplied by the stenosed vessel.

Clinical syndromes: an overview

Deficits in myocardial perfusion may be manifested in the following clinical syndromes:

1. Angina pectoris. This syndrome can be defined pathophysiologically as a state of transient myocardial ischemia without clinically recognizable cell death. It is characterized by chest discomfort that is usually precipitated by activities or events that increase the metabolic demand for oxygen. The duration of pain varies with the individual but typically lasts 3 to 5 minutes; it is relieved by rest or nitroglycerin. At the time of the first episode of anginal pain the extent of the coronary artery obstructive process is generally well developed. As the disease progresses, the anginal pain may change from its stable, predictable nature to "unstable" angina. In this state, pain may be present even at rest, and despite aggressive medical therapy, relief may be inconsistent. This stage of coronary insufficiency is sometimes referred to as "preinfarction" angina.

2. Acute myocardial infarction. Myocardial infarction is defined as myocardial ischemia of sufficient intensity and duration to produce clinically recognizable death (necrosis) of tissue. The most common symptom is severe, persistent pain that may be accompanied by intense anxiety, nausea, vomiting, dyspnea, and diaphoresis. Ancillary clinical and laboratory evidence of dead heart muscle can confirm the presence of the condition. The patient may or may not be able to cite a precipitating factor, although approximately two thirds have premonitory symptoms. A myocardial infarction can be classified by ECG as a subendocardial or transmural infarct, depending on the extent of damage to the myocardial wall.

3. Heart Failure. In this state, cardiac output fails to meet metabolic demands. Heart failure may involve either ventricle initially, but since the ventricles are in series, one ventricle does not fail for long without the other ventricle also becoming affected, leading to decompensation of both

ventricles. Pulmonary edema is a medical emergency caused by severe left heart failure (Table 4-1). Cardiogenic shock, referred to as "power failure," is frequently caused by massive myocardial damage, leaving the ventricle so disabled that it cannot generate an adequate contraction. This profound failure resulting from myocardial infarction is usually irreversible.

4. Cardiomegaly. Cardiomegaly refers to enlargement of the heart and may result from dilation, hypertrophy, or both. Patients with long-standing angina or recurrent infarctions show multiple scars and areas of replacement

Table 4-1. Treatment of acute pulmonary edema

Therapeutic goal	Therapy	Principle	Precaution
Improve gaseous exchange	Morphine sulfate, 8-15 mg IV	Morphine decreases anxiety, reduces venous return, and decreases musculo-skeletal and respiratory activity	Monitor vital signs; hypoxic depression of respiratory system seriously aggravated by morphine; morphine antagonist (Nalline) and respiratory stimulants available
	IPPB, intermittent positive pressure apparatatus delivering 100% O_2 via well-fitted nonrebreathing face mask, using airway pressure of 4-9 cm H_2O	IPPB decreases alveolar fluid, reduces ventilatory rate, increases arterial oxygen, facilitates uniformity of ventilation in all lung segments	Oxygen always administered with humidification to avoid airway drying and inspissation of bronchial secretions; antifoaming agents (20%-50% alcohol) may be used; remember that face mask is frightening to "suffocating" patient
	Aminophylline, IV at rate of about 20 mg/min, to total dose of 240-480 mg*	Aminophylline dilates bronchioles; also increases cardiac output, lowers venous pressure by relaxing smooth muscles of blood vessels	This drug injected slowly IV; otherwise headache, palpitation, dizziness, nausea, and fall in blood pressure occur; sedation required to relax anxious patient; cardiac arrhythmias may also occur
	Arterial line inserted for arterial blood gas determination	Normal blood gas values: pH: 7.38-7.42; Po_2: 90-100 mm Hg; Pco_2: 35-45 mm Hg; %O_2 saturation: 95%-100%	Keep arterial line open with heparin flush

*Aminophylline in suppository form has been used effectively for this stage of pulmonary edema and may be safer than IV administration.

Continued

Table 4-1. Treatment of acute pulmonary edema—cont'd

Therapeutic goal	Therapy	Principle	Precaution
Decrease intravascular volume	Diuretic therapy selecting one of the following: Furosemide (Lasix), 40-120 mg IV Ethacrynic acid (Edecrin), 50 mg IV	These rapidly acting diuretics given IV begin work within minutes; decrease in intravascular volume improves ability of lungs to exchange gases and decreases cardiac work	Monitor blood pressure and intake and output; given in excessive amounts these diuretics can lead to a profound diuresis with volume and electrolyte depletion; local infiltration of ethacrynic acid
	Phlebotomy of 300-500 ml	Same as preceding	If pulmonary edema has already precipitated circulatory collapse, phlebotomy will aggravate shock
Improve cardiac performance	All of the preceding Digitalis, IV administration of rapidly acting preparation (Appendix A)	See preceding Increase force of contraction and efficiency of heart	See preceding Monitor for arrhythmias; in presence of hypoxia in an acutely dilated heart, digitalis-induced arrhythmias likely to occur
Decrease venous return	Sitting (Fowler's) position	Sitting up increases lung volume and vital capacity, decreases venous return and work of breathing	In presence of hypotension, Fowler's position avoided or used cautiously
	IPPB	IPPB effectively reduces venous return by replacing normal negative intrathoracic pressure of spontaneous inspiration with positive pressure, varied as needed and impending venous flow; reduces work of breathing to a degree	High-pressure settings avoided, since excessive reduction of peripheral venous return can cause circulatory collapse; also see preceding
	Tourniquets applied to three extremities with greater pressure than that of estimated venous pressure, but below arterial diastolic pressure; peripheral arterial pulses maintained at all times; tourniquets rotated so that each extremity is free, in sequence for 15 min†	Pooling of blood in the extremities retards venous return, reduces capillary-alveolar transudation, decreases cardiac work	Prolonged constriction of extremities causes pain and loss of function; resultant dramatic edema of extremities may be upsetting to patient; at conclusion of acute phase, tourniquets released one at a time, at 15-min intervals, to avoid flooding pulmonary circulation

†Rotating tourniquets are generally used only if other measures are unavailable or when all of the measures above have been tried without success.

fibrosis in the heart. The heart appears to adapt to these changes by dilation. In part because of dilation and in part because the work load on the heart muscle is shifted from damaged areas to residual normal muscle, these remaining normal components undergo hypertrophy. As a result, heart size determined by x-ray examination, heart dimensions measured by angiography, and heart mass all incrase.

5. Abnormal electrocardiogram. Even though the patient may be totally asymptomatic, certain changes on the ECG may be strongly indicative of coronary insufficiency (Chapter 5). The resting ECG may be normal in the presence of coronary artery disease; therefore it is often helpful to obtain an ECG during and after stress in order to establish the presence of coronary insufficiency. (See Chapter 3 and Fig. 3-10.) The most significant change is the development of S-T segment depression, seen more often in the lateral precordial leads (V_4 to V_6) and less often in leads V_2, II, III, and aV_F. Frequently during an anginal attack, a patient will show these changes also. When the pain has subsided, the S-T segments will return to normal. Prinzmetal's angina, also called "atypical angina," is characterized electrocardiographically by S-T elevation, may occur unrelated to exertion, and may not respond promptly to nitroglycerin. In some instances, at least, transient coronary artery spasm is thought to play a role (See Figs. 6-92 and 6-108.)

6. Arrhythmias. Disorders of impulse formation, abnormal conduction, or both frequently signal the presence of coronary artery disease and may be caused by inadequate oxygenation, heart failure, areas of scar formation, acute infarction, and similar disorders. The patient experiencing arrhythmias may complain of palpitations, dizziness, fatigue, or syncope (Chapter 6).

7. Sudden death. In this text, sudden death is defined as death occurring within an hour of the onset of symptoms. In patients without obvious preexisting disease, sudden death is usually ascribed to ventricular fibrillation precipitated by acute myocardial infarction. However, ventricular fibrillation may result without the occurrence of infarction. The majority of these sudden deaths occur before the patient reaches the hospital.

8. Mitral insufficiency. The normal competence of the mitral valve depends on a structurally and functionally intact mitral apparatus. The components of this apparatus include the posterior left atrial wall, the anulus, the leaflets, the chordae tendineae, and the papillary muscles and their base within the left ventricular wall. It is now recognized that coronary heart disease is probably the most common cause of mitral insufficiency. Ischemic injury to the papillary muscle and its base or frank rupture of the papillary muscle or its chordae may lead to mitral insufficiency. Murmurs caused by mitral insufficiency may develop during an angina attack or may be a stable consequence of fibrotic changes secondary to old infarction. Mitral insufficiency may develop acutely in the setting of myocardial infarction and may contribute to or cause acute left heart failure and pulmonary edema.

9. Ventricular aneurysm. With transmural myocardial infarction the hydraulic stress on the necrotic portion of the ventricular wall may cause this re-

gion to bulge during systole and to become extremely thin as the necrotic material is absorbed. If this occurs during scarring or before a substantial scar has developed, the resulting scar may develop as an outward balloon or bulge that communicates with the ventricular chamber through a "neck." Ventricular aneurysms usually develop during the weeks that follow acute infarction. Their hemodynamic consequence can be related to their size, to the amount of residual normal muscle, and to their location, which sometimes involves the papillary muscles. For reasons that are not completely apparent, patients with ventricular aneurysms are particularly prone to recurrent ventricular arrhythmias. Once a scar has developed, aneurysms seldom rupture. Hence they are detected by x-ray examination, typical ECG changes, or incidently during angiography.

10. Ventricular rupture. Just as hydraulic stresses on necrotic myocardium may lead to aneurysms, they may, in rare instances, produce myocardial rupture. Rupture of the heart occurs as a complication of acute myocardial infarction. When it occurs, it usually develops within 10 days after the onset of infarction symptoms. Rupture may occur through the free wall of the ventricle, producing acute cardiac tamponade. More often, rupture occurs internally through necrotic muscle near the apical end of the interventricular septum. The development of a holosystolic murmur at the apex and left sternal border in a patient with acute infarction should always raise the possibility of septal rupture. Heart failure usually develops or worsens concurrently with this event. The diagnosis can be established by relatively simple catheter techniques, some of which can be performed at the bedside.

Angina pectoris

The diagnosis of angina pectoris may be made from the characteristic history, since there are frequently few abnormalities found on physical examination and, as noted previously, the ECG may be normal at rest. Therefore it is important to allow the patient to describe what he is feeling without influencing him by the use of suggestive terms. Time and patience are necessary to explore all aspects of the patient's life-style, habits and emotions in order to obtain a clear picture of the nature of his pain.

Although the term "angina pectoris" is literally interpreted as "chest pain," it should perhaps be referred to as a discomfort, since some patients may deny chest "pain." They often refer to vague "sensations," "feelings," or "aches." (See Appendix B.) This unpleasant feeling has been described in a variety of ways, including a sense of pressure, burning, squeezing, heaviness, smothering, and, very frequently, "indigestion." Since the discomfort of angina usually centers in the retrosternal region, patients will often illustrate the nature and location of their symptoms by placing a clenched fist against their sternum. Frequently the ache of angina pectoris is not confined to the chest but may radiate to the neck, jaw, epigastrium, both shoulders, or arms. Most often it radiates to the left shoulder and left arm. Occasionally angina pectoris may produce discomfort exclusively in an area of radiation without affecting the retrosternal region.

Attacks of angina are typically preceded by an elevation of blood pressure, heart rate, or both. During the attack, pulse rate and blood pressure usually increase further, presumably as a consequence of anxiety and as a physiologic response to pain. In some instances, however, blood pressure and pulse may fall dramatically as a result of vagally mediated reflexes analogous to vasodepressor syncope or fainting. The patient may remain motionless; at times he may experience a feeling of impending doom. The clenched fist over the sternum may graphically depict the constricting nature of the discomfort but of more importance than location of the pain is its duration and the circumstances under which it occurs. Angina pectoris usually lasts only a few minutes if the precipitating factor is relieved. Attacks are frequently induced by effort and tend to occur during rather than after exertion. Exertion during cold weather or following meals is particularly likely to produce pain. Disturbing thoughts, smoking, stressful situations, worry, anger, hurriedness, and excitement are common precipitating factors. Patients may describe the following typical situations as producing chest pain: running to catch a bus, climbing a long flight of stairs, carrying a bag to or from a plane, driving in heavy traffic, nightmares, painful stimuli, sexual intercourse, and straining at stool.

Angina typically lasts from 1 to several minutes and usually no more than 5 minutes. It is relieved by rest, nitroglycerin, or any influence that decreases arterial pressure or heart rate.

Various types of anginal pain occur. Walk-through angina is a type of anginal pain where the patient, despite chest pain, is able to continue his activity until the pain gradually disappears. Angina decubitus is chest pain occurring at rest in the supine position. Nocturnal angina may awaken a patient from sleep, usually because of dreams, with the same sensation as he had on exertion.

MEDICAL MANAGEMENT

The first principle in the medical management of angina pectoris is to minimize the discrepancy between the demand of the heart muscle for oxygen and the ability of the coronary circulation to meet this demand. Accordingly, the patient must learn to pace himself so that the rate of performing physical activity is kept below the threshold of discomfort. Moderate exercise performed below the angina threshold should be encouraged. Additional general measures include a diet designed to achieve the individual's ideal weight and the cessation of smoking. Hypertension, if present, should be treated. Pharmacologic treatment of angina is directed at two objectives: first, relief of symptoms when they occur and, second, prevention of angina. For the first objective, nitroglycerin taken sublingually is the treatment of choice. For prevention, beta adrenergic blocking agents such as propranolol (Inderal) are prescribed to attenuate the heart rate and contractile response to physical or emotional activity. Long-acting nitrates such as isosorbide dinitrate (Isordil) or nitrol paste exert an action for 2 to 4 hours and are very effective. Recent reports indicate that other vasodilators that act principally on the arterial system, such as hydralazine or prazosin, may attenuate the hypertensive response to exertion and aid in preventing angina. Other general measures include sedation, relief of anxiety, and supervised exercise programs designed to enhance physical condition and thereby to reduce the blood pressure and heart rate response to exercise.

SURGICAL TREATMENT

Coronary artery surgery in the past 7 years has become recognized as an effective treatment for angina pectoris caused by severe coronary artery disease. Using the saphenous vein or internal mammary artery as a graft to bypass the occlusion in one or more of the coronary arteries, dramatic relief from anginal pain is achieved in 80% of patients. Bypass grafting is made surgically feasible by the pattern of disease in the coronary arteries. In most cases the occlusion principally involves the proximal one third to one half of the artery. Distal vessels are usually patent, thus allowing anastomosis. The pypass graft is illustrated in Fig. 4-1.

Coronary arteriograms that verify greater than 75% occlusion of one or more arteries, coupled with the failure of aggressive medical treatment to successfully and consistently control disabling pain, are usually acceptable indications for bypass grafting. Each patient is evaluated individually with risks in mind. Operative risk is increased with impaired contractility, cardiac enlargement, or heart failure. Another relative contraindication includes

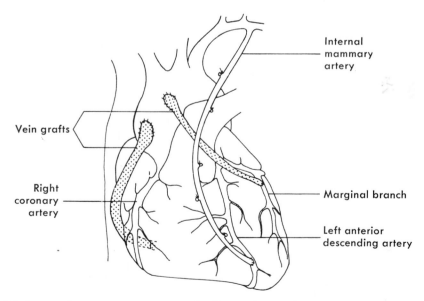

Fig. 4-1. Internal mammary artery attached as end-to-end anastomosis to anterior desecending artery; separate vein grafts to distal right coronary and marginal branch of circumflex coronary arteries. (Adapted from Kirklin, J. W., editor: Advances in cardiovascular surgery, New York, 1973, Grune & Stratton, Inc., by permission.)

occlusion of both the proximal and distal portions of the affected coronary artery. With significant distal disease, long-term patency of the graft is greatly reduced.

Despite encouraging results, coronary artery bypass at present can only offer palliation. Protection from future myocardial infarctions and the prolongation of life cannot be guaranteed in light of present data.

Acute myocardial infarction

Chest pain is the principal symptom in a majority of patients with acute myocardial infarction. The pain is frequently severe, but there may be minimal discomfort, and occasionally there is none. The pain is usually substernal in location and, like angina, may radiate to the epigastric region, jaw, shoulders, elbows, or forearms. The quality of the pain is usually described as heaviness, tightness, or constricting sensation, but occasionally as indigestion or a burning sensation. It usually persists for 30 minutes or longer and often does not subside until potent analgesics have been administered. It is important to recognize that in its classic presentation the symptoms of myocardial infarction differ in severity and duration from those typical of angina. On the other hand, the symptoms of myocardial infarction may be subtle, and very often the severity and duration of the pain cannot be used to distinguish between prolonged angina, coronary insufficiency, and myocardial infarction.

In addition to chest pain, patients with myocardial infarction may experience shortness of breath, sweating, weakness or extreme fatigue, nausea, vomiting, and severe anxiety. On physical examination the patients may show evidence of overactivity of the sympathetic nerves, including tachycardia, sweating, and hypertension. Alternatively, evidence of vagal hyperactivity may predominate, with bradycardia and hypotension. Many patients look surprisingly normal. Hypotension with tachycardia and peripheral cyanosis suggest markedly reduced cardiac output and shock. In some patients, blood pressure is maintained but an S_3 gallop rhythm and pulmonary rales indicate acute left ventricular failure. Murmurs related to mitral insufficiency or a ruptured septum may develop, and a pericardial friction rub may be heard. The heart sounds are usually diminished in intensity and, particularly with anterior infarction, a paradoxic systolic lift inside the apical region can be felt.

Ancillary but nonspecific findings of infarction include low-grade fever, elevation of the white blood cell count, and elevation of the erythrocyte sedimentation rate. The ECG may show the typical findings of infarction (discussed elsewhere), or it may show nonspecific changes of the S-T segment or T wave. Rarely if ever are serial ECGs normal in a patient with documented infarction.

With necrosis of heart muscle, enzymes normally confined within the cell leak out and appear in peripheral blood; glutamic-oxaloacetic transaminase (SGOT), lactic acid dehydrogenase (LDH) and creatine phosphokinase (CPK) are the enzymes measured most frequently. The enzymes LDH and CPK appear in more than one form and are referred to as isoenzymes. The isoenzymes of LDH and CPK are distributed differently in different tissues so that elevations of the "heart" isoenzyme levels are more specific evidence of heart muscle necrosis than elevation of the total CPK or LDH levels. Elevated levels of CPK-MB and LDH_1, which are the predominant heart isoenzymes, are typically observed in myocardial infarction.

In the past 3 to 4 years a new development in methods of establishing the diagnosis of myocardial infarction has received considerable attention. This technique utilizes radionuclide imaging and depends on the fact that technetium 99m stannous pyrophosphate concentrates in necrotic heart muscle. This isotope is taken up by necrotic cells within 12 to 18 hours after the onset of infarction; uptake persists for 4 to 5 days and then typically decays. Even very small areas of infarction can be identified by appropriate scanning equipment from the "hot spot" produced on the scintigram. Technetium imaging is generally regarded as a very sensitive technique for confirming myocardial damage, more sensitive than QRS changes.

The mortality among patients with acute myocardial infarction is approximately 30% to 40%. However, a substantial number of these deaths occur suddenly and prior to hospitalization. Mortality among patients who survive to reach the hospital is approximately 20%, and most of these deaths occur within the first 3 to 4 days. It is useful to distinguish between those patients with uncomplicated and those with complicated acute myocardial infarction, since nearly all deaths occur in the latter group, whereas those in the former group have an excellent prognosis and are candidates for early mobilization and discharge. The conditions that identify the group with complications include the following:

1. *Persistent pain.* Pain that persists or recurs is frequently associated with unusually high enzyme level elevations or secondary rises and suggests that ischemia persists and that infarction is in a process of evolution.

2. *Serious arrhythmia.* Nearly all patients with acute infarction experience transient alterations of rhythm. The alterations considered serious include ventricular fibrillation or ventricular tachycardia, second- or third-degree heart block, and the onset of atrial flutter or fibrillation. In addition, sinus tachycardia of less than 100 beats/minute that persists for more than 24 to 48 hours in the absence of fever should alert those caring for the patient to the possibility of heart failure.

3. *Pulmonary edema.* Pulmonary edema produces a sense of breathlessness, wet rales, and typical changes on the chest x-ray film. It is nearly always accompanied by a significant rise in pulmonary artery and wedge pressure and indicates acute left ventricular failure.

4. *Persistent hypotension.* The arterial systolic blood pressure may drop below 90 mm Hg without accompanying signs of shock. Often this is an early and transient finding associated with bradycardia and other signs

of vagal overactivity. Alternatively, it may reflect inadequate blood volume. When hypotension persists despite an adequate heart rate and central venous pressure, it usually signifies a markedly reduced cardiac output.

In a recent report patients with acute myocardial infarction were classified as having complicated or uncomplicated disorders on the basis of the presence or absence of any of the preceding signs during the first 4 days of hospitalization. No patient among over 500 whose condition was uncomplicated through the fourth day either died subsequently in the hospital or suffered a serious late complication. On this basis patients with uncomplicated conditions during the first 4 days would appear to be candidates for early mobilization and early discharge. This possibility was tested by McNeer et al., and among patients with uncomplicated disorders discharged on the seventh hospital day there were no serious complications or deaths at home during early follow-up.

MEDICAL MANAGEMENT

Our objective here is to discuss the medical management of patients with acute myocardial infarction. An overview is presented now because subsequent sections of this book provide details regarding arrhythmias, heart failure, shock, and the use of specific pharmacologic agents, pacemakers, and so forth.

In the early stages of acute myocardial infarction, pain, anxiety, and alterations of rhythm dominate the clinical picture. After establishing a route for intravenous therapy and ECG monitoring, morphine should be given in doses that are sufficient to eliminate or greatly reduce chest pain. Morphine is also a sedative, and while reducing chest pain usually relieves anxiety as well. Patients with excessive bradycardia and a pulse rate below 50 to 55 beats/minute, particularly if this is accompanied by hypotension and ectopic beats, should be treated with atropine.

The greatest threat to life in the early hours after myocardial infarction is ventricular fibrillation. In a majority of patients, episodes of fibrillation are preceded by ventricular premature beats. The high prevalence of premature beats and the fact that fibrillation is sometimes not signaled by these changes have led most physicians in recent years to advocate the use of prophylactic antiarrhythmic therapy. Lidocaine is given as an initial bolus (75 to 100 mg) followed by a continuous intravenous infusion. Conclusive studies are now available that indicate that the use of prophylactic lidocaine is safe and that the incidence of primary ventricular fibrillation is greatly reduced in patients who have been treated prophylactically.

Oxygen is administered to all patients because decreases in arterial Po_2 caused by ventilation perfusion inequalities are so common. Recent studies have shown that the incidence of thromboembolic complications in patients with infarction is reduced approximately 50% by anticoagulation. In view of this finding and the low rate of complications from anticoagulation per se, many physicians now advocate routine anticoagulation with intravenous heparin followed by warfarin in patients without a contraindication to anticoagulants.

In patients who have persistent or recurrent pain despite the measures previously noted, efforts should be made to favorably affect the balance between coronary supply and demand and hence to diminish ischemia. For example, if sinus tachycardia persists and signs of left ventricular failure are absent, propranolol in doses of 0.05 to 0.10 mg/kg can be given to reduce heart rate. In controlled studies this treatment has been shown to eliminate pain and reduce S-T segment elevation. Other patients with persistent or recurrent pain have elevated arterial blood pressure. In these patients, reducing blood pressure with propranolol or with nitroprusside has a favorable effect. Finally, in patients with left ventricular failure and elevated pulmonary artery and wedge pressures, vasodilators such as nitroprusside or nitroglycerin will "unload" the ventricle and often reduce pain and S-T segment elevation.

It has been evident for a number of years that myocardial infarction is a dynamic process and that the ultimate fate of ischemic but still viable heart muscle is not determined until several hours or perhaps days after the onset of symptoms. It is also evident that acute and late complications of infarction are determined at least in part by the ultimate size of the infarction. These considerations and the recognition, as noted previously, that the balance between supply and demand can be influenced, have led to considerable efforts in the last 5 years to protect ischemic muscle and to reduce infarct size (Fig. 4-2). All

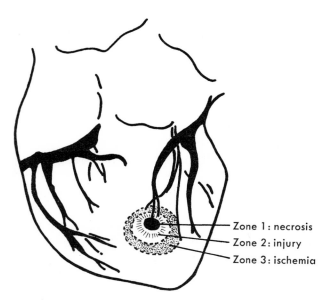

Zone 1: necrosis
Zone 2: injury
Zone 3: ischemia

Fig. 4-2. Tissue damage after myocardial infarction. Zone 1, necrotic tissue; zone 2, injured tissue; zone 3, ischemic tissue.

these efforts have been hampered by the lack of a reliable and quantifiable index of the volume of ischemic muscle in patients. Despite this problem, favorable clinical results, directionally appropriate changes of indices of muscle death, and reduction in anticipated mortality have been reported, with therapy directed at reducing infarct size. Most of the interest in this area has focused on the use of hyaluronidase or solutions containing glucose-insulin-potassium, propranolol, and vasodilators. At this point all such efforts are investigational, and their widespread application on a routine basis should await the results of appropriately designed clinical trials.

Heart failure and shock are serious complications of infarction. The pathophysiology and treatment of these conditions are discussed in a subsequent section of this chapter. A pericardial rub is heard in about 25% of patients with transmural infarction, usually on the third to fifth day. Pericarditis with effusion and fever develops in about 2% to 5% of patients with infarction from 1 to 4 weeks after the acute event. This is referred to as Dressler's syndrome or postmyocardial infarction syndrome and is thought to result from an autoimmune response. Pericarditis, early or late, is generally treated symptomatically. Use of aspirin, indomethacin, or even steroids may be required, and anticoagulation should be discontinued unless there is an overriding reason to continue its use, such as an overt pulmonary embolus.

Prolongation of the P-R interval and Wenckebach cycles are common with posterior infarction. They usually regress or can be treated with atropine. Third-degree A-V block or conditions associated with a high incidence of progression to complete block, such as Mobitz type II second-degree block or new bifascicular bundle branch block (especially associated with P-R prolongation) are regarded as indications that a temporary transvenous pacemaker should be inserted. Use of the pacemaker is then primarily determined by the ventricular rate.

Heart failure

Heart failure may be defined as a state in which cardiac output is insufficient to meet the metabolic needs of the body. This state can occur when cardiac output is normal, increased, or decreased. However, most patients with heart failure have a decreased cardiac output. Congestive failure indicates circulatory congestion resulting from heart failure and is manifested by retention of fluid and formation of edema.

The term "low-output failure" indicates failure of the heart as a pump to supply the tissues with adequate perfusion. The basis for the inadequate perfusion lies in the heart; the tissue demands may be normal but these are not met by the failing heart. A number of cardiac disorders can result in low-output failure. For example, a myocardial infarction that affects a large area of the left ventricle or stenosis or insufficiency of the cardiac valves can impair the heart's ability to pump. Constrictive pericarditis or pericardial effusion can restrict the ability of the heart to fill and empty. Finally, heart block caused by excessively slow ventricular rate may lead to heart failure.

Less commonly, heart failure occurs when peripheral demands exceed even the capacity of a normal heart to adequately perfuse the tissues. This is called high-output failure and can occur in severe anemia, in thyrotoxicosis, and in patients who have arteriovenous fistulas.

The basic defect in heart failure is a decrease in the pumping capacity of the heart. Patients with early or mild heart disease may show no significant abnormalities at rest because of reserve in cardiac function. Despite a normal cardiac output at rest, cardiac output with exercise will be subnormal, with the patient demonstrating decreased exercise tolerance.

PATHOPHYSIOLOGY

As the heart begins to fail, a large number of compensatory mechanisms are set in motion in an effort to maintain cardiac output at a level that is adequate to meet the metabolic needs of the body. Most of these adaptations employ mechanisms that are the same as those activated in normal persons during exercise or during periods of increased stress. The principal initial adjustments are a reflex increase in sympathetic nerve discharge and a decrease in parasympathetic activity. These autonomic alterations, affecting the heart, arteries, and veins, result in maintenance of arterial pressure despite a possible decrease in stroke volume. Venous tone increases, which in turn increases venous pressure and helps to maintain venous return. The resulting increase in end-diastolic volume* helps to maintain stroke volume. The mechanism underlying this adaptation is the fact that cardiac muscle increases its strength of contraction when it is stretched. Starling's law of the heart states that a direct proportion exists between the diastolic volume of the heart, that is, the length of cardiac muscle fibers during diastole, and the force of contraction of the following systole. Increased fiber length immediately prior to contraction increases the strength of the contraction. Consequently, the ultimately distended heart, within certain limits, contracts forcefully enough to maintain arterial perfusion. Furthermore, the contraction is not only more powerful but occurs more frequently as well.

An increase in heart rate, or tachycardia, may by itself increase cardiac output when mechanisms to improve stroke volume are exhausted. But above a certain rate, cardiac output may actually begin to decrease. This rate is about 170 to 180 beats/minute for most normal young individuals. However, in trained athletes the rate may be 200 to 220 beats/minute and in patients with myocardial disease the rate limit may be 120 to 140 beats/minute. This decrease in cardiac output above a certain heart rate is caused by a shortening of diastole, thereby limiting the time for adequate filling of the ventricles and for coronary blood flow. This filling occurs predominantly during diastole, especially of the left ventricle. Slow heart rates allow more complete diastolic

---

*Normally after contraction, some blood remains in the ventricles. The volume of blood ejected during each ventricular contraction is the difference between the volume of blood contained in the ventricle at the end of diastole (end-diastolic volume) and the volume remaining at the end of systole (end-systolic volume).

filling; however, when the rate decreases below 40 to 50 beats/minute, no further increase of stroke volume occurs and cardiac output drops.

When cardiac output falls, from whatever cause, the kidney retains salt and water as an early compensatory mechanism. This is the result in part of sympathetic stimulation, which produces renal vasoconstriction and a reduction in renal blood flow. Sympathetically mediated activation of the renin-angiotensin system triggers aldosterone release and further promotes sodium retention. An expansion of intravascular blood volume follows and results in an increased end-diastolic volume. The maintenance of right ventricular end-diastolic volume and pressure at elevated levels raises systemic venous and capillary pressures, ultimately resulting in transudation of fluid from the vascular bed and edema formation (Table 4-1).

A major long-term hemodynamic adjustment to heart failure is ventricular hypertrophy. This is presumably caused by a chronic increase in the systolic force or tension developed by the myocardial fibers. Although the contractility of hypertrophied myocardium is less than normal per unit of muscle and is associated with an imbalance between energy production and energy utilization, the hypertrophied myocardium may maintain compensation because the total mass of myocardium is increased. If the pumping capacity of the ventricle is restored by hypertrophy, tachycardia and edema may no longer be present.

LEFT HEART FAILURE

The heart comprises two pumps in series, the right ventricle and the left ventricle. Certain events may alter the function of one of these pumps without significant initial impairment to the other. In acute myocardial infarction, for example, the primary insult is usually to the performance of the left ventricle. When the ability of the left ventricle to pump blood is compromised without similar compromise in the right ventricle, a temporary imbalance of output between the two sides of the heart results. The right heart continues to pump blood into the lungs. At the same time the left heart is unable to move the blood adequately into the systemic circulation. The result is an accumulation of blood in the lungs that increases the pressures in all the pulmonary vessels. Consequently, one of the cardinal symptoms associated with acute left ventricular failure is dyspnea. If dyspnea occurs when the patient is recumbent, it is called orthopnea and is usually relieved by sitting up. When the patient is lying down there is decreased vital capacity because the volume of blood in the pulmonary vessels is increased in the recumbent position.

Paroxysmal nocturnal dyspnea is almost a specific sign of left ventricular failure. The patient awakens suddenly at night, extremely breathless, and seeks relief by sitting up or running to an open window for "fresh air." The mechanism for this type of dyspnea is uncertain but represents a form of acute pulmonary edema. When the patient goes to sleep the metabolic needs of the body may decrease. As a result, the cardiac output that had previously been inadequate may now be adequate to supply the body needs. Fluid that had been pocketed away is mobilized into the vascular system, increasing the blood volume. This action in turn may increase the pressure in the lungs and lead to nocturnal pulmonary congestion. The second and more plausible mechanism is a redistribution of fluids to the lungs when the patient assumes a recumbent position.

As the heart's compensatory mechanisms fail, the already elevated diastolic filling pressure continues to increase, but without an increase in stroke volume. This occurrence necessarily increases the left atrial pressure. In order to maintain flow, pressure in the pulmonary veins and capillaries must also increase. When pressure in the capillaries exceeds intravascular osmotic pressure (approximately 30 mm Hg), fluid will rapidly leak into the interstitial regions of the lung tissue. Pulmonary edema greatly reduces the amount of lung tissue available for the exchange of gases and consequently results in a dramatic clinical presentation characterized by extreme dyspnea, cyanosis, and severe anxiety. This is called acute pulmonary edema.

In the early stages of pulmonary edema the patient appears restless and vaguely uneasy. Wheezing, orthopnea, and pallor develop as left heart failure progresses. A third heart sound (S$_3$) may be heard as the distensiblity of the ventricle decreases. Tachycardia and increased systemic arterial pressure are common as neural reflexes attempt to correct the imbalance. If these physiologic compensations fail, hypotension occurs, respirations become bubbling (rales), and copious, bloodtinged, frothy sputum is expectorated. As the accumulation of pulmonary interstitial and intraalveolar fluid progresses, arterial hypoxemia and cyanosis occur in varying degrees. This deterioriation in pulmonary function is reflected in the patient's mental status. Anxiety progresses to mental confusion and eventually to stupor and coma. The patient is literally drowning in his own secretions. The situation is critical and demands immediate emergency action.

RIGHT HEART FAILURE

Usually right heart failure follows left heart failure. In the adult, right heart failure without left heart failure may be caused by pulmonary hypertension secondary to lung disease or recurrent pulmonary emboli and is referred to as *cor pulmonale*. Pressure increases in the pulmonary vasculature during right heart failure leading to a rise of pressure in the right heart. This impedes venous return and consequently, peripheral organs become congested. This is manifested in two ways: (1) distention of the neck veins, which appear full when the head is raised (normally these empty when the head is elevated to a 45-degree angle), and (2) development of body edema (Table 4-2). When the accumulation of fluid becomes extensive and generalized with edema of the tissues throughout the body, the patient is said to have anasarca.

TREATMENT

Treatment of patients with heart failure requires an understanding of the condition(s) leading to this clinical state and of the mechanisms producing heart failure and congestion regardless of the primary cardiac problem.

Table 4-2. Edema formation

Organ	Edema	Description
Skin	Dependent edema, pitting type	Increases venous pressure forces fluid through capillary walls into subcutaneous tissues; in ambulatory patients edema localized in dependent parts of body (hands and feet); patients in bed may lose edema of legs and feet, have it only in presacral region
Liver	Hepatomegaly	Increased pressure in hepatic veins causes accumulation of fluid in liver, which becomes enlarged and tender
Pleural cavity	Pleural effusion; hydrothorax	Venous congestion forces fluid into pleural cavity
Pericardial cavity	Pericardial effusion	Fluid accumulation in pericardial cavity

When heart failure results from such specific mechanical problems as aortic or mitral valve stenosis or insufficiency, persistent uncontrolled arrhythmias, severe anemia, hypertension, or a congenital cardiac lesion, the primary focus of therapy is directed at correcting the cause of heart failure. It is also important to recognize that regardless of cause, infections, arrhythmias, anemia, thyrotoxicosis, and pregnancy may all place an added burden on the heart sufficient to precipitate heart failure. Appropriate treatment of these conditions may help convert the patient's state of decompensation.

We have previously defined heart failure as a condition in which the cardiac output is not sufficient to meet the metabolic demands of the body. Essentially all the situations noted previously that aggravate heart failure do so by increasing the metabolic demands on a heart not capable of responding with an adequate output. In the absence of these conditions a favorable response in patients with heart failure can usually be obtained by rest. Indeed, bed rest is the first principle of treating heart failure. Defining the level of physical activity that a patient can tolerate without precipitating failure is a major objective of subsequent follow-up and treatment.

In addition to providing for rest and defining the level of physical activity a patient can tolerate, a second focus of therapy is directed at improving cardiac performance and cardiac output. Obviously, if severe aortic stenosis or other structural defects are limiting, little can be accomplished through medical management and surgery. On the other hand, digitalis, which increases the contractility of heart muscle, has a favorable effect on cardiac performance and output. It is used routinely in most instances of heart failure with beneficial results. The evidence of benefit from digitalis in acute myocardial infarction, particularly in the early phases, is minimal, and because of an increased sensitivity to toxic manifestations of digitalis excess, its use in this situation is still controversial. Vasodilator agents are a recent and important addition to the treatment of heart failure. This class of agents includes nitrates, nitroprusside, hydralazine, and prazosin. Some are designed for intravenous use and some for oral use. Some act predominantly on the arterial system and others exert significant actions on veins as well. The principle behind the use of these agents is to decrease arterial resistance. This decrease is accompanied by an increase in cardiac output, a drop in left atrial and pulmonary venous pressure, and a decrease in left ventricular end-diastolic volume and pressure. These agents have proved very useful in the treatment of acute heart failure in myocardial infarction, in heart failure associated with severe mitral insufficiency, and in chronic heart failure resulting from myocardial disease. They can be used in addition to digitalis with additive effects. (See Appendix A.) The benefits of vasodilator therapy are greatest when left atrial and pulmonary pressures are elevated. However, vasodilators lack utility and may even be detrimental in patients with normal or reduced left ventricular filling pressures.

The third aim in treating patients with heart failure is directed at achieving and maintaining an appropriate blood volume. As noted before, several compensatory mechanisms invoked when cardiac output is insufficient affect sodium and water balance by the kidney. The net effect of these influences is sodium and water retention and a diminished ability to excrete a sodium load. A normal sodium intake of 5 to 8 gm/day is not tolerated by patients with heart failure and should be reduced to 2 gm or even less. Diuretics promote the renal excretion of sodium and hence of water by one or more of several specific actions. Thiazide diuretics inhibit sodium transport primarily in the distal or cortical segment of the nephron. Loop diuretics such as ethacrynic acid and furosemide are very potent and act on the cortical and medullary segments of the nephron. Spironolactone is a diuretic that specifically antagonizes the effect of aldosterone on the collecting duct. Triamterene has an action on sodium transport identical to spironolactone, but its action does not depend on blocking aldosterone. In general, thiazides and loop diuretics also cause potassium loss, whereas spironolactone and triamterene do not. These agents vary in potency, but with appropriate selection and dosage they can promote a diuresis in patients with edema caused by heart failure and with prolonged use can diminish the tendency of patients with heart failure to retain salt and water.

Mild to moderate heart failure in patients with acute infarction is usually managed successfully with bed rest, morphine, careful attention to fluid balance with optimization of pulmonary artery wedge pressure, and use of vasodilators and diuretics when indicated.

Cardiogenic shock

When oxygen and other nutrients become unavailable to the cells of the body, shock may occur. Shock is a descriptive term denoting a clinical picture that develops in the presence of inadequate tissue perfusion. It occurs in about 15% of patients hospitalized with acute myocardial infarction. The clinical picture is characterized by (1) a systolic blood pressure less than 90 mm Hg or at least 30 mm Hg lower than the prior basal level and (2) signs of impaired tissue perfusion such as pallor, cyanosis of varying degrees, cool and clammy skin, mental confusion or obtundation, and urine output less than 20 ml/hour. Shock may be caused by a variety of conditions unrelated to myocardial infarction: severe dehydration, hyperinsulinism that produces severe hypoglycemia, severe trauma, massive hemorrhage, overwhelming infection, and so forth. In the treatment of shock, it is essential that the cause of the shock be determined. In this discussion, cardiogenic shock is said to be present when the preceding clinical characteristics are present in a patient with acute myocardial infarction. Patients with hypotension related to pain or vasovagal reactions responsive to atropine are specifically excluded from the group defined as having cardiogenic shock. Although cardiac arrhythmias such as excessive tachycardia or bradycardia can cause the picture of shock, the following remarks are intended to describe abnormalities noted among patients in whom these rhythm disturbances either are not present or have been corrected and the picture of shock persists.

HEMODYNAMIC ASSESSMENT

In recent years a number of coronary care units, particularly those with a research interest, have employed a method by which the hemodynamic status of the patient can be measured at the bedside without increasing risk or discomfort for the patient. With the aid of fluoroscopy or a pressure recorder or both, a balloon-tip, flow-directed catheter is inserted into the brachial vein and directed into the right ventricle and pulmonary artery (Fig. 4-3 *A* and *B*). This catheter provides a guide for more precise management of heart failure and especially cardiogenic shock by furnishing a way to measure the pulmonary artery end-diastolic pressure (PAEDP) and pulmonary capillary wedge pressure (PCWP). Since there is a direct relationship between the PAEDP, the PCWP, and the pressure in the left ventricle immediately before systole (left ventricular end-diastolic pressure ([LVEDP]), an elevated PAEDP or PCWP reflects the elevated LVEDP that occurs when the left ventricular contractility is impaired sufficiently to prevent normal emptying. A PAEDP or PCWP measurement greater than 12 mm Hg is considered abnormal. The balloon-tip catheter, furthermore, may aid in establishing the cause of heart failure or shock, as well as in evaluating the effectiveness of the therapy. For example, in a state of hypotension caused by hypovolemia, infusing normal saline solution, whole blood, or low molecular weight dextran elevates the systemic pressure. In this case the PAEDP and PCWP, initially low, will return to normal when the blood volume has been restored. If the PAEDP is elevated because of congestive heart failure that has caused pulmonary edema, for example, effective therapy should lower the pressure readings that were initially elevated.

The use of the central venous pressure (CVP) to measure right atrial pressure (RAP) is no longer considered sufficiently accurate because the relationship between the RAP and LVEDP is inconsistent. Therefore PAEDP and PCWP, rather than CVP, should be accepted as major guides in the treatment of heart failure and shock.

As the clinical features of heart failure worsen, they may be paralleled by

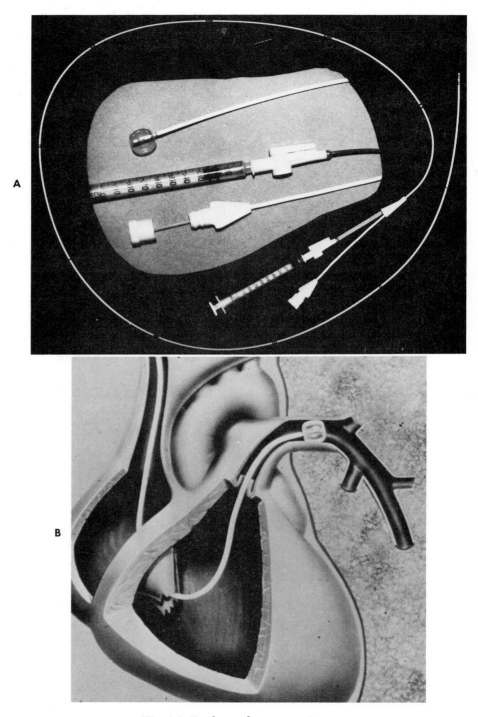

Fig. 4-3. For legend see opposite page.

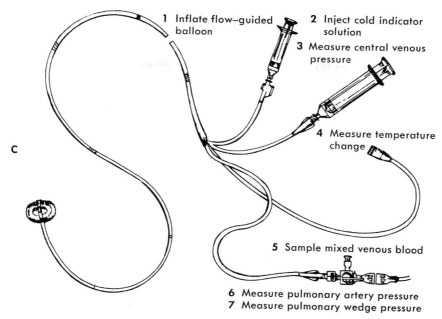

1 Inflate flow–guided balloon
2 Inject cold indicator solution
3 Measure central venous pressure
4 Measure temperature change
5 Sample mixed venous blood
6 Measure pulmonary artery pressure
7 Measure pulmonary wedge pressure

Fig. 4-3. A, The Swan-Ganz flow-directed catheter. **B,** The Swan-Ganz flow-directed catheter with *partially inflated* balloon is passed through the superior vena cava and into the right atrium, where the balloon is then inflated to its maximum recommended capacity. Continued catheter advancement propels the balloon-tipped catheter into the right ventricle, pulmonary artery, and finally into the wedged position that is evidenced by a characteristic change in pressure wave form. **C,** The Swan-Ganz flow-directed thermodilution catheter (**A** and **C** with permission of Edwards Laboratories, Division of American Hospital Supply Corp., Santa Ana, California.)

an elevation of the PAEDP and PCWP, a decrease in cardiac output, a drop in arterial and right atrial oxygen tension, and a widening of the oxygen difference in volume percent between arterial and venous blood samples, commonly referred to as the A-V oxygen difference.

To complement the picture of pump failure, a fall in arterial oxygen tension, a sign of abnormal lung function, occurs. The fall is thought to result at least in part from elevation of left atrial pressure. Changes in pulmonary function include (1) abnormalities of diffusion, particularly of oxygen; (2) a redistribution of pulmonary blood flow into the less well ventilated upper lobes; and (3) right-to-left shunting. Not only is the arterial oxygen tension reduced in patients with acute infarction and shock, but it also fails to increase to expected values with the administration of oxygen until pulmonary congestion has cleared.

It should be noted that a wider A-V oxygen difference and a lower cardiac output can be suspected when the right atrial oxygen saturation is reduced. If arterial oxygen saturation remains constant, reduced right atrial oxygen saturation reflects increased tissue extraction of oxygen during the passage of blood from the arterial to the venous circulation. Widened A-V oxygen difference depicts this increased extraction and indicates reduced cardiac output; the tissues need to extract more oxygen during each passage of the blood, since the total number of "passages" (cardiac output) is reduced. This observation suggests that the determinations of right atrial oxygen saturation can be a useful index of circulatory failure in patients with acute infarction. In addition to the bedside techniques for measuring PAEDP, PCWP, and LVEDP, the simple test of determining whether the right atrial oxygen saturation is above or below 65% has proved to be a useful guide to therapy. The use of this variable is based on the Fick equation for measuring cardiac output:

$$\text{Cardiac output} = \frac{\text{Oxygen consumption}}{\text{A-V oxygen difference}}$$

A specially designed cardiac catheter with a thermister (temperature) electrode has been used to measure cardiac output using the principle of themodilution. The procedure involves injecting a known amount of cold solution into the right atrium or superior vena cava. The temperature change is perceived by the termister electrode in the pulmonary artery. Cardiac output is inversely proportional to the temperature change, that is, the greater the cardiac output the less the temperature change. The use of such a catheter facilitates measurement of the cardiac output and eliminates the need for a systemic arterial blood sample to determine cardiac output (Fig. 4-3, C).

Cardiac output varies inversely with the A-V oxygen difference, since oxygen consumption under basal conditions is stable. Right atrial oxygen saturation may be reduced by (1) hypoventilation, (2) ventilation perfusion abnormalities, (3) diffusion abnormalities, or (4) intrapulmonary shunting. Giving 100% oxygen will correct the effects of the first three. Normal cardiac chamber oxygen values are found in Fig. 4-4.

TREATMENT

The current term to describe the problem of patients in cardiogenic shock with or without congestive heart failure is "power failure." Most studies indicate mortality of at least 80% in patients with cardiogenic shock during the course of acute myocardial infarction; unfortunately, current therapeutic measures have not affected these figures.

Although the primary therapeutic goals are to increase cardiac contractility and to maintain renal blood flow, there is no clear-cut regimen for the treatment of cardiogenic shock that can be applied to all patients, since therapy depends on the specific findings in the individual patient. For the physician to direct treatment intelligently, as much clinical and hemodynamic information as possible should be available. Therapy, as well as the natural

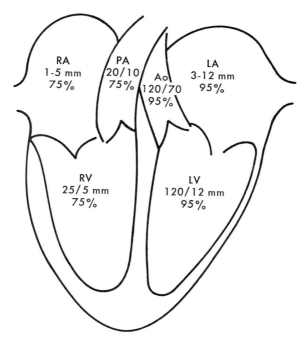

Fig. 4-4. Normal average cardiac pressures (mm Hg) and normal oxygen content (%) in each chamber.

evolution of the shock state, may change these values, and therefore measurements should be repeated as often as necessary. Clinical management of the patient in cardiogenic shock is divided into general and specific measures, as follows:

A. **General therapeutic measures**
1. Have patient assume a supine position with a pillow. Trendelenburg position is not recommended for treating cardiogenic shock.
2. Relieve pain with intravenous morphine sulfate in low doses, 5 to 10 mg initially, just sufficient to be effective. Large doses of morphine sulfate should be avoided if possible. Observe for lowering of arterial pressure.
3. Insert a Foley catheter to measure hourly urine output as an index of kidney function. Maintain urine output at a minimum of 20 ml/hour to prevent renal failure.
4. Insert an intra-arterial needle or catheter to monitor arterial blood pressure, blood gas levels, pH, cardiac output, A-V oxygen difference, and peripheral resistance. Total peripheral vascular resistance is calculated according to the following formula:

$$\frac{\text{Mean aortic pressure} - \text{Mean right atrial pressure (mm Hg)}}{\text{Cardiac output (L/minute)}}$$

5. Use balloon-tip, flow-directed catheter to monitor PAEDP and PCWP as a reflection of left ventricular performance.

B. **Specific therapeutic goals**
  1. Correct arrhythmias and establish appropriate heart rate. If the heart rate is above normal but not in the abnormal tachycardia range, no special therapy is necessary. However, if the rate is abnormally slow, the use of atropine must be considered. The use of atropine in patients with myocardial infarction is presently being evaluated. For the symptomatic patient (ventricular ectopic systoles, hypotension, and so forth) with sinus bradycardia, atropine is clearly indicated. For the asymptomatic patient with sinus bradycardia, it would appear best not to administer atropine, but merely to monitor the patient closely. When atropine is indicated, initial doses should be in the range of 0.4 to 0.6 mg IV, repeating with 0.2 to 0.4 mg if the initial dose does not produce the desired effect. If atropine does not raise the heart rate sufficiently to eliminate the symptoms accompanying the slower rate, or if the cause for the low heart rate is complete heart block, electrical pacing should be considered.
  2. Correct hypovolemia. One correctable cause of shock is hypovolemia. Elderly patients with myocardial infarction are prime candidates for relative hypovolemia, especially if they have been receiving diuretics or a low-sodium intake. The initial stages of acute myocardial infarction are associated with a reduced fluid intake because of pain, analgesic therapy, nausea, and vomiting. Further routes of fluid loss are profuse sweating, diarrhea secondary to medication, vigorous treatment with diuretics, and phlebotomy. Consequently, patients showing evidence of low cardiac output syndrome with hypotension and oliguria may be given a trial of fluid loading, particularly if PAEDP and PCWP are low. Patients with evidence of severe pulmonary congestion are not suitable for this therapy. With low PAEDP and PCWP values, normal saline solution, whole blood, or low molecular weight dextran may be infused until the PCWP reaches 15 to 18 mm Hg. Current experience indicates that the PCWP value should be kept slightly elevated in patients with cardiogenic shock.
  3. Correct hypoxemia. Hypoxia with PO_2 values below the level of 70 to 75 mm Hg while the patient is receiving nasal oxygen indicates that the patient should probably be intubated and given intermittent positive pressure breathing or volume assistance and 100% oxygen.
  4. Correct acidosis. When circulatory impairment exists, the metabolic activity of the perfused cells of the body changes, and lactic acid and other metabolic products are released into the vascular system and ineffectively metabolized. Consequently, systemic acidosis develops. This state is indicated by a low blood pH and contributes to poor tissue perfusion. This complication is treated with intravenous sodium bicarbonate, taking precautions not to produce sodium overload.
  5. Improve cardiac contractility. Use of digitalis in the management of cardiogenic shock is not well supported by existing data. Recent experimental studies show that the positive inotropic effect of digitalis preparations improves contractility but significantly increases myocardial oxygen demand. Other agents that enhance the state of cardiac contractility have been employed in cardiogenic shock. In patients with adequate filling pressures and normal or increased peripheral resistance, dopamine hydrochloride can cause a significant increase in cardiac output. Dopamine has a strong inotropic effect with minimal effect on cardiac rate and causes renal vasodilation.
  6. Improve circulation. Clinical estimates of the degree of increased peripheral resistance usually present in the shock syndrome can be made from the amount of increase in venous pressure, the amount of decrease in pulse pressure, the decrease in cutaneous blood flow with cold and cyanotic extremities, the poorly palpable peripheral pulses despite bounding central pulsations, and the clinical appearance of the patient. If these findings continue to persist, a dangerously in-

appropriate prolonged period of peripheral vasoconstriction may exist. If the patient exhibits signs of the shock syndrome with a low or normal calculated peripheral resistance, an infusion of a drug with combined alpha and beta adrenergic properties may be considered. Metaraminol (Aramine) and norepinephrine (levarterenol, Levophed) are used to increase arterial blood pressure and improve perfusion of ischemic areas of myocardium that are functionally depressed. The elevated pressure may open existing or latent coronary collateral channels, which require a relatively high pressure to maintain blood flow through them, bypassing concomitant areas of arterial atherosclerosis. Consequently, these drugs may improve myocardial function and increase cardiac output. However, at the same time they increase cardiac afterload—resistance against which the ventricle pumps—and thus increase myocardial oxygen consumption. Therefore the use of these agents should be aimed at producing a balance between coronary perfusion and ventricular afterload.

To deal with patients who exhibit clinical signs of shock with an increased peripheral resistance, several groups of investigators are evaluating agents that produce vasodilation, decreased peripheral resistance, and, thereby, increased cardiac output. Such agents include nitroprusside and intravenous nitroglycerin. Current studies show promise for these drugs in patients with an increased PCWP and signs of left heart failure. They should not be used if arterial pressure is below 90 mm Hg.

A technique currently receiving great recognition in the management of cardiogenic shock is mechanical circulatory assistance in the form of intra-aortic counterpulsation, a unique intervention utilizing the physiologic effects of an intra-aortic balloon. The balloon is deflated during ventricular systole and thus partially empties the aorta. The effect is to potentiate forward stroke volume but to reduce developed ventricular pressure and hence myocardial oxygen consumption. In diastole the balloon is inflated, thus restoring arterial pressure and coronary perfusion. Counterpulsation improves cardiac output, reduces evidence of myocardial ischemia, and frequently relieves pain and reduces S-T segment elevation. Patients with shock usually demonstrate a favorable hemodynamic and systemic metabolic response to balloon pumping. A minority of patients can be weaned off the pump, but most revert to the picture of shock when pumping is stopped. Thus balloon pumping per se has a minimal effect on mortality associated with shock, despite its temporary utility. However, several groups have reported that when patients in shock use the pump and then undergo coronary arteriography in 12 to 24 hours to define likely surgical candidates, significant rates of salvage can be obtained by surgery. In a recent report by Resnekov the pump was used for 35 patients who were studied by catheterization. Of these, 28 (80%) were believed to be surgical candidates, and 21 of this group (55%) were discharged alive after surgery. Others have reported survival rates among shock patients with balloon pumping and surgery to range from 40% to 50%. This should be compared to a mortality of 80% to 90% in comparable patients treated medically only. Thus balloon pumping as a support device while diagnostic and subsequent surgical therapy are contemplated has a much more favorable outcome than pumping alone. Based on these data, counterpulsation probably is indicated for the treatment of shock in institutions where an experienced pump team, catheter laboratory, and coronary surgery program are established.

REFERENCES

Braunwald, E., and Maroko, P. R.: The reduction of infarct size—an idea whose time (for testing) has come, Circulation **50**:206, 1974.

Chatterjee, K., and Parmley, W. W.: The role of vasodilator therapy in heart failure, Prog. Cardiovasc. Dis. **19**:301, 1977.

Ewy, G. A.: Anticoagulation in patients with acute myocardial infarction, Pract. Cardiol. **4**:25, 1978.

Harrison, T. R., and Reeves, T. J.: Principles and problems of ischemic heart disease, Chicago, 1968, Year Book Medical Publishers, Inc.

Harvey, W. P.: Some pertinent physical findings in the clinical evaluation of acute myocardial infarction, Circulation **39**:(Suppl. 4): 175, 1969.

Holzer, J., et al.: Effectiveness of dopamine in patients with cardiogenic shock, Am. J. Cardiol. **32**:79, 1973.

Lamberti, J. J., et al.: Mechanical circulatory assistance for the treatment of complications of coronary artery disease, Surg. Clin. North Am. **56**:83, 1976.

Loeb, H. S., et al.: Acute hemodynamic effects of dopamine in patients with shock, Circulation **44**:163, 1971.

McNeer, J. F., et al.: Hospital discharge one week after acute myocardial infarction, N. Engl. J. Med. **298**:229, 1978.

Mueller, H., and Ayers, S.: Propranolol in the treatment of acute myocardial infarction, Circulation **49**:1078, 1974.

Mueller, H., and Ayers, S.: The effects of intraaortic balloon counterpulsation on cardiac performance and metabolism in shock associated with acute myocardial infarction, J. Clin. Invest. **50**:1885, 1971.

The Pathfinder family of Swan-Ganz flow-directed right heart catheters, Santa Anna, Calif., 1973, Edwards Laboratories, Division of American Hospital Supply Corp.

Ratshin, R. A., Rackley, C. E., and Russell, R. O.: Hemodynamic elevation of left ventricular function in shock complicating myocardial infarction, Circulation **45**:127, 1972.

Resnekov, L.: Management of acute myocardial infarction, Cardiovasc. Med. **2**:949, 1977.

Rogers, W. J., et al.: Reduction of hospital mortality rate of acute myocardial infarction with glucose-insulin-potassium infusion, Am. Heart J. **92**:441, 1976.

Romhilt, D. W., and Fowler, N. O.: Physical signs in acute myocardial infarction, Heart Lung **2**:74, 1973.

Rotman, M., et al.: Pulmonary artery diastolic pressure in acute myocardial infarction, Am. J. Cardiol. **33**:357, 1974.

Shubin, H., and Weil, M. H.: Practical considerations in the management of shock complicating acute myocardial infarction. A summary of current practice, Am. J. Cardiol. **26**:603, 1970.

Waugh, R. A.: Immediate and remote prognostic implications of fascicular block during acute myocardial infarction, Circulation **47**:765, 1973

Willerson, J. T., et al.: Radionuclide imaging in acute myocardial infarction, Cardiovasc. Med. **3**:69, 1978.

CHAPTER FIVE

INTRODUCTION TO ELECTROCARDIOGRAPHY

This chapter describes some basic principles of electrocardiography, indicates the use of the normal electrocardiogram, and introduces certain abnormalities commonly encountered in patients with cardiac disease manifesting electrocardiographic changes. Additional electrocardiographic disorders are presented in Chapter 6.

Basic considerations

The electrocardiogram (ECG) is simply defined as a graphic tracing of the electrical forces produced by the heart. In the evaluation of patients with heart disease, this test is a frequently used and highly important diagnostic procedure. The ECG, however, has limitations, and consequently, it is important to evaluate the tracing in conjunction with the clinical examination of the patient. For example, electrocardiographic abnormalities may occur in normal healthy persons and in the absence of organic heart disease. Conversely, organic heart disease may occur with normal electrocardiographic patterns. Moreover, numerous extrinsic factors not related to the heart per se may alter the final recording. Such factors include disease, drugs, and stress, as well as skin resistance, distance of the chest wall from the heart, skeletal muscle tremors, electrical interference, faulty equipment, and improper method of taking the ECG.

STANDARDIZATION

The ECG comprises a series of horizontal and vertical lines that are used to measure amplitude and duration of the various deflections, segments, and intervals. The horizontal lines are 1 millimeter (mm) apart; the vertical lines are also 1 mm apart on the amplitude scale, as well as 0.04 second apart on the time scale. Furthermore, each fifth horizontal and vertical line is darker than the others, forming a large square incorporating 25 smaller squares.

Conventionally, the ECG is *standardized* so that a 1 millivolt (mv) impulse will cause a deflection of 10 mm or two large squares (Fig. 5-1). If the amplitude of the deflection recorded from the heart is too large for the ECG paper, the standardization must be halved so that 1 mv results in a deflection of 5 mm or one large square. If the standardization is halved, this must be noted on the ECG paper.

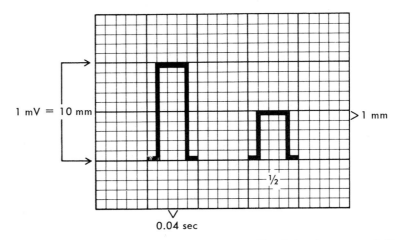

Fig. 5-1. Normal standardization of the ECG. One millivolt (mv) causes a deflection of 10 millimeters (mm). For large deflections the standard must be halved so that 1 mv = 5 mm. This must be noted on the ECG.

DEFLECTIONS

Any wave or complex recorded in the ECG is inscribed as a *positive* (above the base line) or *negative* (below the base line) deflection. When a deflection is partly above the base line and partly below it, and the positive and negative components are approximately equal, the complex is called *diaphasic* or *biphasic*. As previously mentioned, the amplitude of deflections is recorded in millimeters or millivolts. Measurement of positive deflections is made from the upper edge of the base line to the peak of the wave; negative deflections are measured from the lower edge of the base line to the lowest point of the wave.

The six major deflections of the normal ECG are designated by the letters P, Q, R, S, T, and U (Fig. 5-2). These waves are produced by the electrical energy caused by the movement of charged particles across the membranes of myocardial cells (depolarization and repolarization).

ELECTROPHYSIOLOGIC PRINCIPLES

At the time the resting potential of a cardiac cell is recorded, the cell membrane is impermeable to sodium and relatively permeable to potassium, the latter being the major determinant of intracellular diastolic potential. Measurements of intra- and extracellular ionic concentrations during diastole show a high intracellular potassium concentration and a low extracellular potassium concentration, whereas similar measurements of sodium show the reverse with high extracellular and low intracellular sodium levels. Accordingly, the inside of the cell is negatively charged with respect to the outside. The cell, therefore, in a resting state, *polarized*, can be represented

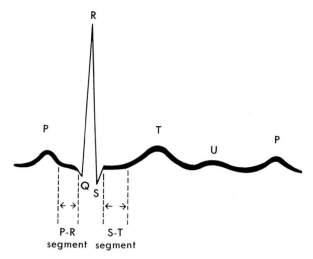

Fig. 5-2. The deflections in a normal ECG are the P wave (atrial depolarization), QRS complex (ventricular depolarization), and T wave (ventricular repolarization). The U wave is sometimes present and always follows the T wave. The P-R segment is the interval between the end of the P wave and the beginning of the QRS complex. The S-T segment is the interval between the end of the QRS complex and the beginning of the T wave. Sometimes atrial repolarization, the Ta wave, can be recorded (see Fig. 5-5).

by negative and positive charges lining, respectively, the inside and outside of the cell membrane (Fig. 5-3, *A*). If an electrode of an ECG machine (galvanometer) were attached to this polarized cell, no electrical potential would be registered, and there would be no deviation from the isoelectric base line (Fig. 5-3, *A*).

When a cell is stimulated, a change in membrane permeability permits the sodium ions to rapidly migrate across the cell membrane into the cell so that the inside of the cell becomes positive with respect to the outside. This process is called *depolarization*. When a large group of cells is suddenly depolarized, an electrical field is generated between the depolarized and polarized areas of the myocardium. The *P wave* represents *atrial depolarization*, and the *QRS complex* represents *ventricular depolarization* (Fig. 5-3, *B*, *C*, and *D*).

A slower movement of ions across the membrane restoring the cell to the polarized state is termed *repolarization*. Movement of potassium ions out of myocardial cells primarily accounts for repolarization. In late diastole, after most of the repolarization has occurred, potassium and sodium reverse positions to restore concentrations to the polarized state. The *Ta wave*, representing *atrial repolarization*, generally lies buried in the QRS complex and S-T segment. The *S-T segment* is an isoelectric line extending from the end of the QRS complex to the beginning of the T wave, during which early ventricular

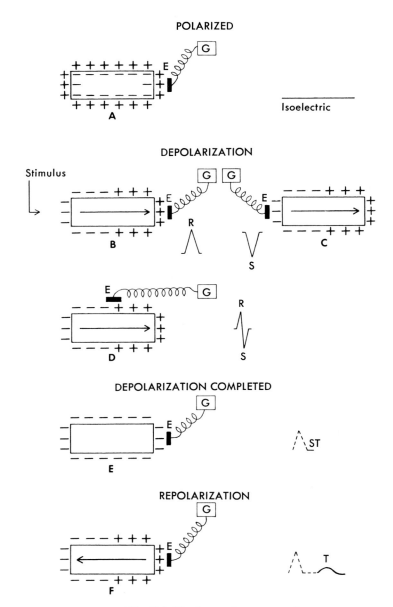

Fig. 5-3. For legend see opposite page.

repolarization is beginning very slowly (Fig. 5-3, *E*). The *T wave* represents *ventricular repolarization* (Fig. 5-3, *F).*

Waves and complexes
P WAVE

As previously mentioned, the P wave represents atrial depolarization, and begins as soon as the impulse leaves the sinoatrial (S-A) node and initiates atrial depolarization. Since the S-A node is situated in the right atrium, right atrial activation begins first and is followed shortly therafter by left atrial activation. As left atrial activation begins, before the end of right atrial activation, the two processes overlap. This close overlap of the forces results in a gently rounded P wave. As will be discussed later in this chapter, the P wave may be normally positive, negative, or diphasic, depending on which lead of the ECG is recorded. Whatever the case, the amplitude of the P wave should not exceed 2 or 3 mm in any lead (Fig. 5-4).

Although not usually visible on the ECG, the Ta wave of atrial repolarization occurs in an opposite direction to that of the P wave and is recorded after the first portion of the P wave and continues through the P-R interval. It is usually not identified unless the P wave occurs independently of

---

Fig. 5-3. A, A schematic illustration of a polarized (resting) myocardial muscle cell maintaining a negative charge on the inside of the cell membrane and a positive charge on the outside of the membrane. An electrode *(E)* facing the right side of the polarized cell and attached to an ECG machine *(G,* galvanometer) will record no current, and an isoelectric line results. **B,** The cell is stimulated from the left, and depolarization proceeds from left to right in the direction of the arrow. The depolarized left end of the cell becomes immediately electrically negative, whereas the right end of the cell is still polarized and electrically positive. There now exists a difference of electrical potentials (negative and positive ions), and an electric current is flowing. The electrode facing the positive side of this current and attached to an ECG machine will record a positive deflection, and in the case of ventricular depolarization, this deflection is called an R wave. **C,** The same myocardial cell is stimulated again from the left; however, the electrode is facing the negative side of the current, and will, therefore, record a negative deflection. In the case of ventricular depolarization, this deflection is called an S wave. **D,** Once again the cell is activated from the left. The electrode facing the center of the cell will first write a positive and then a negative deflection. In the case of ventricular depolarization, this deflection is called an RS complex. **E,** With the completion of depolarization, the outer surface of the myocardial cell becomes electrically negative; the flow of electric current ceases, and the R wave returns to the isoelectric line. The short period following complete ventricular depolarization is recorded as the S-T segment. **F,** In the previous illustrations, the myocardial muscle cell was depolarized from left to right. Now the cell returns to the resting state, repolarization, in the opposite direction, from right to left. The right end of the cell becomes positive first and an electrode facing this site will inscribe a positive deflection. In the case of ventricular repolarization, this deflection is termed a T wave.

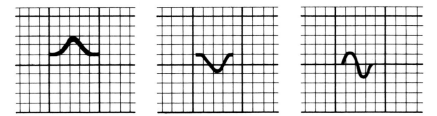

Fig. 5-4. The P wave is gently rounded in contour, may be normally positive, negative, or diphasic in different ECG leads, and should not exceed 2 or 3 mm.

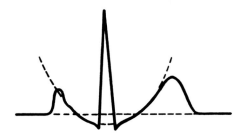

Fig. 5-5. Atrial repolarization as a cause of S-T segment deviation. Note that the P-Q (P-R) and S-T segments can be connected by a smooth curve, and that the direction of the deviation is opposite in direction to the P wave. (Adapted from Hurst, J. W., et al.: The heart: arteries and veins, ed. 3, New York, 1974, McGraw-Hill Book Co.)

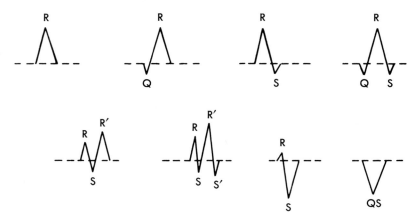

Fig. 5-6. Components of the QRS complex.

the QRS, as in complete A-V block. When the P wave is large, the Ta wave is also generally large and may be seen to extend beyond the QRS complex, resulting in a distortion of the initial portion of the S-T segment. This may cause a depression of the S-T segment that may be mistaken for pathologic significance. In order to make a correct interpretation in the setting of a depressed S-T segment, one must (1) observe the configuration of the atrial repolarization wave (smooth curve with upward concavity), (2) recognize a similar deviation of the base line before the QRS is recorded, and (3) recognize a large P wave (Fig. 5-5).

QRS COMPLEX

The QRS complex representing ventricular depolarization may have various components, depending on which lead of the ECG is recorded. These components are illustrated in Fig. 5-6 and described as follows:

R wave: The first positive deflection
Q wave: An initial negative deflection preceding an R wave
S wave: The negative deflection following an R wave
R′ wave: The second positive deflection
S′ wave: The negative deflection following the R′ wave
QS wave: The totally negative deflection

The QRS complexes should be examined as follows:
1. The general *configuration* of the complex, including the presence and location of any slurred component (see Chapter 6 discussion of bundle branch block and Wolff-Parkinson-White syndrome)
2. The presence of abnormal *Q waves* (discussed under myocardial infarction in this chapter)
3. The *duration* of the complex (see Chapter 6 discussion of QRS interval
4. The *amplitude* of the components
The timing of the *intrinsicoid deflections* in precordial leads V_1 to V_6

Amplitude. The *amplitude* of the QRS complex has wide normal limits; however, it is generally agreed that if the total amplitude (above and below the base line) is 5 mm or less in all three standard leads, it is abnormally low. Such low voltage may be seen in patients with cardiac failure, diffuse coronary disease, pericardial effusion, myxedema, primary amyloidosis, and any other conditions producing widespread myocardial damage. Additionally, it may be found in patients with emphysema, generalized edema, and obesity. The minimal normal QRS amplitude in precordial leads varies from right to left across the chest, being generally accepted as 5 mm in V_1 and V_6, 7 mm in V_2 and V_5, and 9 mm in V_3 and V_4.

Upper limits for normal QRS voltage (amplitude) have been difficult to set. Diagnostic evaluation is imperative when QRS amplitudes reach the following upper limits: V_1 an R wave of 5 mm; V_1, V_2 an S wave of 30 mm; V_5, V_6 an R wave of 30 mm; and in the limb leads an R or S wave of 20 mm.

Intrinsicoid deflection. Ventricular activation time is the interval between the beginning of the QRS complex and the onset of the *intrinsicoid deflection.*

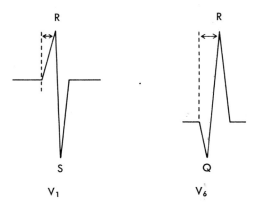

Fig. 5-7. The time of onset of the intrinsicoid deflection is measured from the beginning of the QRS complex to the peak of the R wave.

The time of onset of the intrinsicoid deflection is measured from the beginning of the QRS complex to the peak of the R wave, and it is measured in the precordial leads (Fig. 5-7). In right-sided precordial leads (V_1 or V_2) the time of onset for the intrinsicoid deflection is normally 0.03 second or less. In left-sided precordial leads (V_5 or V_6) the time of onset is normally 0.05 second or less in adults. If the time of onset for the intrinsicoid deflection exceeds 0.03 or 0.05 second, respectively, it is taken to indicate that the impulse arrived late at the epicardial surface of the ventricle under the electrode. Such delay may be caused by thickening or dilation of the ventricular wall or a block in the conducting system to the ventricle involved (bundle branch block).

S-T SEGMENT

The interval that occurs between the end of the QRS complex and the beginning of the T wave is called the S-T segment. It represents the time during which the ventricles are completely depolarized and ventricular repolarization may begin. Usually, the S-T segment is isoelectric (see Fig. 5-2), but it may normally deviate between −0.5 and +1.0 mm from the base line in the standard and unipolar leads (ECG leads are presented in the next section). In some instances, upward displacement of 2 or 3 mm may be normal, provided the S-T segment is concave upward and the succeeding T wave is tall and upright. This is called "early repolarization." *Downward displacement in excess of 0.5 mm is abnormal.* In all situations, depression caused by a depressed P-R segment must be considered. Even more important may be S-T segments, elevated or depressed, that vary temporarily (see discussions of myocardial infarction, pericarditis).

Elevation of the S-T segment is measured from the upper edge of the isoelectric line to the upper edge of the S-T sement; depression is measured

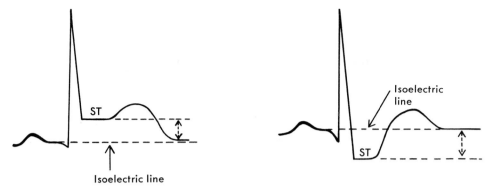

Fig. 5-8. Elevation of the S-T segment is measured from the upper edge of the isoelectric line to the upper edge of the S-T segment; depression is measured from the lower edge of the isoelectric line to the lower edge of the S-T segment.

from the lower edge of the isoelectric line to the lower edge of the S-T segment (Fig. 5-8).

T WAVE

The T wave, normally slightly rounded and slightly asymmetric, represents the recovery period (repolarization) of the ventricles. Upright T waves are measured from the upper level of the base line to the summit of the T wave, whereas inverted T waves are measured from the lower level of the base line to the lowest point of the T wave. Diphasic T waves are measured by adding the amplitudes above and below the base line. T waves normally do not exceed 5 mm in any standard lead or 10 mm in any precordial lead.

U WAVE

The U wave is a small wave of low voltage sometimes observed following a T wave and in the same direction as its preceding T wave, that is, when the T wave is upright, the U wave normally will be upright. It is best observed in the chest leads, even though it is present, but barely detectable, in the limb leads.

Relatively little is known about the U wave. Although the cause and clinical significance of the U wave is uncertain, the appearance of U waves or an increase in their magnitude is seen in certain disorders (see Chapter 6 discussion of hypokalemia).

Electrocardiogram leads

As previously mentioned, the deflections on the ECG are produced by the electrical energy owing to the movement of charged ions across the membranes of myocardial cells (depolarization and repolarization). This movement of charged particles results in a flow of electrical current. The "pressure" behind the flow of electrical current is called *electrical potential*, which creates an electrical field. This electrical field extends to the body surface, where electrical potential can be measured by the electrocardiograph.

By convention there are 12 lead recordings in the ECG. Each lead has a positive and negative pole (electrode), and the location of these poles determines the *polarity* of the lead. A hypothetic line joining the poles of a lead is known as the *axis* of the lead. Moreover, every lead axis is oriented in a certain direction, depending on the location of the positive and negative electrodes.

Six of the twelve ECG leads measure cardiac forces in the *frontal plane* (I, II, III, a V_R, aV_L, and aV_F); the remaining six leads V_1 to V_6) measure the cardiac forces in the *horizontal plane*. The frontal plane is measured by the standard limb leads and the augmented leads.

STANDARD (BIPOLAR) LIMB LEADS (I, II, III)

The standard limb leads, designated leads I, II, and III, were developed by Willem Einthoven (1860-1927), physiologist and inventor of the string galvanometer. Using the principle that the heart is situated in the center of the electrical field it generates, Einthoven placed the electrodes of the three standard leads as far away from the heart as possible, that is, on the extremities—the right arm, left arm, and left leg.* These three electrodes, therefore, are considered to be electrically equidistant from the heart. Consequently, the heart may be viewed as a point source in the center of an equilateral triangle, whose apices are the right arm, left arm, and left leg. This is called Einthoven's triangle (Fig. 5-9, *A*).

The standard bipolar limb leads measure the *difference* between two recording sites. The actual potential under either of the electrodes is not known, as it is for the unipolar leads. For lead I, the negative electrode is placed on the right arm and the positive electrode on the left arm. For lead II, the negative electrode is on the right arm and the positive electrode on the left leg. For lead III, the left arm electrode is negative, and the left leg electrode is positive (Fig. 5-9, *A*). This is summarized as follows:

Lead	Location
I	Right arm (−) to left arm (+)
II	Right arm (−) to left leg (+)
III	Left arm (−) to left leg (+)

Because of the established relationship of the standard limb leads to each other, at any given instant during the cardiac cycle the sum of the electrical potentials recorded in leads I and III equals the electrical potential recorded

---

*The right leg serves as a ground electrode, thereby providing a pathway of least resistance for electrical interference in the body. Actually, the ground electrode can be placed at any location on the body.

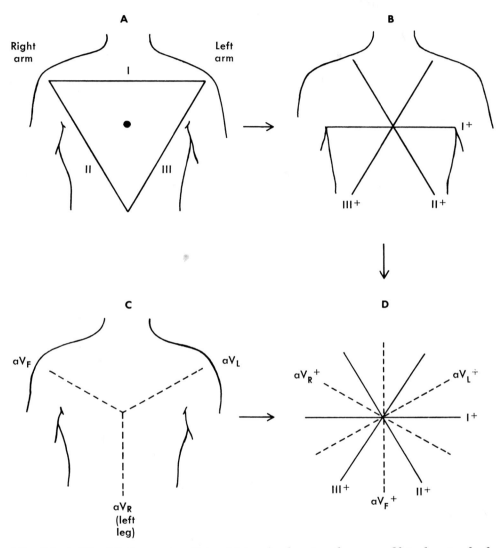

Fig. 5-9. A, The Einthoven equilateral triangle showing the axes of bipolar standard limb leads I, II, and III. The heart is at the center or zero point. **B,** The axes of the standard limb leads are shifted to the center of the triangle (zero point of the electrical field), forming a triaxial figure. **C,** The axes of the unipolar augmented leads. **D,** The axes of the standard and augmented limb leads are combined to form a hexaxial figure. Each lead is labeled at its positive pole.

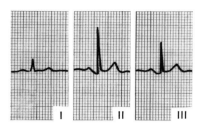

Fig. 5-10. Einthoven's law states: Lead I + Lead III = Lead II. The deflections in the ECG leads demonstrate this law.

in lead II. This is *Einthoven's law,* and it applies to a triangle of any shape. The law stated mathematically is as follows:

$$\text{Lead I} + \text{Lead III} = \text{Lead II}$$

Einthoven's law may be used to detect errors in electrode placement. Furthermore, it may clarify perplexing findings in one or another lead. If, for example, the deflections of lead II are obscured by muscular or electrical interference or by a wandering base line, the characteristics of the other two leads may be used to determine the presence of a Q wave or S-T segment deviation in lead II. Einthoven's law is also helpful in evaluating serial tracings. For example, if in a given tracing the T wave in lead I appears to be lower than in the previous tracing, changes must be present in the T waves of the other two limb leads as well, so that $T_1 + T_3 = T_2$ (Fig. 5-10).

To avoid confusion about polarity the ECG machine records a positive deflection in the bipolar leads when in lead I the left arm is in the positive portion of the electrical field, in lead II the left leg is in the positive portion of the electrical field, and in lead III the left leg is in the positive portion of the electrical field.

Triaxial reference figure. The three lead axes of the equilateral triangle can be shifted without changing their direction, so that their midpoints intersect at the same point. Thus the *triaxial reference figure* is formed with each of the lead axes seqarated from one another by 60 degrees (Fig. 5-9, *B*).

AUGMENTED (UNIPOLAR) LEADS (aV$_R$, aV$_L$, aV$_F$)

All unipolar leads are called V leads and consist of extremity (limb) leads and precordial (chest) leads. The augmented leads aV$_R$, aV$_L$, and aV$_F$ use the same electrode locations as the standard limb leads. Therefore the positive electrode is attached to the right arm (aV$_R$), left arm (aV$_L$), or left leg (aV$_F$). The negative electrode, however, is formed by combinining leads I, II, and III, whose algebraic sum is zero. Since the electrical center of the heart is at zero potential, the augmented leads measure the difference in potential between the limbs and the center of the heart.

The axis for each augmented lead is a line drawn from the extremity,

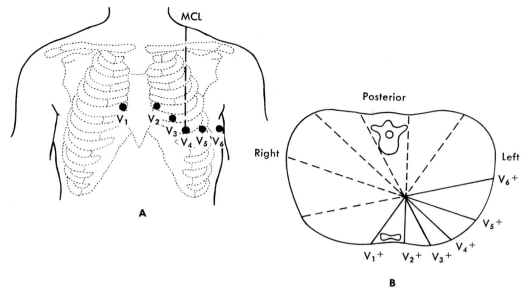

Fig. 5-11. A, Electrode positions of the precordial leads: V_1, fourth intercostal space at the right sternal border; V_2, fourth intercostal space at the left sternal border; V_3, halfway between V_2 and V_4; V_4, fifth intercostal space at the midclavicular line; V_5, anterior axillary line directly lateral to V_4; V_6, midaxillary line directly lateral to V_5. **B,** The precordial reference figure. Leads V_1 and V_2 are called right-sided precordial leads; leads V_3 and V_4, mid-precordial leads; and leads V_5 and V_6, left-sided precordial leads.

where the positive electrode is placed, to the zero point of the electrical field of the heart, which is at the center of the equilateral triangle (Fig. 5-9, *C*). These three unipolar lead axes also form a triaxial reference system with the axes 60 degrees apart.

    Hexaxial reference figure. When the triaxial figure of the standard leads and the triaxial figure of the augmented leads are combined, they form a *hexaxial reference figure* in which each augmented lead is perpendicular to a standard limb lead (Fig. 5-9, *D*). The hexaxial figure is a useful reference for plotting mean cardiac forces in the frontal plane.

PRECORDIAL (UNIPOLAR) LEADS (V_1 TO V_6)

    In the horizontal plane, precordial leads are utilized to determine how far anteriorly or posteriorly from the frontal plane the electrical forces of the heart are directed. The standard precordial ECG consists of six unipolar leads, V_1 through V_6. In Fig. 5-11, *A*, the V leads are shown with reference to their electrode positions on the anterior chest wall. These chest electrodes represent a positive pole (unipolar). Any electrical force traveling toward one

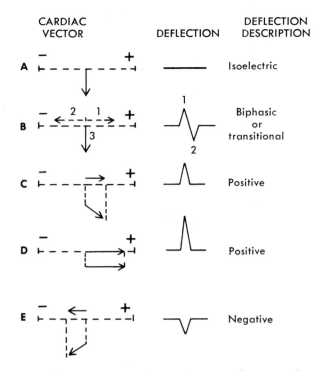

Fig. 5-12. Vectors and their electrocardiographic recordings. Each arrow represents the vector generated by an electrical force. This force produces an electrocardiographic deflection, shown on the right. **A,** Because the vector is perpendicular to the axis of the recording lead, no projection appears on that lead. The absence of a deflection establishes an uninterrupted isoelectric line. **B,** The mean vector (number 3) is perpendicular to the axis of the recording lead when the positive and negative forces are equal (the net area of the deflection is zero). A biphasic or transitional deflection is recorded because the initial forces moved rightward (vector 1) at the same distance that the later forces moved leftward (vector 2). The instantaneous vectors have equal magnitude but opposite direction. **C,** The vector projects on the positive side of the axis of the recording lead to inscribe a small positive deflection. **D,** When the vector is parallel with the lead axis, the projection onto the recording lead has its maximal magnitude. **E,** The vector projects on the negative side of the lead axis, and a small negative deflection is recorded.

of these leads will produce a positive deflection and traveling away from it will produce a negative deflection. For descriptive purposes, leads V_1 and V_2 are called right-sided precordial leads; leads V_3 and V_4, midprecordial leads; and leads V_5 and V_6, left-sided precordial leads.

Precordial reference figure. A transverse representation of the chest wall and the V leads results in the precordial reference figure (Fig. 5-11, *B*). This figure is a useful reference for plotting mean cardiac forces in the horizontal plane.

The vector approach to electrocardiography

The electrical potentials generated during the cardiac cycle can be described and measured. To adequately characterize such an electrical potential or force, both the magnitude and the direction of the force must be specified; this can be done by a *vector*. Briefly stated, a vector is a quantity (of electrical force) that has known magnitude and direction. A *vector* may be illustrated graphically by an *arrow;* the length of the arrow represents the *magnitude* of the force and the *direction* of the arrow indicates the *direction* of the force. The *arrowhead* depicts the location of the positive field.

Representing electrical forces of the heart by vectors more easily explains the relationship between the electrical activity generated by the heart and the recording of this electrical activity by a specific lead. When an electrical force (and therefore the vector that represents it) establishes a direction *parallel* to the lead that records it, this electrical force causes the *largest deflection* to be inscribed by that lead. An electrical force perpendicular to the recording lead produces no deflection in that lead. Forces in between these extremes generate deflections according to their directions: the more nearly parallel the force (and vector) to the recording lead, the larger the deflection produced in that lead; the more nearly perpendicular the force to the recording lead, the smaller the deflection. When the positive and negative forces on a lead are equal, the net area of the deflection is zero. This results in a biphasic or transitional deflection (Fig. 5-12).

SEQUENCE OF ELECTRICAL EVENTS IN THE HEART

In the normal heart, depolarization of the ventricle is a sequential process. The process can be represented by *instantaneous vectors*, each of which corresponds to all the heart's electrical forces at a given moment. A diagram of successive instantaneous vectors depicting ventricular depolarization is shown in Fig. 5-13, *A*. Initial depolarization passes from left to right across the interventricular septum. During the second phase, depolarization of subendocardial muscle occurs near the apex. The last phase of depolarization occurs in the posterior free wall of the left ventricle.

The deflection recorded by any given lead results from the projection of the cardiac vector generated during depolarization onto the axis of the lead. Thus arrow 1 (Fig. 5-13, *B*), depicting depolarization of the septum, usually causes a small negative deflection in lead I, resulting in a Q wave and a larger positive deflection in lead III, resulting in an R wave. Arrow 2, illustrating depolarization of the apical region of the heart, usually produces a very small positive deflection (R wave) in lead I because of its leftward orientation and an R wave in lead III. Late depolarization of the heart, being from right to left in the posterior free wall of the left ventricle, causes a large positive deflection in lead I (the major part of the R wave) and an S wave in lead III. Following the completion of depolarization of ventricles, the electrical wave returns to the base line. Therefore the three arrows have generated a small initial Q wave followed by a large R wave in lead I and an R wave followed by an S wave in lead III (Fig. 5-13, *C* and *D*).

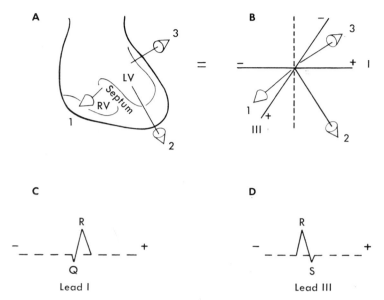

Fig. 5-13. **A,** Depolarization of the ventricles illustrated by instantaneous vectors. Arrow 1 depicts depolarization of the septum from left to right and is directed to the right and somewhat anteriorly. Arrow 2 illustrates depolarization of the apical region of the heart and is directed to the left and inferiorly. Arrow 3 represents depolarization of the posterior aspect of the left ventricle and is directed to the left and posteriorly. **B,** The instantaneous vectors representing ventricular depolarization are inscribed on lead I and lead III. **C** and **D,** Arrow 1 causes a small negative deflection in lead I, resulting in a Q wave, and a larger positive deflection in lead III, resulting in an R wave. Arrow 2 produces a small positive deflection (R wave) in lead I and an R wave in lead III. Arrow 3 causes a large R wave in lead I and S wave in lead III.

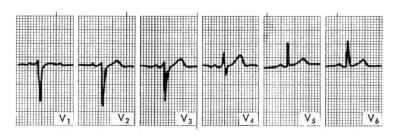

Fig. 5-14. Normal precordial lead ECG.

As previously discussed, each ECG lead has a different orientation to the heart. Therefore the instantaneous vectors of ventricular depolarization will produce a different deflection in each lead. This is also true of ventricular repolarization and atrial depolarization.

In this chapter, detailed consideration will be given to the vectors of the QRS complex. However, the positions of the P wave and T wave in the frontal plane are also important. Normally the P wave is upright in leads I and II and may be biphasic, flat, or inverted in lead III; inverted in lead aV_R; upright, biphasic, or inverted in lead aV_L; and upright in lead aV_F.

Normally the T wave is upright in leads I and II, flat, biphasic, or inverted in lead III, and inverted in lead aV_R. In lead aV_L, the T wave may be upright, flattened, or biphasic, according to the QRS pattern. It may also be inverted, provided the T wave in lead aV_R is also inverted. In lead aV_F the T wave is usually upright; however, it can be normally flattened, biphasic, or inverted, provided the T wave in lead aV_R is also inverted.

In the horizontal plane the P wave is normally upright in all precordial leads; the normal QRS complex is transitional at some point between V_3 and V_4. The precordial transition zone is characterized by the transition from the RS complexes, recorded by the leads oriented to the right ventricle, to the QR complexes, recorded by the leads oriented to the left ventricle (Fig. 5-14). The normal T wave is upright in leads V_2 through V_6. The T wave may be flat or inverted in V_1 and still be normal.

THE MEAN CARDIAC VECTOR

The mean cardiac vector, which is the average of all the instantaneous vectors, can be expressed more accurately on the hexaxial reference figure. Furthermore, since the hexaxial reference system divides the frontal plane into 30-degree intervals, the leads have been classified as follows: all degrees in the upper hemisphere of the hexaxial figure are labeled as negative degrees, and all degrees in the lower hemisphere are labeled as positive degrees. Accordingly, commencing at the positive end of the standard lead I axis (labeled 0 degrees and progressing counterclockwise), the leads will be successively at -30, -60, -90, -120, -150, and -180 degrees. Progressing clockwise, the leads will be successively at $+30$, $+60$, $+90$, $+120$, $+150$, and $+180$ degrees* (Fig. 5-15).

The position of the mean cardiac vector provides information about the electrical "position" of the heart, also expressed as the mean electrical axis, and is influenced by the relationship of the heart within the chest, as well as by the anatomy of the heart itself. If the P vector is projected on the hexaxial figure, the mean electrical axis of the P in the frontal plane lies approximately

---

*The conventional labeling of the hexaxial reference figure as positive and negative units should not be confused with the positive and negative poles of the lead axes.

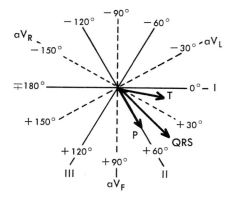

Fig. 5-15. The hexaxial reference system divides the frontal plane into 30-degree intervals. All degrees in the upper hemisphere are labeled as negative degrees, and all degrees in the lower hemisphere are labeled as positive degrees. The mean P vector normally lies along the +60-degree axis. The mean QRS vector normally lies anywhere between 0 and +90 degrees; in the figure the mean QRS vector lies on the +45-degree axis. The mean T vector normally lies between −10 and +75 degrees. In the figure the mean T vector lies on the +15-degree axis. The mean frontal plane QRS axis and T wave axis are usually similarly directed, and the angle between them normally does not exceed 60 degrees.

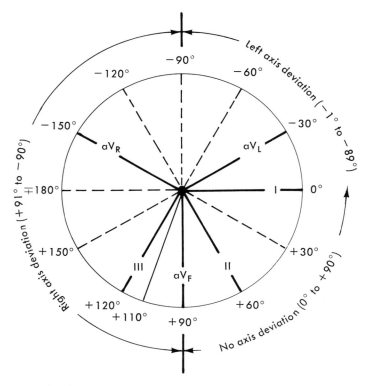

Fig. 5-16. Hexaxial reference figure indicating values for no axis deviation, left axis deviation, and right axis deviation.

along the +60-degree axis (Fig. 5-15). The mean QRS vector lies normally between 0 and +90 degrees, whereas the mean electrical axis of the T wave lies between −10 and +75 degrees. The mean frontal plane QRS axis and T wave axis are usually similarly directed, and the angle between them normally does not exceed 60 degrees (Fig. 5-15).

MEAN QRS AXIS

The remainder of this section will discuss the significance and determination of the mean QRS axis. The principles also may be applied to the mean P and T vectors.

Deviations in the mean electrical axis, even without other ECG abnormalities, may assist in the diagnosis of cardiac disease. As indicated in Fig. 5-16, the mean QRS vector normally lies between 0 and +90 degrees. Right axis deviation occurs when the mean QRS vector lies between +90 and −90 degrees. Right axis deviation with a mean QRS vector between +90 and +110 degrees may be abnormal, as in patients who have block in the posterior division of the left bundle branch (Chapter 6), but is frequently normal, as seen in young adults or asthenic individuals. This vector is illustrated in Fig. 5-17, *A*. *Abnormal right axis deviation* is present when the mean QRS vector lies between +110 and −90 degrees. This usually implies either delayed activation of the right ventricle as seen in right bundle branch block (Chapter 6) or right ventricle enlargement.

"Normal" left axis deviation is present when the mean QRS vector lies between 0 and −30 degrees. For example, this situation can occur in patients who have ascites or abdominal tumors, are pregnant, or are obese. *Abnormal left axis deviation*, however, is present when the mean QRS vector lies between −30 and −90 degrees. This vector is illustrated in Fig. 5-17, *B*. It may indicate delayed activation of the left ventricle as seen in left anterior hemiblock (Chapter 6) or left ventricular enlargement.

Occasionally the electrical position of the heart is described as horizontal, semihorizontal, intermediate, semivertical, or vertical. It has been convenient to refer to a heart with an axis in the neighborhood of 0 to −30 degrees as a *horizontal heart*, and to one with an axis between +60 and +90 degrees as a *vertical heart*. Semihorizontal and semivertical positions are halfway stations between the intermediate position and the horizontal and vertical extremes and are not very useful terms.

Determination of the frontal plane projection of the mean QRS vector. First, recall the following principles: an electrical force perpendicular to a lead axis will record a small or biphasic complex in the ECG lead. An electrical force parallel to a given lead axis will record its largest deflection in that ECG lead. With this in mind, follow the procedure below by referring to Fig. 5-17, *A*.

1. Examine the six frontal plane leads and identify the lead with the smallest or most diphasic deflection.
2. In Fig. 5-17, *A*, this is lead I.
3. The electrical axis must be near perpendicular to lead I, and it must run

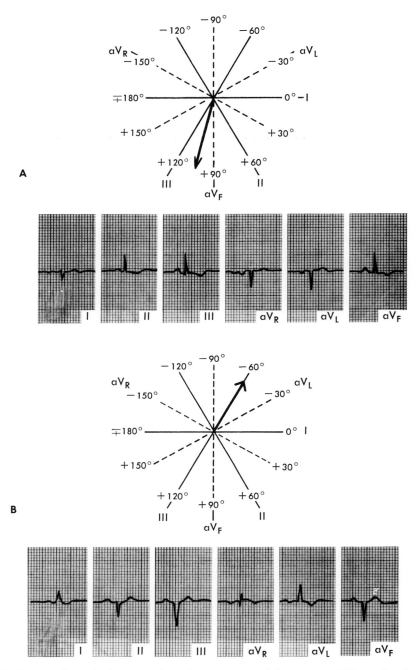

Fig. 5-17, A, A frontal plane ECG and projection of the mean QRS on the hexaxial figure. The mean QRS is located at +105 degrees and this is called right axis deviation. **B,** A frontal plane ECG and projection of the mean QRS on the hexaxial figure. The mean QRS is located at −60 degrees, and this is called left axis deviation.

near parallel to the lead that intersects lead I at right angles. aV_F is perpendicular to lead I.

4. The deflection in lead aV_F, therefore, must be largest in the frontal plane.
5. Since the deflection in lead aV_F is positive, the vector must be directed toward the positive pole of that lead.
6. Examine the six frontal plane leads to see if any other lead deflections are as large as lead aV_F. If the QRS complex is equal in amplitude in two leads, the mean QRS vector is directed halfway between the axes of these leads.
7. In this case the deflection in lead III is equal to that in lead aV_F.
8. The mean electrical axis of the QRS, therefore, lies between lead aV_F and lead III and is located at $+105$ degrees (right axis deviation).

In the example just given, if the deflection in lead aV_F had been greater than that in lead III, then the mean QRS vector would have been more parallel to lead aV_F, that is, at $+100$ or even $+95$ degees, depending on how much larger the deflection in lead aV_F was compared with lead III.

Another example following this procedure is shown in Fig. 5-17,*B*.

1. The smallest, or in this case the diphasic, deflection is seen in lead aV_R.
2. The mean QRS vector thus runs perpendicular to lead aV_R.
3. Since lead III runs perpendicular to lead aV_R, the deflection in lead III must be the largest.
4. The deflection in lead III is negative; therefore the mean axis is directed toward the negative pole of lead III.
5. The mean QRS vector in this figure is located at -60 degrees (left axis deviation).

Determination of the horizontal plane projection of the mean QRS vector

1. Identify the precordial lead with the transitional QRS deflection in Fig. 5-18, *A*.
2. Lead V_4 is transitional.
3. The QRS vector is perpendicular to the transitional lead (V_4).
4. The vector should be directed toward the positive sides of the leads with position deflections, and on the negative sides of the leads with negative deflections, as shown in Fig. 5-18, *C*.
5. When the horizontal plane direction of the mean QRS is noted, an arrowhead may be placed on the mean QRS frontal plane vector to indicate the vector's anterior or posterior direction, as shown in Fig. 5-18, *B*.

It should be noted that the transitional QRS deflection may appear early, that is, between V_1 and V_2, or late, that is, between V_5 and V_6. One explanation for this is that the heart has rotated on its longitudinal axis. In describing the rotation about this axis, one must consider a view of the heart from under the diaphragm. From this viewpoint, if the front of the heart rotates toward the left, this is called *clockwise rotation*. If the front of the heart rotates toward the right, this is called *counterclockwise rotation*. With a counterclockwise rotation the transitional zone will move toward the right (V_1, V_2). With a

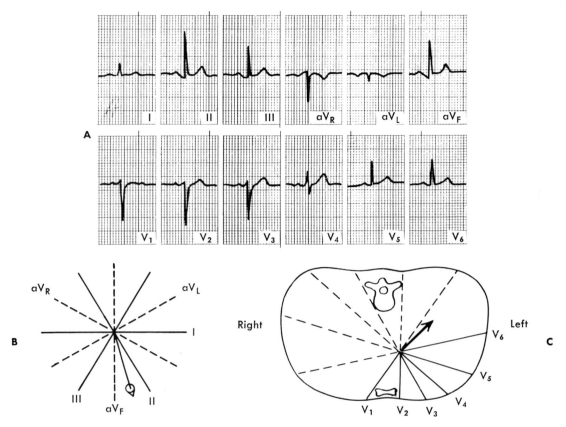

Fig. 5-18. Determination of the mean QRS vector in the frontal and horizontal planes. **A,** Twelve-lead ECG. **B,** The mean QRS vector in the frontal plane is located at +70 degrees. The arrowhead indicates that the mean QRS vector points posteriorly in the horizontal plane. **C,** The horizontal plane projection of the mean QRS is drawn in a posterior direction on the precordial reference figure. This calculation gives information for the direction of the arrowhead in the frontal plane (**B**).

clockwise rotation the transitional zone will shift to the left (V_5, V_6). Such rotations may be normal or abnormal.

Left ventricular enlargement

It is not usually possible in the ECG to differentiate between ventricular dilation and hypertrophy. The term "hypertrophy" is commonly used; however, this presentation will use "enlargement", since it includes both dilation and hypertrophy.

Hypertension, aortic valvular disease, mitral insufficiency, coronary artery disease, and congenital heart disease, for example, patent ductus arteriosus and coarctation of the aorta, commonly produce left ventricular enlargement. Under these circumstances the wall of the left ventricle is thicker or more dilated than normal. Furthermore, this increase in muscle mass results in

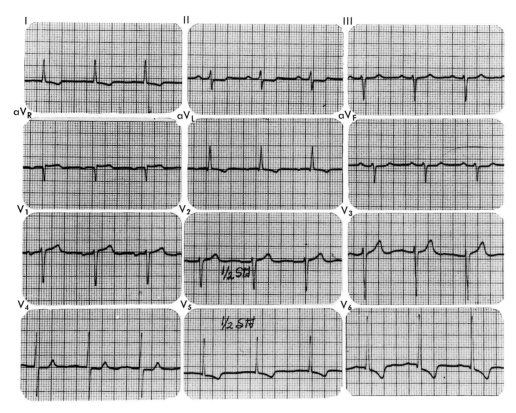

Fig. 5-19. Left ventricular enlargement. This tracing illustrates left ventricular hypertrophy using the Estes criteria: S wave in V_2 and R wave in V_5 and V_6 (note half standard in V_2 and V_5) exceed 30 mm (3 points); S-T segment depression in the absence of digitalis (3 points); terminal negativity of P wave in V_1 (1 point). A score of 5 or more points is interpreted as indicating left ventricular hypertrophy. The "score" for this ECG is 7 points.

increased voltage of those QRS deflections that represent left ventricular potentials. Accordingly, the QRS interval may increase in duration to the upper limits of normal; the intrinsicoid deflection may be somewhat delayed over the left ventricle; and the voltage of the QRS complex will increase—producing deeper S waves over the right ventricle (leads V_1 and V_2) and taller R waves over the left ventricle (leads V_5, V_6, I, aV_L).

Leads oriented to the left ventricle may also demonstrate a "strain" pattern, that is, depressed S-T segments and inverted T waves. "Strain" is a useful, noncommittal term and its mechanism is not understood. It is known, however, to develop in those patients who have long-standing left ventricular enlargement, and the pattern intensifies when dilation and failure set in. Myocardial ischemia and slowing of intraventricular conduction are some of the important factors that probably contribute to the pattern.

In general, the voltage criteria proposed for the diagnosis of left ventricular enlargement are unreliable. However, the best approach so far is the Estes' scoring system as follows (compare with Fig. 5-19):

1. R wave or S wave in limb lead = 20 mm or more; or
   S wave in V_1, V_2, or V_3 = 30 mm or more; } 3
   or R wave in V_4, V_5, or V_6 = 30 mm or more

2. Any S-T segment shift opposite to mean QRS   3
   vector (without digitalis)
   Typical "strain" S-T segment, T wave (with   1
   digitalis)
3. Left axis deviation: −30 degrees or more   2
4. QRS interval: 0.09 second or more (The normal   1
   duration of the QRS interval is 0.06 to 0.10
   second.)
   Intrinsicoid deflection in V_{5-6}; 0.05 second or more   1
5. Left atrial enlargement   3

Definite left ventricular enlargement is present with a *point score of 5 or more. Probable left ventricular enlargement* is present if the *point score is 4.*

It should be noted that left ventricular enlargement may be present without concomitant left axis deviation. Left axis deviation supports the diagnosis of left ventricular enlargement only when the voltage criteria are fulfilled. The voltage criteria just listed, however, include a small percentage of both false positive and false negative diagnoses. Therefore in making an electrocardiographic diagnosis of left ventricular enlargement, it is wise to evaluate such factors as body build, the thickness of the chest wall, and the presence of complicating disease.

Left atrial enlargement

Left atrial abnormality occurs frequently in left ventricular enlargement. However, left atrial enlargement caused by mitral stenosis is not associated with left ventricular enlargement unless there is mitral insufficiency or concomitant aortic valvular disease.

The following criteria are used in the ECG diagnosis of left atrial enlargement (Fig. 5-20):

1. The duration of the P wave is often widened to 0.12 second or more (normal P wave duration is 0.11 second).
2. The contour of the P wave is *notched* and slurred in leads I and II *(P mitrale).* (Notching per se is not abnormal unless the P wave shows increased voltage or duration or both, or the summits are more than 0.03 second apart.)
3. The right precordial leads (V_1, V_2) reflect diphasic P waves with a wide, deep, negative terminal component. The duration (in seconds) and amplitude (in millimeters) of the terminal component are measured and the algebraic product determined. A more negative value than −0.03 sec. is considered abnormal.
4. The mean electrical axis of the P wave may be shifted leftward to between +45 and −30 degrees.

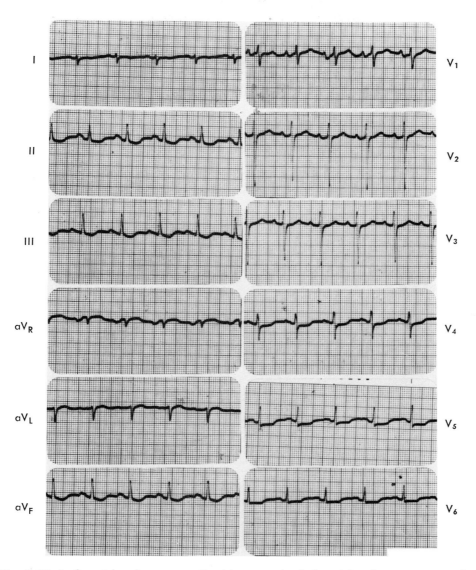

Fig. 5-20. Left atrial enlargement. In this example, left atrial enlargement may be diagnosed by the P terminal force abnormality seen in V_1. The negative portion of the diphasic P wave in approximately 0.04 second in duration and 1 mm in amplitude. The M-shaped broad contour seen prominently in leads I, II, III, and a V_F and the lateral precordial leads are also found in left atrial enlargement. In addition, right axis deviation of approximately +110 degrees exists in this patient with mitral stenosis.

Right ventricular enlargement

Right ventricular enlargement is commonly seen with mitral stenosis, some forms of congenital heart disease, and chronic diffuse pulmonary disease, such as pulmonary hypertension, emphysema, and bronchiectasis. For right ventricular enlargement in the adult to become evident electrocardiographically, however, the right ventricle must enlarge considerably, since the normal adult ECG reflects left ventricular predominance. This accounts for the relative frequency of a normal ECG in the presence of right ventricular enlargement.

Most of the criteria for diagnosing right ventricular enlargement focus on the QRS pattern in the right precordial leads. As the right ventricle enlarges, the height of the right precordial R waves increases, with a concomitant decrease in the depth of the S wave. When right ventricular enlargement becomes fully developed, the normal precordial pattern is completely reversed so that tall R waves (QR or RS) are recorded in V_1 with deep S waves (RS) in V_6.

Prolongation of the QRS interval does not develop unless an intraventricular conduction defect develops with the enlarged right ventricle. The time of onset of the intrinsicoid deflection, however, may be delayed in the right precordial leads because the vectors representing activation of the right ventricle usually occur later in the QRS interval than they do normally and are of increased magnitude.

Right axis deviation is the most common sign of right ventricular enlargement. The diagnosis of right ventricular enlargement, however, should not be made on this finding alone unless other causes for right axis deviation have been ruled out. Furthermore, right ventricular enlargement may occur without abnormal right axis deviation.

A right ventricular "strain" pattern is manifested in S-T, with T changes similar to those seen in left ventricular enlargement. The S-T segment is depressed and the T wave is inverted in the right-sided precordial leads and often leads II, III, and aV_F, as well. This is a nonspecific abnormality.

Right bundle branch block is seen in right ventricular enlargement, especially of the volume-overload variety. In the younger person, right ventricular enlargement is commonly associated with right bundle branch block, either complete or incomplete. In the older age group (40 years and up), coronary artery disease is the most common cause. The surface ECG is less useful than the vectorcardiogram in the assessment of the degree of right ventricular enlargement in cases of incomplete or complete right bundle branch block. Further elaboration on the vectorcardiogram is beyond the scope of this presentation; therefore the reader is encouraged to refer to textbooks on this subject. Moreover, see Chapter 6 for a discussion of right bundle branch block.

A summary of the features of right ventricular enlargement is given here; these should be compared with the example in Fig. 5-21.

1. Reversal of precordial pattern with tall R waves over the right precor-

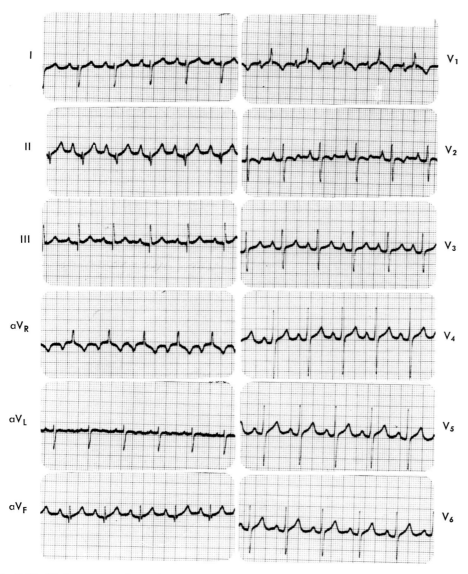

Fig. 5-21. Right ventricular enlargement. The presence of right axis deviation (approximately +160 degrees), an R wave in V_1 that exceeds 5 mm, and an R:S ratio in V_1 that exceeds 1.0 are all diagnostic of right ventricular hypertrophy. In addition, the totally upright R wave in V_1 suggests that the pressure in the right ventricle equals or almost equals the pressure in the left ventricle. The P waves suggest biatrial enlargement.

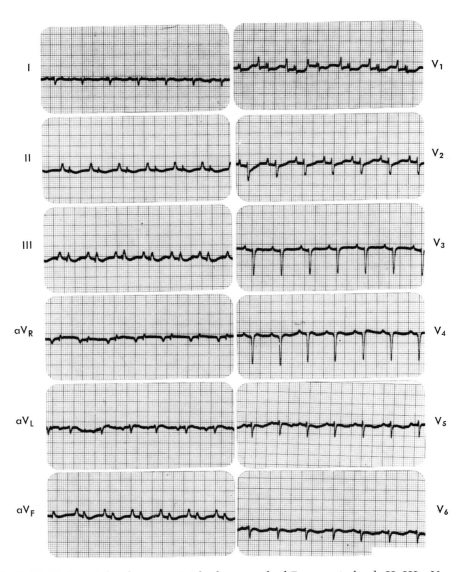

Fig. 5-22. Right atrial enlargement. The large peaked P waves in leads II, III, aV_F, and V_1, with an amplitude that exceeds 2.5 mm in leads II and III, characterize right atrial enlargement in this example. The mean P axis is more positive than +60 degrees, another criterion for right atrial enlargement. The patient has pulmonic stenosis.

dium (V_1, V_2), and deep S waves over the left precordium (V_5, V_6). The R to S ratio in V_1 becomes greater than 1.0.

2. Duration of QRS interval within normal limits (if no right bundle branch block).
3. Late intrinsicoid deflection in V_1, V_2.
4. Right axis deviation.
5. Typical "strain" S-T segment T wave patterns in V_1, V_2, and in leads II, III, and aV_F.

Right atrial enlargement

In the presence of right ventricular enlargement, it is not unusual to find an enlarged right atrium. Moreover, right atrial enlargement is often an indirect sign of right ventricular enlargement.

The following criteria are used in the ECG diagnosis of right atrial enlargement (Fig. 5-22):

1. The duration of the P wave is 0.11 second or less.
2. The contour of the P wave is tall, *peaked (P pulmonale)*, and measures 2.5 mm or more in amplitude in leads II, III, and aV_F.
3. The right precordial leads reflect diphasic P waves, often with increased voltage of the initial component.
4. The mean electrical axis of the P wave may be shifted rightward to +70 degrees or more.

It should be noted that abnormal P waves may occur in healthy patients and, conversely, normal P waves may be identified in the presence of atrial disease. For example, acceleration of the heart rate alone may cause peaking and increased voltage of the P wave.

Myocardial infarction

To diagnose myocardial infarction, the ECG should be used to confirm the clinical impression. Because the ECG may not be diagnostic in many instances, if a patient is suspected clinically of having experienced a myocardial infarction, he should be treated accordingly, regardless of what the ECG shows.

Only Q wave changes (necrosis) are diagnostic of infarction, but changes in the S-T segments (injury) and T waves (ischemia) may be suspicious and provide presumptive evidence. These changes are illustrated in Fig. 5-23.

Q WAVE

The Q wave is one of the most important, and sometimes most difficult, assessments to diagnose myocardial infarction on the ECG. For example, with normal intraventricular conduction, small Q waves are present in leads V_5, V_6, aV_L, and I, particularly with a horizontal heart position or left axis deviation. Furthermore, with a vertical heart position or right axis deviation, small Q waves may be present in leads II, III, and a V_F. Finally, deep wide Q waves or QS complexes are normally present in a V_R and may be present in lead V_1.

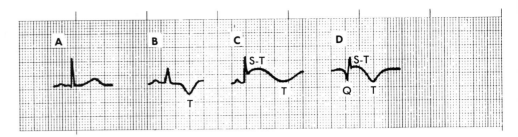

Fig. 5-23. ECG wave changes indicative of ischemia, injury, and necrosis of the myocardium. **A,** Normal left ventricular wave pattern. **B,** Ischemia indicated by inversion of the T wave. **C,** Ischemia and current of injury indicated by T wave inversion and S-T segment elevation. The S-T segment may be elevated above or depressed below the base line, depending on whether or not the tracing is from a lead facing toward or away from the infarcted area and depending on whether epicardial or endocardial injury occurs. Epicardial injury causes S-T segment elevation in leads facing the epicardium. **D,** Ischemia, injury, and myocardial necrosis. The Q wave indicates necrosis of the myocardium.

Major importance is placed on the development of *new* Q waves in ECG leads where they previously were not present.

Accordingly, the *appearance* of abnormal Q waves must be considered in light of the overall picture, considering that pathologic Q waves have the following features:

1. Q waves are 0.04 second or longer in *duration.*
2. Q waves are usually greater than 4 mm in *depth.*
3. Q waves appear in *leads* that do not normally have deep, wide Q waves (aV_R, V_1). Pathologic Q waves are usually present in several leads.

VECTOR ABNORMALITIES

In acute myocardial infarction, electrical and anatomic death of the myocardium occurs in the region of the infarct; hence the initial forces of depolarization tend to point away from the infarcted area, producing Q waves in the ECG leads facing the involved site. The mean T vector also tends to point away from the site of infarction, presumably because of electrical ischemia in the tissues surrounding the infarct. The S-T vector represents the effect of injury current. When the injury current is in the epicardial layers of the myocardium, as in myocardial infarction and pericarditis, the S-T segment is elevated in leads facing the injury and the S-T vector points toward the injured area. When the injury current is located in the subendocardial layers, as in angina pectoris, coronary insufficiency, and subendocardial infarction, the S-T segment is depressed in leads facing the injury and the S-T vector points away from the site of injury (Fig. 5-32). The S-T displacement in subendocardial infarction persists longer than that of angina pectoris and coronary insufficiency.

Thus with an acute myocardial infarction the S-T vector is opposite in

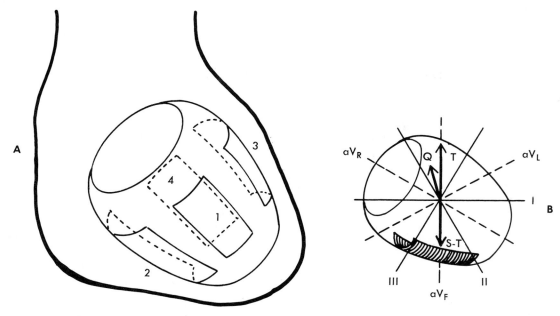

Fig. 5-24. A, Lie of the left ventricle in the chest as viewed frontally. The left ventricle has been divided into four topographic regions where infarctions may occur: (1) anterior, (2) diaphragmatic or inferior, (3) lateral, and (4) posterior (pure). **B,** Vectors of a diaphragmatic myocardial infarction. Hexaxial reference figure is superimposed on the left ventricle as viewed in **B.** The mean vector for the initial 0.04 second of the QRS complex points *away* from the infarcted area and indicates the dead zone. This produces Q waves in the leads "looking at" the infarction. The mean T vector indicates the ischemic zone surrounding the infarct and points *away* from the infarcted area. The S-T vector indicates the injury zone and in the event of myocardial infarction, the S-T vector points *toward* the injured area.

direction to the Q vector and the mean T vector, resulting in S-T segment elevation in those leads that have Q waves and inverted T waves. The relationship of these three vectors to one another is diagrammed in Fig. 5-24, *B.*

LOCALIZATION OF INFARCTION

Localization of infarcts may be prognostically important. Localization is based on the principle that diagnostic signs of myocardial infarction (Fig. 5-23) occur in leads whose positive terminals face the damaged surface of the heart. In order to facilitate localization, the left ventricle has been divided into four topographic regions where infarctions may occur (Fig. 5-24, *A).* Although these locations represent electrical rather than anatomic sites of infarction, anatomic correlations occur with reasonable frequency, particularly for the first myocardial infarction.

An *anterior infarction* produces characteristic changes in leads V_1, V_2, and V_3; a *diaphragmatic* or *inferior infarction* affects leads II, III, and aV_F; a *lateral infarction* involves leads I, aV_L, V_5, and V_6. In strictly *posterior infarction*, there are no leads whose positive terminals are directly over the infarct. However, the changes of the electrical field produced by any infarction still apply; hence in purely posterior infarction the initial forces of the QRS complex and the T wave point anteriorly away from the site of the infarct, and the S-T segment is directed posteriorly. This is recognized in the ECG as tall broad initial R waves, S-T segment depression, and tall upright T waves in leads V_1 and V_2. In other words, a mirror image of the typical infarction pattern of an anterior myocardial infarction is recorded. Stated another way, infarction of the true posterior surface of the heart must be inferred from reciprocal (opposite) changes occurring in the anterior leads. These locations are summarized in Table 5-1.

It should be noted that although diagnostic signs of myocardial infarction appear in leads facing the infarcted heart surface, *reciprocal changes* occur concomitantly in leads facing the diametrically opposed surface of the heart. These changes include no Q wave with some increase of the R wave, depressed S-T segments, and upright tall T waves.

Reciprocal changes, therefore, in an anterior infarction will occur in leads II, III, and aV_F. In a diaphragmatic or inferior infarction, reciprocal changes occur in leads I, aV_L, and some of the precordial leads. In lateral wall infarction, lead V_1 may show reciprocal changes.

Frequently the localization of an infarction is not as strict as just described. If the anterior and lateral walls of the left ventricle are both involved in the process, it would be called an *anterolateral infarction*. If the limb leads indicate an inferior infarction, and diagnostic changes are also present in leads V_5 and V_6, then it would be called an inferior infarction with lateral extension or an *inferolateral infarction*, and so on.

EVOLUTION OF A MYOCARDIAL INFARCTION

The evolution of a myocardial infarction is a sequential process, and it is important to record the time relationships in the diagnosis. Within the first few hours after an infarction, sometimes referred to as the hyperacute state, elevated S-T segments and tall (hyperacute) upright T waves appear in those leads facing the infarction. Q waves may appear early or may not develop for several days. Within several days of the infarct the S-T segment begins to return to base line, whereas the T waves develop progressively deeper inversion. After weeks or months the T waves become shallower and may finally return to normal. The Q waves are most likely to remain as a permanent record of the myocardial scar (Fig. 5-25). Persistent S-T segment elevation (beyond 6 weeks) suggests the possibility of ventricular aneurysm (Table 5-2). The different locations of myocardial infarction in different stages of clinical evolution are shown in Figs. 5-26 to 5-32.

Table 5-1. Location of myocardial infarction

Area of infarction	Leads showing wave changes
Anterior	V_1, V_2, V_3
Diaphragmatic or inferior	II, III, aV_F
Lateral	I, aV_L, V_5, V_6
Posterior (pure)	V_1 and V_2: tall broad initial R wave, S-T segment depression, and tall upright T wave

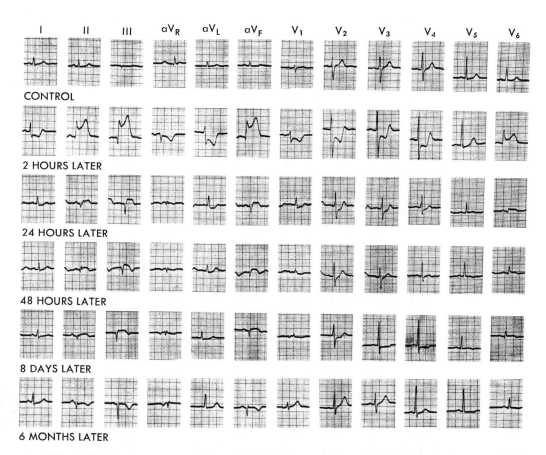

Fig. 5-25. Evolutionary changes in a posteroinferior myocardial infarction. *Control tracing* is normal. The tracing recorded *2 hours* after onset of chest pain demonstrates development of early Q waves, marked S-T segment elevation, and hyperacute T waves in leads II, III, and a V_F. In addition, a larger R wave, S-T segment depression and negative T waves have developed in leads V_1 to V_2. These are early changes indicating acute posteroinferior myocardial infarction. The *24-hour* tracing demonstrates evolutionary changes. In leads II, III, and aV_F the Q wave is larger, the S-T segments have almost returned to base line, and the T wave has begun to invert. In leads V_1 to V_2 the duration of the R wave now exceeds 0.04 second, the S-T segment is depressed, and the T wave is upright. (In this classic example, ECG changes of true posterior involvement extend past V_2; ordinarily only V_1 and V_2 may be involved.) Only minor further changes occur through the *8-day* tracing. Finally, *6 months later* the ECG illustrates large Q waves, isoelectric S-T segments, and inverted T waves in leads II, III, and aV_F, large R waves, isoelectric S-T segment, and upright T waves in V_1 and V_2 indicative of an "old" posteroinferior myocardial infarction.

Table 5-2. Time relationships in the evolution and resolution of a myocardial infarction

ECG abnormality	Onset	Disappearance
S-T segment elevation	Immediately	1 to 6 weeks
Q waves > 0.04 second	Immediately or in several days	Years to never
T wave inversion	6 to 24 hours	Months to years

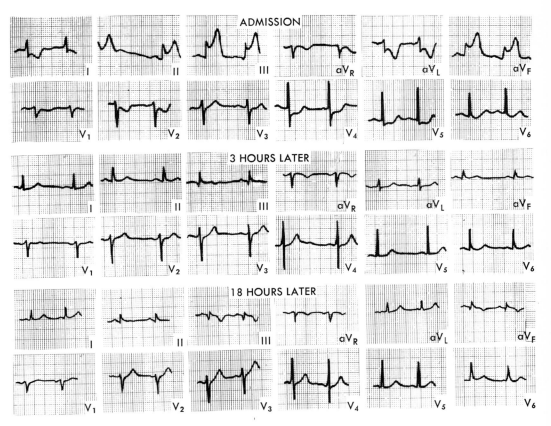

Fig. 5-26. These three 12-lead ECGs obtained at different time intervals from a patient with an unequivocal myocardial infarction demonstrate that at one point during the electrocardiographic evolution of a myocardial infarction, the ECG may appear almost normal. Note the hyperacute T wave changes and unquestionable injury current portrayed in the admission ECG. Hyperacute T waves are normally upright; these enlarged T waves can occur very early after infarction, preceding the more characteristic T wave inversion. Three hours later, the S-T segment has returned almost completely to the baseline, significant Q waves have not yet appeared, and the T waves remain fairly normal. This ECG is at most "nonspecifically" abnormal. Eighteen hours after admission, classic changes in an acute diaphragmatic myocardial infarction have evolved. This illustration serves to deemphasize the value of a single ECG in diagnosing an acute myocardial infarction. The patient quite possibly would have been sent home if the determination for admission to the CCU had been based solely on a single ECG, that is, the second tracing.

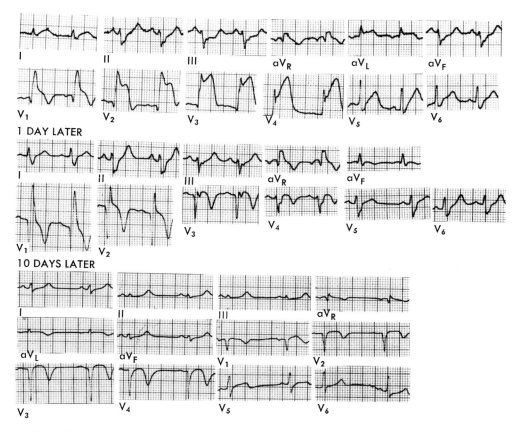

Fig. 5-27. Serial tracings on a patient with an acute anterior myocardial infarction. On admission patient's ECG showed left axis deviation (left anterior hemiblock) and right bundle branch block, thus supporting the presence of bifascicular block (see Chapter 6). Terminal T wave inversion in V_1 to V_2 and profound S-T segment elevation are present in V_1 to V_5. These changes are not masked by the presence of the right bundle branch block. One day later the S-T segments have returned toward the baseline, the Q waves in the anterior precordial leads have enlarged greatly, and there is now T wave inversion in these leads. Left anterior hemiblock and right bundle branch block are still present. In the tracing recorded 10 days later the right bundle branch block and left anterior hemiblock have disappeared, leaving the electrocardiographic changes of an anteroseptal myocardial infarction with Q waves in V_1 to V_3 and T wave inversion in V_1 to V_4.

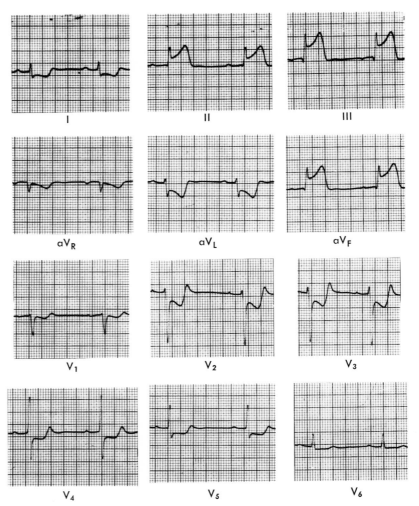

Fig. 5-28. Inferior (diaphragmatic) myocardial infarction, hyperacute stage. Note S-T segment elevation in leads II, III, and aV$_F$, with reciprocal S-T depression in the anterior precordial leads. The T waves in leads II, III, and aV$_F$ are still upright and pointed and indicate the hyperacute stage of myocardial infarction. Note the development of only very small Q waves in leads II, III, and aV$_F$. Subsequent evolution of this ECG will demonstrate the progressive development of significant (greater than 0.04 second) Q waves and T wave inversion in leads II, III, and aV$_F$; the S-T segment will return to an isoelectric position.

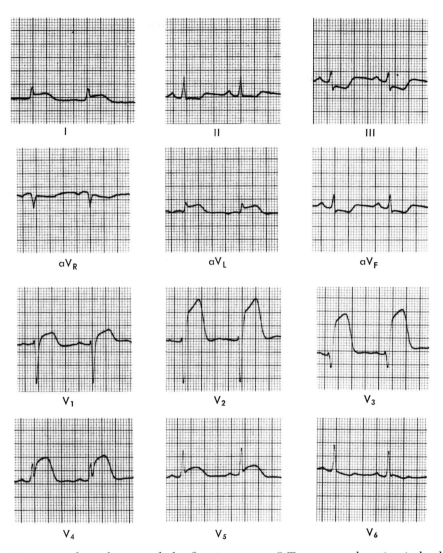

Fig. 5-29. Anterolateral myocardial infarction, acute. S-T segment elevation in leads I, aV_L, and V_1 to V_5 indicate an acute anterolateral myocardial infarction. During the evolution of this tracing, one would expect the development of Q waves and T wave inversion in leads I and a V_L and the precordial leads, with the S-T segment returning to baseline.

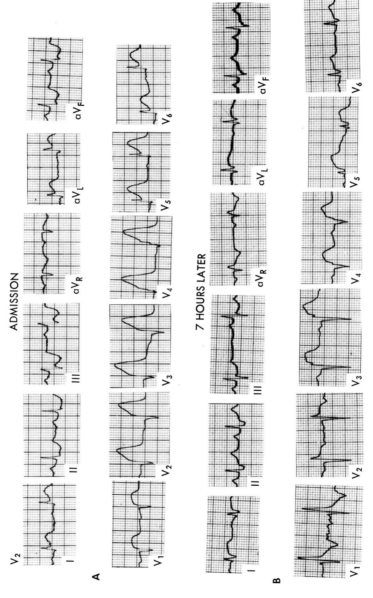

Fig. 5-30. Anterolateral myocardial infarction, acute. The 12-lead electrocardiogram on admission, **A,** Demonstrates S-T segment elevation in leads I, aV$_L$, and V$_1$ to V$_6$, indicating the anterolateral injury current of an acute anterolateral myocardial infarction. **B,** Seven hours later. The patient has developed right bundle branch block with abnormal Q waves in leads I, aV$_L$, and V$_2$ to V$_5$. **C,** Twenty-six hours later. In addition to the right bundle branch block, the patient has now developed left anterior hemiblock. **D** Three months later. The left anterior hemiblock and right bundle, branch block are still present. The Q waves in leads I and aV$_L$ are not as prominent as the Q waves in V$_1$ to V$_5$. Persistent S-T segment elevation for a duration greater than 6 weeks after the myocardial infarction raises the possibility of a left ventricular aneurysm.

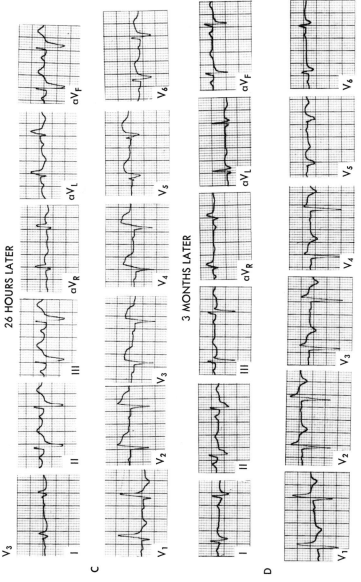

Fig. 5-30, cont'd. For legend see opposite page.

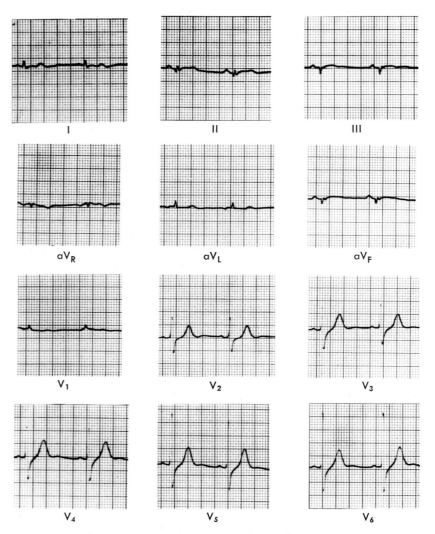

Fig. 5-31. Posteroinferior myocardial infarction, date indeterminant. Q waves in II, III, and aV_F are consistent with an old inferior myocardial infarction. The large R wave in V_1 signifies true posterior infarction as well. Compare with Fig. 5-25 at 6 months.

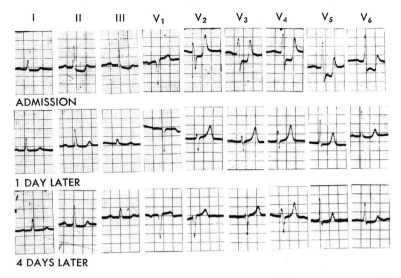

Fig. 5-32. Subendocardial myocardial infarction. Note slight S-T segment depression in leads I, II, and III with marked S-T segment depression in leads V_2 to V_6 on admission. One day later the S-T segments have returned to normal and there is diminution of the height of the R wave in the precordial leads, but no other changes. The tracing 4 days later is essentially unchanged. Note failure to develop the classic Q waves of a transmural myocardial infarction. The patient died and at autopsy had an extensive subendocardial myocardial infarction.

REFERENCES

Beckwith, J. R.: Grant's clinical electrocardiography; the spatial vector approach, New York, 1970, McGraw-Hill Book Co.

Bernreiter, M.: Electrocardiography, ed. 2, Philadelphia, 1963, J. B. Lippincott Co.

Burch, G. E., and Winsor, T.: A primer of electrocardiography, ed. 6, Philadelphia, 1971, Lea & Febiger.

Friedman, H. H.: Diagnostic electrocardiography and vectorcardiography, ed. 2, New York, 1977, McGraw-Hill Book Co.

Hurst, J. W., Logue, R. B., Schlant, R. C., and Wenger, N. K. (editors): The heart: arteries and veins, ed. 3, New York, 1978, McGraw-Hill Book Co.

Lipman, B. S., Massie, E., and Kleiger, R. E.: Clinical scalar electrocardiography, ed. 6, Chicago, 1972, Year Book Medical Publishers, Inc.

Marriott, H. J. L.: Practical electrocardiography, ed. 6, Baltimore, 1977, The Williams & Wilkins Co.

Schamroth, L.: An introduction to electrocardiography, ed. 4, Oxford, England, 1971, Blackwell Scientific Publications.

Schlant, R. C., and Hurst, J. W., (editors): Advances in electrocardiography, vol. 2, New York, 1976, Grune & Stratton, Inc.

CHAPTER SIX

ARRHYTHMIAS

Normal cardiac cycle

Prior to discussing electrocardiographic interpretation of cardiac arrhythmias, a review of the normal electrical events that occur during a cardiac cycle, as well as a discussion of basic electrophysiologic principles is necessary. During sinus rhythm the cardiac impulse originates in the sinus node and then travels to right and left atria. Sinus node discharge and conduction from the sinus node to the atria are not recorded from the body surface and therefore these events are not present in the electrocardiogram (ECG). In response to the sinus node impulse, the atria depolarize and generate the P wave; atrial repolarization (Ta wave) is generally obscured by the QRS complex and is therefore not usually seen. Atrial conduction probably proceeds through both atria in a more-or-less radial fashion (like spreading ripples caused by a rock thrown into still water), eventually reaching the A-V node and His bundle. Some data suggest that conduction through the atria travels preferentially through loosely connected bundles of atrial muscle called the anterior, middle, and posterior internodal pathways, which, it is argued, provide specialized pathways of conduction from the sinus node to the left atrium (via Bachmann's bundle, a division of the anterior internodal pathway) and to the A-V node. However, the functional importance of these pathways in providing specialized tracts for conduction is unsettled. The speed at which the impulse travels (conduction velocity) becomes reduced as the impulse traverses the A-V node, but once again accelerates through the His bundle, bundle branches, and Purkinje fibers. These fibers distribute the impulse rapidly and uniformly over the ventricular endocardium, finally depolarizing the ventricular myocardium (Fig. 6-1). It is important to remember that the surface ECG records only ventricular muscle depolarization (QRS) and repolarization (T wave), atrial depolarization (P wave), and sometimes repolarization (Ta wave). Activity from the sinus and A-V nodes, His bundle, bundle branches, and Purkinje fibers is not recorded in the ECG. Special intracardiac electrodes can be employed to record activity from some of these structures and will be discussed briefly later in this chapter.

It has been postulated that the bundle branches are really composed of three divisions, called fascicles, that are formed by the right bundle branch and two divisions of the left bundle branch, the anterosuperior division, and

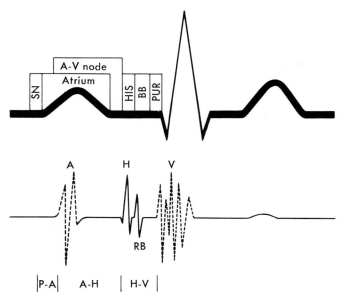

Fig. 6-1. Schematic illustration of a cardiac cycle, demonstrating the normal ECG (top) and a His bundle recording (bottom). The diagram illustrates the approximate time of activation of various structures in the specialized conduction system. It is important to emphasize that conduction has already reached the Purkinje fibers just prior to the onset of the QRS complex. *SN* Sinus node; *HIS*, bundle of His; *BB*, bundle branches; *PUR*, Purkinje fibers; *A*, low right atrial deflection; *H*, His bundle deflection; *RB*, right bundle branch deflection; *V*, ventricular septal muscle depolarization; *P-A*, interval from the onset of the P wave in the surface tracing to the onset of the low right atrial deflection, serving as a measure of intra-atrial conduction; *A-H*, measurement of conduction across the A-V node; *H-V*, measurement of conduction through the His bundle distal to the recording electrode, the bundle branches, and the Purkinje system up to the point of ventricular activation. (Top panel modified from Hoffman, B. F., and Singer, D. H.: Prog. Cardiovasc. Dis. **7:**226, 1964.

the posteroinferior division. The term "hemiblock" has been used to describe block in one of these fascicles. A more accurate term is fascicular block. Although a number of careful anatomic and pathologic studies of human hearts have failed to substantiate the anatomic separation of the left bundle branch into two distinct and specific divisions, the fascicular block concept has been useful to explain observed electrocardiographic and clinical entities (see discussion of bundle branch block).

The electrical activity of the heart is recorded by an electrocardiograph machine onto ECG paper. This graph paper is divided into a series of vertical lines measuring time and horizontal lines measuring voltage (Fig. 6-2). The electrical pattern of a typical cardiac cycle is displayed in Fig. 6-3 and is discussed in Table 6-1. (See also Chapter 5.)

The atrial rate in beats per minute may be determined by dividing the

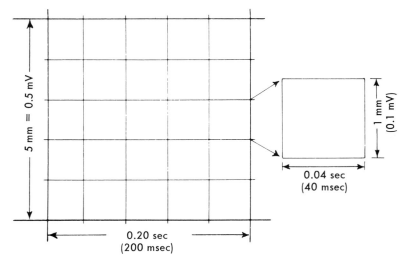

Fig. 6-2. Time and voltage lines of the ECG. The interval between two heavy vertical lines is 0.20 second (200 milliseconds) and between each light line 0.04 second (40 milliseconds). The voltage between each heavy horizontal line is 0.5 mV.

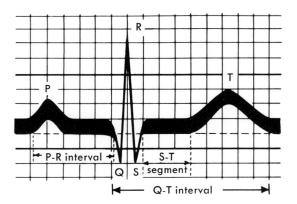

Fig. 6-3. Electrical pattern of cardiac cycle. (Refer to Table 6-1.)

time interval between regularly occurring consecutive P waves (P-P interval) into 60. A similar procedure performed for the interval between ventricular beats (R-R interval) determines the ventricular rate (Fig. 6-4). The rate can be more rapidly determined by dividing the *number* of large (0.2-second) divisions between two consecutive complexes into 300 or *small* squares into 1500. For irregular rhythms, the rate must be averaged over a longer interval; for example, the number of large divisions separating four QRS complexes (three complete cardiac cycles) may be divided into 900. Table 6-2 can be used to calculate the rate of a regular rhythm.

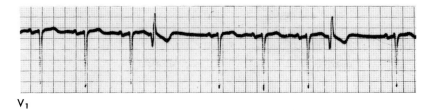

V₁

Fig. 6-4. Calculation of the atrial and ventricular rates. The heart rate is 75 beats per minute, determined by dividing 60 seconds by 0.80 second, the time interval between consecutive P waves and/or consecutive R waves or by dividing four large squares into 300 or 20 small squares into 1500. Two premature ventricular extrasystoles are present. See Table 6-2.

Table 6-1. Meaning and significance of ECG intervals*

Description	Duration	Significance of disturbance
P-R interval: from beginning of P wave to beginning of QRS complex; represents time taken for impulse to spread through the atria, A-V node and His bundle, the bundle branches and Purkinje fibers, to a point immediately preceding ventricular activation	0.12 to 0.20 second	Disturbance in conduction usually in A-V node, His bundle, or bundle branches butcan be in atria as well
QRS interval: from beginning to end of QRS complex; represents time taken for depolarization of both ventricles	0.06 to 0.10 second	Disturbance in conduction in bundle branches and/or in ventricles
Q-T interval: from beginning of QRS to end of T wave; represents time taken for entire electrical depolarization and repolarization of the ventricles	0.36 to 0.44 second	Disturbances usually affecting repolarization more than depolarization such as drug effects, electrolyte disturbances, and rate changes

*Heart rate influences the duration of these intervals, especially that of the P-R and Q-T intervals.

Electrophysiologic principles

Certain specialized cells, such as those in the sinus node, some parts of the atria, A-V node, and His-Purkinje system, are able to discharge spontaneously; they do not require an external or propagated stimulus to fire. This property, known as *automaticity* (also called diastolic depolarization), creates the potential for these cells to depolarize the rest of the heart. Normally the sinus node rules as the pacemaker, since it spontaneously discharges faster than these other latent pacemakers.

Should a latent pacemaker possessing the property of automaticity

Table 6-2. Determination of heart rate from the ECG

Time (second)	No. of small squares	Rate (beats per minute)	Time (second)	No. of small squares	Rate (beats per minute)
0.10	2.5	600	0.60	15.00	100
0.12	3.0	500	0.64	16.00	94
0.15	3.75	400	0.70	17.50	86
0.16	4.0	375	0.72	18.00	83
			0.76	19.00	79
0.20	5.0	300			
0.24	6.0	250	0.80	20.00	75
0.26	6.5	230	0.84	21.00	71
0.28	7.0	214	0.88	22.00	68
			0.92	23.00	65
0.30	7.5	200	0.96	24.00	63
0.32	8.0	188			
0.34	8.5	176	1.00	25.00	60
0.36	9.0	167	1.08	27.00	56
0.38	9.5	158	1.14	28.50	53
0.40	10.0	150	1.20	30.00	50
0.42	10.5	143	1.40	35.00	43
0.44	11.0	136	1.50	37.50	40
0.46	11.5	130	1.60	40.00	38
0.48	12.0	125	1.80	45.00	33
			2.00	50.00	30
0.50	12.5	120			
0.52	13.0	115			
0.56	14.0	107			

discharge more rapidly than the sinus node, it may depolarize atria, ventricles, or both. This may occur in two ways. If the sinus node discharges more slowly than the discharge rate of the latent pacemaker (Fig. 6-12), or if the sinus impulse is blocked before reaching the latent pacemaker site (Fig. 6-58), the latent pacemaker may passively *escape* sinus domination and discharge automatically at its own intrinsic rate. Such escape beats are slower than normal, since the A-V junction and bundle branch–Purkinje system (two probable escape focus sites) generally beat at 40 to 60 times per minute and 30 to 40 times per minute, respectively. However, should a latent pacemaker abnormally accelerate its discharge rate and actively *usurp* control of the heartbeat from the sinus node, a premature beat results. This may happen in the atria, ventricles, or A-V junction. A series of these premature beats in a row produces a tachycardia. A shift in the normal manner of atrial or ventricular activation, such as might be produced by a shift in pacemaker focus, is reflected by a change in P or QRS contour.

Automatic discharge of a pacemaker focus is not sufficient to depolarize a cardiac chamber; the impulse must also be conducted from its site of origin to the surrounding myocardium. The heart possesses the property of *excitability,* which is a characteristic enabling it to be depolarized by a stimulus; this is

Table 6-3. Probable pathogenesis of arrhythmias

Automaticity	Reentry	Automaticity or reentry
Escape beats—atrial, junctional, or ventricular	Paroxysmal atrial tachycardia	Premature systoles—atrial, junctional, or ventricular
Atrial rhythm	Paroxysmal junctional tachycardia	Atrial flutter
Atrial tachycardia with or without AV block	Atrial flutter	Paroxysmal ventricular tachycardia
Junctional rhythm	Atrial fibrillation	
Nonparoxysmal junctional tachycardia	Paroxysmal ventricular tachycardia	
Accelerated idioventricular rhythm	Ventricular flutter	
Parasystole	Ventricular fibrillation	

an integral part of the propagation or conduction of the impulse from one fiber to the next. Many factors may influence the level of excitability but the most important, in the normal state, is how long after depolarization the heart is re-stimulated. Cardiac tissue requires a recovery period following depolarization. If a stimulus occurs too early, the heart has had insufficient time to recover and it will not respond to the stimulus, no matter how intense it is (absolute refractory period, excitability zero). A slightly later stimulus allows more time for recovery (relative refractory period, excitability improving), and a still later stimulus finds the heart completely recovered (no longer refractory, full excitability).

If conduction becomes unevenly depressed, with block in some areas and not in others, some regions of the myocardium (unblocked areas) must necessarily be activated (and recover) earlier than others. Under appropriate circumstances, when the block is only in one direction (unidirectional), this uneven conduction may allow the initial impulse to *reenter* areas previously inexcitable but that have now recovered. Should the reentering impulse then be able to depolarize the entire atria and/or ventricles, a corresponding premature extrasystole results; maintenance of the *reentrant excitation* establishes a tachycardia. A special form of reentry may produce echo or reciprocal beats (Fig. 6-41 *D*).

Thus disorders of impulse *formation* (automaticity) or *conduction* (unidirectional block and reentry) and, at times, combinations of both may initiate arrhythmias.

Only indirect evidence exists to enable a clinical classification of arrhythmias according to pathogenesis. In addition, an arrhythmia may be initiated and perpetuated by different mechanisms. For example, spontaneous diastolic depolarization (automaticity) may trigger a premature atrial or ventricular systole that initiates an arrhythmia caused by reentry. Thus the clinical classification of arrhythmias according to pathogenesis remains speculative to a degree. Antiarrhythmic agents specifically indicated to treat one mechanism or the other do not yet exist. (Table 6-3).

Arrhythmia analysis (Table 6-4)

For proper analysis, each arrhythmia must be approached in a systematic manner. A suggested guide follows:

1. What is the rate? Is it too fast or too slow? Are atrial and ventricular rates the same? Are P waves present?
2. Are the P-P and R-R intervals regular or irregular? If irregular, is it a consistent, repeating irregularity?
3. Is there a P wave (and therefore atrial activity) related to each ventricular complex? Does the P wave precede or follow the QRS complex?
4. Are all P waves and QRS complexes identical and normal in contour? To determine the significance of changes in P or QRS contour, or amplitude, one must know the lead being recorded.
5. Are the P-R, QRS and Q-T intervals normal?
6. Considering the clinical setting, what is the significance of the arrhythmia?
7. How should the arrhythmia be treated?

Table 6-4. Classification of normal and abnormal cardiac rhythms

Rhythms originating in the sinus node	Rhythms originating in the ventricles
Sinus rhythm	Ventricular escape beats
Sinus tachycardia	Premature ventricular systole
Sinus bradycardia	Ventricular tachycardia
Sinus arrhythmia	Idioventricular tachycardia
Sinus arrest	(accelerated idioventricular rhythm)
Sinus exit block	Ventricular fibrillation
Rhythms originating in the atria	A-V block
Wandering pacemaker between sinus node and	First-degree
atrium or A-V junction	Second-degree
Premature atrial systole	Type I (Wenckebach)
Paroxysmal atrial tachycardia	Type II
Atrial flutter	Third-degree (complete)
Atril fibrillation	Bundle branch block
Atrial tachycardia with block	Right
Rhythms originating in the A-V junction (A-V	Left
node–His bundle)	Fascicular blocks (hemiblocks)
Premature A-V junctional systole	Parasystole
A-V junctional escape beats	
A-V junctional rhythm	
Paroxysmal A-V junctional tachycardia	
Nonparoxysmal A-V junctional tachycardia	

Therapy of arrythmias (Table 6-5)
GENERAL THERAPEUTIC CONCEPTS

The therapeutic approach to a patient with a cardiac arrhythmia begins with an accurate electrocardiographic *interpretation* of the arrhythmia and continues with determination of the *etiology* of the arrhythmia (if possible), the nature of the underlying *heart disease* (if any), and the *consequences* of the arrhythmia for the individual patient. Thus one cannot treat arrhythmias as isolated events without having knowledge of the clinical situation; *patients* who have arrhythmias, not arrhythmias themselves, are treated.

The ventricular rate and duration of an arrhythmia, its site of origin, and the cardiovascular status of the patient primarily determine the electrophysiologic and hemodynamic consequences of a particular rhythm disturbance. Electrophysiologic consequences, often influenced by the presence of underlying heart disease such as acute myocardial infarction, include the development of serious arrhythmias as a result of rapid (and slow) rates, initiation of sustained arrhythmias by premature extrasystoles, or the degeneration of rhythms like venticular tachycardia into ventricular fibrillation. Hemodynamic performance of the heart and circulation may be altered by extremes of heart rate or by loss of atrial contribution to ventricular filling. Rapid rates greatly shorten the diastolic filling time and, particularly in diseased hearts, the increased heart rate may fail to compensate for the reduced stroke output; blood pressure, along with cardiac output, declines. Arrhythmias that prevent sequential A-V contraction mitigate the hemodynamic benefits of the atrial booster pump whereas atrial fibrillation causes complete loss of atrial contraction and may reduce cardiac output.

When a patient develops a tachyarrhythmia, slowing the ventricular rate is the initial and frequently the most important therapeutic maneuver. Since medical therapy frequently involves a time-consuming and potentially dangerous biologic titration of drugs such as digitalis or quinidine, electrical direct current (DC) cardioversion may be preferable, depending on the clinical situation. Therapy may differ radically for the very same arrhythmia in two different patients because the consequences of the tachycardia on the individual patients differ. For example, a supraventricular tachycardia at 200 beats per minute may produce little or no symptoms in a healthy young adult and therefore require little or no therapy; the very same arrhythmia may precipitate pulmonary edema in a patient with mitral stenosis or syncope in a patient with aortic stenosis, shock in a patient with an acute myocardial infarction, or hemiparesis in a patient with cerebrovascular disease. In these situations the tachycardia requires prompt electrical conversion.

The etiology of the arrhythmia may influence therapy markedly. Electrolyte imbalance (potassium, magnesium, calcium), acidosis or alkalosis, hypoxemia, and many drugs may produce arrhythmias. Because heart failure may cause arrhythmias, digitalis may effectively suppress arrhythmias during heart failure when all other agents are unsuccessful or prevent more severe arrhythmias by reversing early congestive heart failure. Similarly, an

Table 6-5. Cardiac arrhythmias

Type of arrhythmia	P waves			QRS complexes		
	Rate	Rhythm	Contour	Rate	Rhythm	Contour
Sinus rhythm	60 to 100	Regular†	Normal	60 to 100	Regular	Normal
Sinus bradycardia	<60	Regular	Normal	<60	Regular	Normal
Sinus tachycardia	100 to 180	Regular	May be peaked	100 to 180	Regular	Normal
Paroxysmal atrial tachycardia	150 to 250	Very regular except at onset and termination	Abnormal; difficult to see	150 to 250	Very regular except at onset and termination	Normal
Atrial flutter	250 to 350	Regular	Sawtooth	75 to 175	Generally regular in absence of drugs or disease	Normal
Atrial fibrillation	400 to 600	Grossly irregular	Base line undulations; no P waves	100 to 160	Grossly irregular	Normal
Atrial tachycardia with block	150 to 250	Regular; may be irregular	Abnormal	75 to 200	Generally regular in absence of drugs or disease	Normal
A-V junctional rhythm	40 to 100§	Regular	Normal	40 to 60	Fairly regular	Normal; may be abnormal but <0.12 second
Paroxysmal junctional tachycardia	150 to 250	Very regular except at onset and termination	Retrograde; difficult to see	150 to 250	Very regular except at onset and termination	Normal
Nonparoxysmal A-V junctional tachycardia	60 to 100§	Regular	Normal	70 to 130	Fairly regular	Normal; may be abnormal but <0.12 second
Ventricular tachycardia	60 to 100§	Regular	Normal	110 to 250	Fairly regular; may be irregular	Abnormal, >0.12 second

*In an effort to summarize these arrhythmias in a tabular form, generalizations have to be made, particularly complete discussion.

†P waves initiated by sinus node discharge may not be precisely regular because of sinus arrhythmia.

‡Often, sinus tachycardia fails to respond to carotid sinus massage.

§Any independent atrial arrhythmia may exist or the atria may be captured retrogradely.

‖ Constant if atria captured retrogradely.

Ventricular response to carotid sinus massage	Physical examination			Treatment
	Intensity of S_1	Splitting of S_2	A waves	
Gradual slowing and return to former rate	Constant	Normal	Normal	None
Gradual slowing and return to former rate	Constant	Normal	Normal	None, unless symptomatic; atropine
Gradual slowing‡ and return to former rate	Constant	Normal	Normal	None, unless symptomatic; treat underlying disease
Abrupt slowing caused by termination of PAT, or no effect	Constant	Normal	Normal; difficult to see	Vagal stimulation, digitalis, propranolol, DC shock
Abrupt slowing and return to former rate; flutter remains	Constant; variable if A-V block changing	Normal	Flutter waves	DC shock, digitalis, quinidine, propranolol
Slowing; gross irregularity remains	Variable	Normal	No A waves	Digitalis, quinidine, DC shock
Abrupt slowing and return to former rate; tachycardia remains	Constant; variable if A-V block changing	Normal	More A waves than C-V waves	Stop digitalis if toxic; digitalis, if not toxic
None; may be slight slowing	Variable ‖	Normal	Intermittent cannon waves ‖	None; unless symptomatic; atropine
Abrupt slowing caused by termination of PJT, or no effect	Constant but decreased	Normal	Constant cannon waves	See paroxysmal atrial tachycardia above
None; may be slight slowing	Variable ‖	Normal	Intermittent cannon waves ‖	None, unless symptomatic; stop digitalis if toxic
None	Variable ‖	Abnormal	Intermittent cannon waves ‖	Lidocaine, procainamide, DC shock, quinidine

under therapy. Some of the exceptions are indicated by the footnotes, but the reader is referred to the text for a

Continued.

Table 6-5. Cardiac arrhythmias — cont'd

Type of arrhythmia	P waves			QRS complexes		
	Rate	Rhythm	Contour	Rate	Rhythm	Contour
Accelerated idioventric- ular rhythm	60 to 100§	Regular	Normal	50 to 110	Fairly regu- lar; may be irregular	Abnormal, >0.12 second
Ventricular fibrillation	60 to 100§	Regular	Normal; dif- ficult to see	400 to 600	Grossly ir- regular	Base line un- dulations; no QRS complexes
First-degree A-V block	60 to 100¶	Regular	Normal	60 to 100	Regular	Normal
Type I sec- ond-degree A-V block	60 to 100¶	Regular	Normal	30 to 100	Irregular**	Normal
Type II-sec- ond-degree A-V block	60 to 100¶	Regular	Normal	30 to 100	Irregular**	Abnormal, >0.12 second
Complete A-V block	60 to 100§	Regular	Normal	<40	Fairly regular	Abnormal, >0.12 second
Right bundle branch block	60 to 100	Regular	Normal	60 to 100	Regular	Abnormal, >0.12 second
Left bundle branch block	60 to 100	Regular	Normal	60 to 100	Regular	Abnormal, >0.12 second

¶Atrial rhythm and rate may vary, depending on whether sinus bradycardia or tachycardia, atria tachycardia,
**Regular or constant if block is unchanging.

arrhythmia secondary to hypotension may respond to leg elevation or vasopressor therapy. Mild sedation or reassurance may be successful in treating some arrhythmias related to emotional stress. Precipitating or contributing disease states such as infection, hypovolemia, anemia, and thyroid disorders should be sought and treated. Aggressive management of premature atrial or ventricular systoles, which often presage or precipitate the occurrence of sustained tachyarrhythmias, may prevent later occurrence of more serious tachyarrhythmias.

Since therapy always involves some risk, one must decide, particularly as the therapeutic regimen escalates, that the risks of not treating the arrhythmia continue to outweigh the risks of the therapy. The antiarrhythmic agents lidocaine, procainamide, quinidine, propranolol, disopyramide, and diphenylhydantoin exert negative inotropic effects on the myocardium, and, when given parenterally, they may produce hypotension. Bretylium is the

Ventricular response to carotid sinus massage	Physical examination			Treatment
	Intensity of S_1	Splitting of S_2	A waves	
None	Variable ‖	Abnormal	Intermittent cannon waves ‖	None, unless symptomatic; lidocaine, atropine
None	None	None	Cannon waves	DC shock
Gradual slowing caused by sinus slowing	Constant, diminished	Normal	Normal	None
Slowing caused by sinus slowing and and increase in A-V block	Cyclic decrease and then increase after pause	Normal	Normal; increasing A-C interval; A waves without C waves	None, unless symptomatic; atropine
Gradual slowing caused by sinus slowing	Constant	Abnormal	Normal; constant A-C interval; A waves without C waves	Pacemaker
None	Variable ‖	Abnormal	Intermittent cannon waves ‖	Pacemaker
Gradual slowing and return to former rate	Constant	Wide	Normal	None
Gradual slowing and return to former rate	Constant	Paradoxical	Normal	None

etc. is the atrial mechanism.

only antiarrhythmic agent with a positive inotropic action. Antiarrhythmic agents may slow conduction velocity, depress the activity of normal (sinus) as well as abnormal (ectopic) pacemaker sites, and cause arrhythmias. It should be remembered that doses of all drugs may need to be adjusted according to the size of the patient, routes of excretion or degradation, presence of impaired organ function (heart, liver, kidney), degree of absorption (if given orally), adverse side effects, interaction with other drugs, electrolyte imbalance, hypoxemia, and the like.

The remainder of this chapter will be devoted to a discussion of cardiac arrhythmias (see Tables 6-4 and 6-5). An analysis similar to that presented in the discussion of arrhythmia analysis will be employed. For most arrhythmias the normal limits in seconds of the various intervals are stated, with the actual values of the examples presented contained in parentheses.

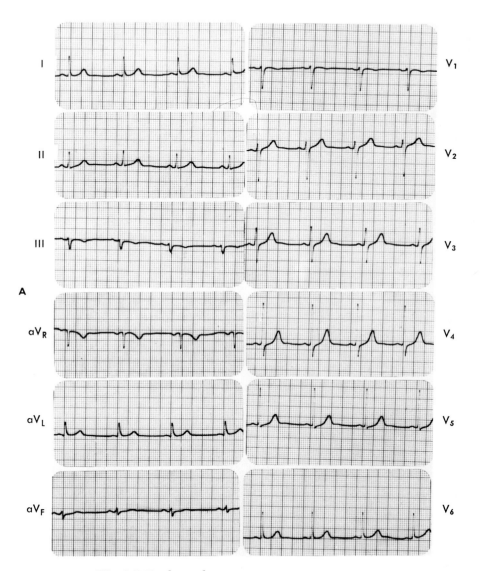

Fig. 6-5. For legend see opposite page.

NORMAL SINUS RHYTHM (Fig. 6-5, *A* and *B*)

Normal sinus rhythm is arbitrarily limited to rates of 60 to 100 beats per minute. The P wave is upright in leads I and II and negative in lead aV$_R$ with a vector in the frontal plane between 0 and +90 degrees. In the horizontal plane the P vector is directed anteriorly and slightly leftward and may therefore be negative in V$_1$ and V$_2$ but is positive in V$_3$. The P-P interval characteristically varies slightly but by less than 0.16 second. The P-R interval is greater than 0.12 second and may vary slightly with rate. The sinus node responds readily to autonomic stimuli; parasympathetic (cholinergic) stimuli slow and sympathetic (adrenergic) stimuli speed the rate of discharge. The resulting rate depends on the net effect of these two opposing forces.

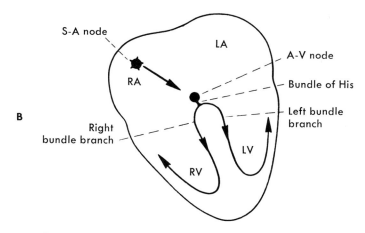

Fig. 6-5. A, Normal sinus rhythm. The ECG is normal. Schematic illustration in **B**.

Rate: 60 to 100 (60 to 65).
Rhythm: Fairly regular.
P waves: Precede each QRS with normal, unchanging contour. Note P wave contour in each of the 12 leads.
P-R interval: 0.12 to 0.20 second (0.14).
QRS: 0.06 to 0.10 second (0.08).
Significance and treatment: For significance and treatment of this and the following arrhythmias, see discussion under each arrhythmia.

SINUS TACHYCARDIA (Figs. 6-6 and 6-7)

Sinus tachycardia, because of enhanced discharge of the sinus node from vagal inhibition or sympathetic stimulation, maintains a rate between 100 to 180 beats per minute but may be higher with extreme exertion and in infants. It has a gradual onset and termination, and the P-P interval may vary slightly from cycle to cycle. P waves have a normal contour, but may develop a larger amplitude and become peaked. Carotid sinus massage and Valsalva or other vagal maneuvers gradually slow a sinus tachycardia, which then accelerates to its previous rate. More rapid sinus rates may fail to slow in response to a vagal maneuver.

Significance. Sinus tachycardia is the normal reaction to a variety of physiologic stresses such as fever, hypotension, thyrotoxicosis, anemia, anxiety, exertion, hypovolemia, pulmonary emboli, myocardial ischemia, congestive heart failure, or shock. Inflammation such as pericarditis may produce sinus tachycardia. Sinus tachycardia is usually of no physiologic significance; however, in patients with organic myocardial disease, reduced cardiac output, congestive heart failure, or arrhythmias may result. Since heart rate is a major determinant of oxygen requirements, angina or perhaps an increase in the size of an infarction may accompany persistent sinus tachycardia in patients with coronary artery disease.

Treatment. Therapy should be directed toward correcting the underlying disease state that caused the sinus tachycardia. Elimination of tobacco, alcohol, coffee, tea, or other stimulants, for example, vasoconstrictors in nose drops, may be helpful. If sinus tachycardia is not secondary to a correctable physiologic stress, treatment with sedatives, reserpine, or guanethidine is occasionally useful. The only presently available medication that consistently slows a sinus tachycardia directly is propranolol, administered orally, 10 to 60 mg, four times daily. Verapamil (Isoptin) may also slow the rate of sinus node discharge but at present is available in the United States only as an investigational drug.

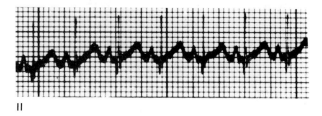

II

Fig. 6-6. Sinus tachycardia in an infant. Note peaked P waves in lead II.

Rate: 100 to 180, occasionally may exceed 200 (182).
Rhythm: Regular.
P waves: Precede each QRS complex with normal unchanging contour; often they are tall, peaked.
P-R interval: Normal, constant (0.08 second).
QRS: Normal (0.06 second).

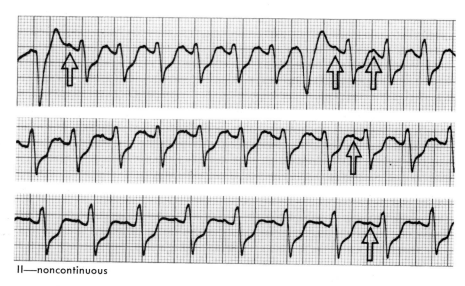

II—noncontinuous

Fig. 6-7. Sinus tachycardia. Patient has a preexisting bundle branch block. Clear P waves *(arrows)* can be seen in the pause that follows the two ventricular extrasystoles (top tracing). The heart rate gradually slowed following edrophonium (Tensilon) administration (middle and bottom tracings).

Rate: 100 to 180, occasionally may exceed 200 (125 in top tracing); gradually slows (100 in bottom tracing).
Rhythm: Regular.
P waves: Normal, but hidden by preceding T waves *(arrows)*.
P-R interval: Normal, constant (0.16 second).
QRS: Generally normal; in this example, abnormal, prolonged (0.14 second) because of the presence of a preexisting left bundle branch block.

SINUS BRADYCARDIA (Figs. 6-8 and 6-9)

Sinus bradycardia exists in the adult when the sinus node discharges at a rate less than 60 beats per minute. P waves have a normal contour and occur before each QRS complex with a constant P-R interval of greater than 0.12 second. Sinus arrhythmia is frequently present.

Significance. Sinus bradycardia results from excessive vagal or decreased sympathetic tone. Eye surgery, meningitis, intracranial tumors, cervical and mediastinal tumors and certain disease states such as myocardial infarction, myxedema, obstructive jaundice, and cardiac fibrosis may produce sinus bradycardia. In most instances, sinus bradycardia is a benign arrhythmia and may actually be beneficial by producing a longer period of diastole and increased ventricular filling. It occurs commonly during sleep, vomiting, or vasovagal syncope and may be produced by carotid sinus stimulation or by the administration of parasympathomimetic drugs. Sinus bradycardia occurring in patients with myocardial infarction, more commonly diaphragmatic or posterior, may compromise optimal myocardial function and predispose to premature systoles and sustained tachyarrhythmias. More recent data suggest sinus bradycardia actually is beneficial in some patients with acute myocardial infarction because it reduces oxygen demands, may help to minimize the size of the infarction, and may lessen the frequency of some arrhythmias. Patients with acute myocardial infarction who have sinus bradycardia generally have lower mortality than patients who have sinus tachcardia.

Treatment. Treatment of sinus bradycardia per se usually is not needed. If the patient with an acute myocardial infarction is asymptomatic, it is probably best not to try to speed the sinus rate. If the cardiac output is inadequate, or if arrhythmias are associated with the slow rate, atropine (0.5 mg IV as an initial dose repeated if necessary) or isoproterenol (1 to 2 μg per minute IV) is usually effective. The latter should be used cautiously. In some patients who experience congestive failure as a result of chronic sinus bradycardia, electrical pacing may be needed.

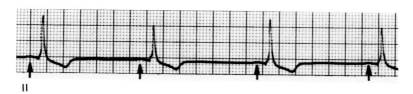

II

Fig. 6-8. Sinus bradycardia. Patient is receiving methyl dopa for hypertension. Normal rate was restored following discontinuation of methyl dopa therapy. Low amplitude P waves indicated by arrows.

Rate: Less than 60; usually 40 to 60 (41).
Rhythm: Fairly regular.
P waves: Precede each QRS with a normal contour.
P-R interval: Normal contract (0.16 second).
QRS: Generally normal; in this example, borderline prolonged (0.11 second).

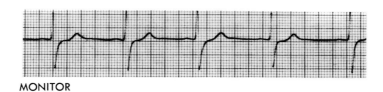

MONITOR

Fig. 6-9. Sinus bradycardia. Patient has an acute diaphragmatic (inferior) myocardial infarction.

Rate: Less than 60; usually 40 to 60 (50 to 58).
Rhythm: Fairly regular.
P waves: Precede each QRS with a normal contour.
P-R interval: Normal, constant (0.16 second).
QRS: Generally normal; in this example, borderline prolonged (0.11 second).

SINUS ARRHYTHMIA (Figs. 6-10 to 6-12)

Sinus arrhythmia is characterized by a phasic variation in cycle length of greater than 0.16 second during sinus rhythm. It is the most frequent form of arrhythmia and occurs as a normal phenomenon. The P waves do not vary in morphology, and the P-R interval is greater than 0.12 second and remains unchanged, since the focus of discharge is fixed within the sinus node. Occasionally the pacemaker focus may wander within the sinus node, producing P waves of slightly different contour (but not retrograde) and a changing P-R interval (but not less than 0.12 second). Sinus arrhythmia commonly occurs in the young or aged, especially with slower heart rates or following enhanced vagal tone from digitalis or morphine administration. Sinus arrhythmia appears in two basic forms. In the respiratory form the P-P interval cyclically shortens during inspiration as a result of reflex inhibition of vagal tone or enhancement of sympathetic tone or both. Breath holding eliminates the cycle length variation. Nonrespiratory sinus arrhythmia is characterized by a phasic variation unrelated to the respiratory cycle.

Significance. Symptoms produced by sinus arrhythmia are rare, but on occasion, if the pauses between beats are excessively long, palpitations or dizziness may be experienced. Marked sinus arrhythmia can produce a sinus pause sufficiently prolonged to induce syncope if not accompanied by an escape rhythm.

Treatment. Treatment is usually not necessary. Increasing the heart rate by exercise or drugs will abolish sinus arrhythmias. Symptomatic individuals may experience relief from feelings of palpitations through the use of sedatives, tranquilizers, atropine, ephedrine, or isoproterenol administration, as in the treatment of sinus bradycardia.

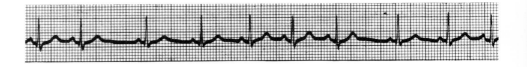

II

Fig. 6-10. Respiratory sinus arrhythmia. The phasic variation corresponds to a respiratory rate of approximately 18 per minute.

Rate: Sinus rate increases with inspiration and decreases with expiration (70 to 110).
Rhythm: Irregular with a repetitive phasic variation in cycle length according to respiratory cycles. Cycle lengths vary by more than 0.16 second. Breath holding eliminates the rate variations.
P waves: Precede each QRS with a normal, fairly constant contour.
P-R interval: Normal, constant (0.12 second).
QRS: Normal (0.08 second).

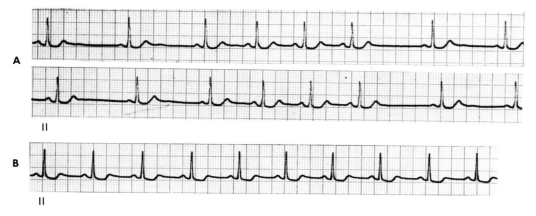

Fig. 6-11. Nonrespiratory sinus arrhythmia. In this instance, it was caused by digitalis toxicity, **A.** One week following discontinuation of digitalis the nonrespiratory sinus arrhythmia disappeared, **B.**

Rate: Rate increases and decreases independently of respiration, **A** (47 to 80). Rate constant (78) in **B.**

Rhythm: Irregular with a repetitive phasic variation in cycle length which continues during breath holding, **A.** Regular, **B.**

P waves: Precede each QRS with a normal, fairly constant contour.

P-R interval: Normal, constant (0.12 second).

QRS: Normal (0.06 second).

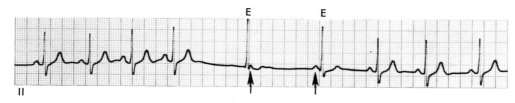

Fig. 6-12. Respiratory sinus arrhythmia. The first four P waves are fairly regular; the P-R interval is 0.16 second and constant. Then the sinus node slows and the next two P waves occur much later *(arrows)*. The marked sinus slowing allows a latent pacemaker—possibly located in the His bundle or high in the fascicles—to escape sinus domination, depolarize automatically, and discharge the ventricles (*E*, junctional escapes). A slight change in QRS contour is apparent in these beats. The sinus node then speeds up to resume control. This slightly complex arrhythmia is completely normal in an otherwise healthy person.

Rate: Rate increases with inspiration and decreases with expiration (55 to 80).

Rhythm: Irregular with a repetitive phasic variation in cycle length according to respiratory cycles.

P waves: Normal, fairly constant contour.

P-R interval: Normal, constant (0.16 second) during sinus-conducted beats.

QRS: Normal (0.08 second) during sinus-conducted beats.

SINUS ARREST (Figs. 6-13 and 6-14)

Failure of sinus node discharge results in absence of atrial depolarization and periods of ventricular asystole if escape beats produced by latent pacemakers do not discharge. Sinus arrest may be produced by involvement of the sinus node or the sinus node artery by acute myocardial infarction, digitalis toxicity, excessive vagal tone, or degenerative forms of fibrosis.

Significance. Transient sinus arrest may have no clinical significance by itself if latent pacemakers promptly escape to prevent ventricular asystole. Prolonged ventricular asystole results should the latent pacemakers fail to escape. Other arrhythmias may be precipitated by the slow rates.

Treatment. Atropine (0.5 mg IV initially, repeated if necessary) or isoproterenol (1.0 to 2.0 μg per minute IV) may be tried as the first therapeutic approach. If these drugs are unsuccessful, atrial or ventricular pacing may be required. In patients who have a chronic form of sinus node disease, characterized by marked sinus bradycardia or sinus arrest (sick sinus syndrome), permanent pacing is often necessary. Some of these patients experience sinus bradycardia alternating with periods of supraventricular tachycardia (bradycardia-tachycardia syndrome). These patients are best treated by a combination of drugs (to slow the ventricular rate during the supraventricular tachycardia) and permanent demand pacemaker implantation (to avoid the slow rate when the tachycardia terminates).

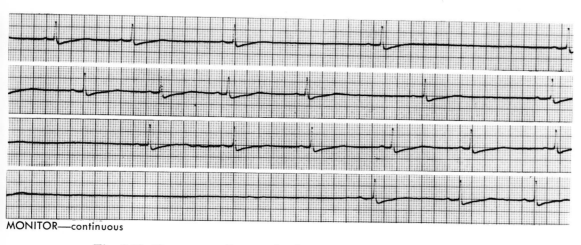

MONITOR—continuous

Fig. 6-13. Sinus arrest. Patient also has an acute inferior myocardial infarction. Asystolic intervals are not interrupted by escape beats.

Rate: Varying, slow (maximum rate of 55).
Rhythm: Irregular; periods of asystole not a multiple of basic sinus cycle length.
P waves: Precede each QRS with a normal contour; may be altered by escape beats.
P-R interval: Constant, generally normal; in this example, slightly prolonged (0.21 second); may be altered by escape beats.
QRS: Generally normal (0.09 second).

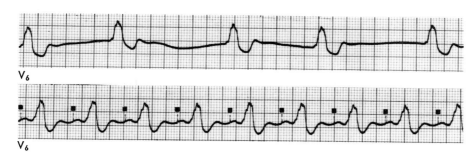

Fig. 6-14. Sinus arrest (top) and right atrial pacing (bottom). Patient also has a left bundle branch block. A supraventricular escape focus controls the rhythm in the top panel, but atrial activity is not apparent. **Atrial pacing** (stimuli indicated by filled squares, bottom tracing) results in atrial capture, producing a P wave and an unchanged QRS contour.

Rate: Varying, slow (36 to 50) (top); normal (81) (bottom).
Rhythm: Irregular (top); regular (bottom).
P waves: Not seen (top); follows pacemaker stimulus (bottom).
P-R interval: Not measurable (top); normal, constant (0.16 second) (bottom).
QRS: Generally normal, in this example, left bundle branch block (0.20 second).

SINOATRIAL EXIT BLOCK (Figs. 6-15 and 6-16)

Sinoatrial (S-A) block is a conduction disturbance during which an impulse formed within the S-A node is blocked from depolarizing the atria. S-A exit block is indicated on the ECG by the absence of the normally expected P wave(s). The length of the pause between P waves is a multiple of the basic P-P interval, approximately two, less commonly three or four times the normal P-P interval (type II exit block). Type I (Wenckebach) S-A exit block may also occur, in which case the P-P interval progressively shortens prior to the pause and the duration of the pause is less than two P-P cycles.

Significance. S-A exit block may be caused by excessive vagal stimulation, by acute infections such as diphtheria or rheumatic carditis, by atherosclerosis involving the S-A nodal artery, or by fibrosis involving the atrium. Occlusion of the S-A nodal artery owing to acute myocardial infarction may result in an atrial infarction and produce S-A exit block. Medications such as quinidine, procainamide, and digitalis may lead to S-A exit block. S-A block is usually transient and often of no clinical importance except to prompt a search for the underlying cause. Syncope may result if the S-A block is prolonged and unaccompanied by an A-V junctional or ventricular escape rhythm. Digitalis produces type II S-A exit block (but type I A-V block).

Treatment. Therapy for symptomatic S-A exit block is directed toward increasing sympathetic tone and decreasing parasympathetic tone. Thus atropine and isoproterenol are useful, as described under sinus bradycardia. If the clinical situation demands therapy and pharmacologic measures are not effective, atrial or ventricular pacing may be indicated.

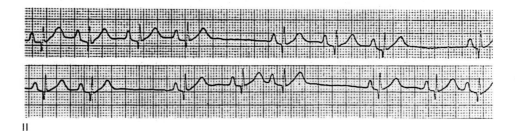

II

Fig. 6-15. Sinoatrial (S-A) exit block (type II). The longer P-P intervals are approximately twice the shorter P-P intervals, indicating an intermittent 2:1 sinus exit block of the type II variety.

Rate: Varying, slow (43 to 68).
Rhythm: Irregular; pauses are twice as long as the shorter intervals.
P waves: Contour normal, precede each QRS complex; intermittent loss of P wave.
P-R interval: Normal, constant (0.16 second).
QRS: Normal (0.08 second).

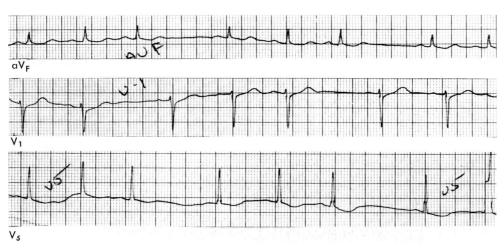

aV_F

V_1

V_5

Fig. 6-16. Sinoatrial (S-A) exit block (type I or Wenckebach). The following four characteristics of this tracing allow the diagnosis of a Wenckebach exit block from the sinus node: (1) A pause in atrial activity occurs. (2) The P-P interval progressively shortens up until the pause. (3) The duration of the pause is less than twice the shortest P-P interval. (4) The P-P interval following the pause exceeds the P-P interval preceding the pause.

Rate: Varying, slow (50 to 88).
Rhythm: Four features mentioned in legend.
P waves: Contour normal, precede each QRS complex; intermittent loss of P wave.
P-R interval: Normal, constant (0.20 second).
QRS: Normal (0.08 second).

WANDERING PACEMAKER (Figs. 6-17 and 6-18)

Wandering pacemaker, a variant of sinus arrhythmia, involves the passive transfer of the dominant pacemaker focus from the sinus node to latent pacemakers with the next highest degree of automaticity, usually in the A-V junctional tissue. Thus only one pacemaker is operative at a time. As with other forms of sinus arrhythmia, the change occurs in a gradual fashion over the duration of several beats. The ECG displays a cyclic increase of the R-R interval, a P-R interval that gradually shortens and may become less than 0.12 second, and a change in P wave configuration until it becomes negative in lead I or II or becomes buried in the QRS complex. A slight change in QRS configuration may occur owing to aberrant conduction. These changes occur in reverse as the pacemaker shifts back to the sinus node. Rarely a wandering pacemaker may appear without changes in rate.

Significance. Wandering pacemaker is a normal phenomenon that is often seen in the very young or in the aged, and particularly in athletes. Persistence of an A-V junctional rhythm for long periods of time, however, usually indicates underlying heart disease.

Treatment. Treatment of a wandering pacemaker usually is not indicated. Sympathomimetic agents such as ephedrine or isoproterenol or parasympatholytic agents such as atropine can be used if necessary (see discussion of sinus bradycardia).

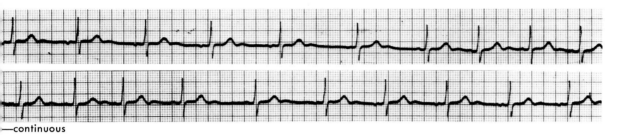

—continuous

Fig. 6-17. Wandering atrial pacemaker. As the heart rate speeds, the P waves become upright and then gradually become inverted again as the heart rate slows.

Rate: Varying, slow (47 to 75).
Rhythm: Irregular with a repetitive phasic variation in cycle length as in sinus arrhythmia.
P waves: Vary contour, indicating shift in pacemaker site. May become negative in lead I or II if retrogradely activated (become negative).
P-R interval: Varies and may become 0.12 second or less if pacemaker origin shifts close to A-V junction (0.16 second).
QRS: Generally normal but may be slightly aberrant when pacemaker shifts to A-V junction (normal, 0.08 second).

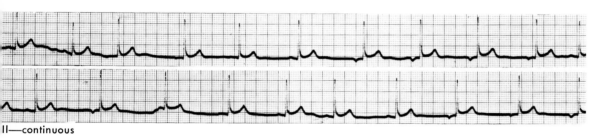

II—continuous

Fig. 6-18. Wandering atrial pacemaker. As the heart rate slows, the P waves become inverted and then gradually revert toward normal as the heart rate speeds. The P-R interval shortens to 0.14 second with the inverted P wave and is 0.16 second with the upright P wave.

Rate: Varying, slow (52 to 72).
Rhythm: Irregular with a repetitive phasic variation in cycle length as in sinus arrhythmia.
P waves: Vary contour, indicating shift in pacemaker site. May become negative in lead I or II if retrogradely activated (become negative).
P-R interval: Varies and may become 0.12 second or less if pacemaker origin shifts close to A-V junction (0.14, 0.16 second).
QRS: Generally normal, but may become slightly aberrant when pacemaker shifts to A-V junction (normal, 0.08 second).

PREMATURE ATRIAL SYSTOLES (Figs. 6-19 to 6-22)

Premature systoles are the most common cause of an intermittent pulse. They may originate from any area of the heart most frequently from the ventricles less often from the atria and from the A-V junctional region, and rarely from the sinus node. Although premature systoles arise from normal hearts, they are more often associated with organic disease, particularly in older patients.

The diagnosis of premature atrial systoles is indicated by a premature P wave that may have a contour similar, but not identical, to the sinus P wave and a P-R interval greater than 0.12 second. Variations in the basic sinus rate at times may make the diagnosis of prematurity difficult, but differences in the contour of the P wave are usually quite apparent and indicate a different focus of origin. When a premature atrial systole occurs early in diastole, conduction may not be completely normal. The A-V junction may still be refractory from the preceding beat and will prevent propagation of the impulse (blocked premature atrial systole) or cause conduction to be slowed (prolonged P-R interval). As a general rule, a short R-P interval is followed by a long P-R interval. On occasion, when the A-V junction has sufficiently repolarized to conduct normally, the supraventricular QRS complex may be aberrant in configuration, because the ventricle has not completely repolarized (see discussion of supraventricular arrhythmia with abnormal QRS complexes, p. 223).

The length of the pause following any premature beat or series of premature beats is determined by the interaction of a number of factors. If the premature atrial systole occurs when the sinus node is not refractory, the impulse may conduct to the sinus node, discharge it prematurely, and cause the next sinus cycle to begin from that point. The interval between the two normal beats flanking a premature atrial systole that has reset the timing of the basic sinus rhythm is less than twice the normal cycle, and the pause after the premature atrial systole is said to be "noncompensatory." The interval following the premature atrial systole is generally longer than one sinus cycle, however. Less commonly the premature atrial systole may find the sinus node refractory, in which case the timing of the basic sinus rhythm is not altered, and the interval between the two normal beats flanking the premature atrial systole is twice the normal P-P cycle. The interval following this premature atrial discharge is therefore said to be a "full compensatory pause." A compensatory pause is one of sufficient duration to make the interval between the two normal beats on each side of the premature beat twice the basic cycle length. However, sinus arrhythmia may lengthen or shorten this pause.

Significance. Premature atrial systoles may occur in a variety of situations for example, during infection, inflammation, or myocardial ischemia, or they may be provoked by a variety of medications, by tension states, or by tobacco and caffeine. Premature atrial systoles may precipitate or presage the occurrence of a sustained supraventricular tachycardia.

Treatment. In the absence of organic heart disease, treatment may not be

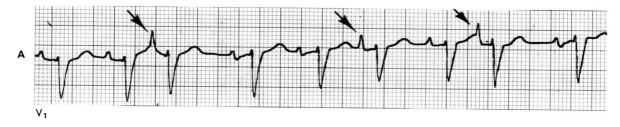

A

V_1

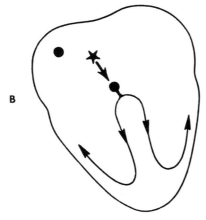

B

Fig. 6-19. A, **Premature atrial systoles depressing sinus node discharge.** Sharply pointed P waves *(arrows)* represent premature atrial systoles that, when they occur early (first and third), delay return of sinus node. Contour of P waves following earlier premature atrial systoles differs from normal P wave, indicating a shift in pacemaker focus or a change in intra-atrial conduction. **B,** Schematic illustration presented.

Rate: Determined by basic rate and number of atrial extrasystoles.
Rhythm: Irregular because of premature beats; may be a regular irregularity as in bigeminy or trigeminy (irregular).
P waves: Premature atrial systole has different contour; may be buried in preceding T wave (sharply pointed) *(arrows).*
P-R interval (of atrial systole): Depending on degree of prematurity, may be conducted with a normal or prolonged P-R interval or the atrial systole may be completely blocked (0.16 second).
QRS: Generally normal; may be aberrantly conducted (normal, 0.08 second).

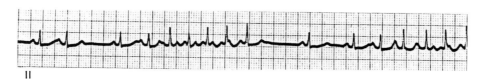

II

Fig. 6-20. **Single and multiple premature atrial systoles** can be seen hidden within preceding T waves and appear to initiate short bursts of an atrial tachyarrhythmia, probably atrial flutter-fibrillation.

Rate: Determined by basic rate and number of atrial systoles.
Rhythm: Irregular because of premature systoles; may be a regular irregularity as in bigeminy or trigeminy (irregular).
P waves: Premature atrial systole has different contour; may be buried in preceding T wave.
P-R interval (of atrial systole): Depending on the degree of prematurity, may be conducted with a normal or prolonged P-R interval or the atrial extrasystole may be completely blocked (0.14 second).
QRS: Generally normal; may be aberrantly conducted (normal, 0.08 second).

PREMATURE ATRIAL SYSTOLES (Figs. 6-19 to 6-22—cont'd)

necessary, unless the patient complains of symptoms such as palpitations or has recurrent tachycardias or an excessive number of atrial extrasystoles. If treatment is indicated as in the patient with acute myocardial infarction, initial therapy should probably be with digitalis, combined with quinidine or procainamide if digitalis alone is not successful. Sedation and/or omission of alcohol, caffeine, or smoking may be helpful in some patients.

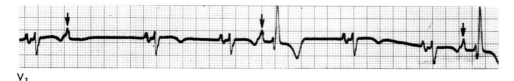

V₁

Fig. 6-21. Nonconducted premature systoles and premature atrial systoles initiating functional right bundle branch block. Sinus-initiated P waves are abnormal and suggest left atrial enlargement. Premature atrial systoles *(arrows)* can be seen hidden in the preceding T waves. The first two premature atrial systoles are blocked and generate a pause in the ventricular rhythm. The second two premature atrial systoles conduct to the ventricle with a prolonged P-R interval and initiate a functional right bundle branch block.

Rate: Determined by basic rate and number of premature systoles (slow, because of nonconducted premature atrial systoles).
Rhythm: Irregular because of premature atrial systoles (irregular).
P waves: Premature atrial systoles have different contour and may be buried in preceding T wave *(arrows)*.
P-R interval (of premature atrial systoles). First two premature atrial systoles are completely blocked; third and fourth premature atrial systoles conduct with a prolonged P-R interval (0.21 second).
QRS: Generally normal, may be aberrantly conducted (third and fourth premature atrial systoles initiate aberrantly conducted QRS complex with a right bundle branch block pattern).

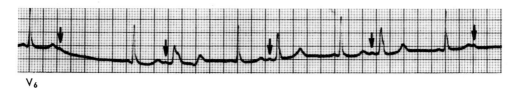

V₆

Fig. 6-22. Nonconducted premature atrial systoles and premature atrial systoles that produce a functional left bundle branch block. Premature atrial systoles can be seen in the terminal portion of the preceding T waves and look like a U wave *(arrows)*. Fairly early premature atrial systoles block whereas slightly later premature atrial systoles conduct to the ventricles with an increase in P-R interval and varying degrees of left bundle branch block.

Rate: Determined by basic rate and number of premature atrial systoles (slow, because of nonconducted atrial extrasystoles).
Rhythm: Irregular because of premature atrial systoles (irregular).
P waves: Premature atrial systoles have different contour and may be buried in the preceding T wave *(arrows)*.
P-R interval (of premature atrial systole): Later premature atrial systoles (second, third, and fourth) conduct whereas early premature atrial systoles (first, fifth, and sixth) fail to reach the ventricles.
QRS: Generally normal, may be aberrantly conducted (second, third, and fourth premature atrial systoles produce varying degrees of left bundle branch block).

PAROXYSMAL ATRIAL OR JUNCTIONAL TACHYCARDIA (Figs. 6-23 to 6-25)

Paroxysmal atrial (PAT) or junctional (PJT) tachycardia is characterized by a rapid, regular, atrial or junctional tachycardia of sudden onset and termination, occurring at rates generally between 150 and 250 beats per minute. Uncommonly the rate may be as low as 110 beats per minute and occasionally, especially in children, the rate may exceed 250 beats per minute. The clinical presentation, ECG characteristics, and treatment for both PAT and PJT are virtually identical and suggest that both rhythms may be the same or at least very closely related. In the same patient an alteration in A-V conduction time can change P-R relationship from one in which P waves precede the QRS by a normal interval (PAT) to one in which the P waves occur during or after the QRS (PJT). Sometimes the rapid rate obscures distinct P waves entirely and the tachycardia must be called, nonspecifically, paroxysmal supraventricular tachycardia (PSVT). Therefore all comments made regarding PAT are equally applicable to PJT.

PAT recorded at the onset begins abruptly, usually following premature atrial systole that conducts with a prolonged P-R interval; the abrupt termination is sometimes followed by a brief period of asystole. The R-R interval may shorten over the course of the first few beats at the onset or lengthen over the course of the last few beats preceding termination of the tachycardia. The "clockwork" regularity ascribed to PAT may not always be present. Variation in cycle length is usually because of variation in A-V conduction time and occurs with sufficient frequency to prevent excluding the diagnosis of PAT when slight rate of rhythm variations exist:

Significance. PAT and PJT may occur at any age unassociated with underlying heart disease. However, when organic disease is present, it is often coro-

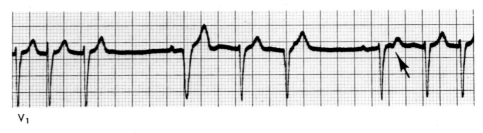

V_1

Fig. 6-23. Paroxysmal supraventricular tachycardia. Paroxysmal atrial or junctional tachycardia suddenly terminates, begins briefly, stops, and then restarts again following a premature atrial systole *(arrow)* that conducts with a prlonged P-R interval.

Rate: 150 to 250; most commonly near 200 (150).
Rhythm: Quite regular except at the onset and termination.
P waves: Contour differs from sinus P wave but P waves are frequently difficult to see because of superimposed preceding T wave. P waves may require special leads to demonstrate. Because failure to identify P waves, the tachycardia must often be called, nonspecifically, paroxysmal supraventricular tachycardia.
P-R interval: Usually constant if P waves can be seen.
QRS: Usually normal (0.08 second).

nary artery disease; thyrotoxicosis is frequently associated with PAT and must be considered. The arrhythmia may be related to specific inciting causes such as overexertion, emotional stimuli, and coffee and smoking; it may follow a specific pattern or its onset may be unrelated to any particular event.

Symptoms frequently accompany the attack and range from feelings of palpitations, nervousness, and anxiety to angina, frank heart failure, or shock, depending on the duration and rate of the PAT and the presence of organic heart disease. PAT may cause syncope because of the rapid ventricular rate, reduced cardiac output, and cerebral circulation or because of asystole when the PAT terminates, owing to PAT-induced depression of sinus node automaticity. The prognosis for patients without heart disease is usually quite good.

Treatment. Treatment of the acute attack depends on the clinical situation and how well the PAT is tolerated, the natural history of the attacks in the individual patient, and the presence of associated disease. For some patients, rest, reassurance, and sedation may be all that are required to abort an attack.

1. Vagal maneuvers, including carotid sinus massage, Valsalva, and gagging, serve as the first line of therapy and either terminate PAT or leave it unaffected (actually, slight slowing may occur during vagal stimulation). These maneuvers should be retried after *each* pharmacologic approach.

2. Cholinergic drugs, particularly edrophonium chloride (Tensilon), short-acting cholinesterase inhibitor, may terminate PAT when administered initially at a dose of 3 to 5 mg IV and, if unsuccessful, repeated at a dose of 10 mg IV. Its action is rapid in onset and short in duration, with minimal side effects. Edrophonium should be used cautiously or not at all in patients who are hypotensive or who have lung disease, especially asthmatics.

3. Pressor drugs may terminate PAT by inducing reflex vagal stimulation mediated via baroreceptors in the carotid sinus and aorta when the systolic blood pressure is acutely elevated to levels of about 180 mm Hg.

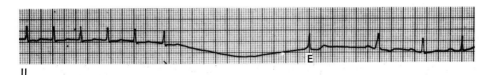

II

Fig. 6-24. Paroxysmal supraventricular tachycardia (atrial or junctional). Paroxysmal atrial or junctional tachycardia suddenly terminates following carotid sinus massage and produces a short period of asystole that is ended by an A-V junctional escape beat *(E)*. Sinus rhythm then returns.

Rate: 150 to 250; most commonly near 200 (130).
Rhythm: Regular, except at onset and termination.
P waves: Not seen during tachycardia.
P-R interval: Usually constant when P waves can be identified.
QRS: Usually normal (0.06 second).

One of the following drugs, diluted in 5 to 10 ml of 5% dextrose and water, may be given IV over 1 to 3 minutes: phenylephrine (Neo-Synephrine), 0.5 to 1.0 mg; methoxamine (Vasoxyl), 3 to 5 mg; or metaraminol (Aramine), 0.5 to 2.0 mg. Pressor drugs should be used cautiously or not at all in the elderly or in patients with organic heart disease, significant hypertension, hyperthyroidism, or acute myocardial infarction. A new drug, verapamil, may become the treatment of choice to terminate acute PAT, but this drug is limited to investigational use at present. (See Appendix A.)

4. If these approaches are unsuccessful, IV digitalis administration may be attempted next, using one of the following short-acting digitalis preparations: ouabain, 0.25 to 0.50 mg IV, followed by 0.1 mg every 30 to 60 minutes if needed, keeping the total dose less than 1.0 mg within a 24-hour period; digoxin (Lanoxin), 0.5 to 1.0 mg IV, followed by 0.25 mg every 2 to 4 hours, with a total dose less than 1.5 within a 24-hour period; or deslanoslide (Cedilanid-D), 0.8 mg IV, followed by 0.4 mg every 2 to 4 hours, restricting the total dose to less than 2.0 mg within a 24-hour period. Oral digitalis administration to terminate an acute attack is generally not indicated. Vagal maneuvers, previously ineffective, may terminate PAT following digitalis administration and therefore should be repeated.

5. Propranolol (Inderal) given IV at a rate of 0.5 to 1 mg per minute for a total dose of 0.5 to 3 mg may be tried if digitalis administration is unsuccessful. Propranolol must be used cautiously, if at all, in patients with heart failure or chronic lung disease because its adrenergic beta-receptor blocking action depresses myocardial contractility and may produce bronchospasm.

Prior to administering digitalis or propranolol, it is advisable to reassess the clinical status of the patient and consider whether DC cardioversion may be advisable at this stage. DC shock, administered to patients who have received excessive amounts of digitalis, may be dangerous and result in serious postshock ventricular arrhythmias (see Chapter 8 for discussion).

6. Particularly if signs or symptoms of cardiac decompensation occur, DC electrical shock should be attempted next. DC shock, synchronized to the QRS complex to avoid precipitation of ventricular fibrillation, successfully terminates PAT with energies in the range of 10 to 50 watt-seconds; higher energies may be required in some instances. Short-acting barbituates like methohexital (Brevital), 50 to 120 mg given IV at a rate of 50 mg per 30 seconds, may be used to provide anesthesia, or diazepam (Valium), 5 to 15 mg given IV at a rate of 5 mg per minute, may be used to provide sedation and amnesia. Doses must be individualized and in general should be reduced for patients with heart failure, hypotension, or liver disease. During DC cardioversion a physician skilled in airway management should be in attendance, and IV

route established, and all equipment and drugs necessary for emergency resuscitation immediately accessible. One hundred percent oxygen is administered throughout the procedure, employing manually assisted ventilation if necessary.

If DC shock becomes necessary in patients who have received large amounts of digitalis, one should begin with 1 to 5 watt-seconds and gradually increase the energy level in increments of approximately 25 to 50 watt-seconds as long as premature ventricular systoles do not result. If premature ventricular systoles occur but can be suppressed with lidocaine or diphenylhydantoin, the next higher energy level may be tried.

7. In the event that digitalis has been given in large doses and DC shock is contraindicated, right atrial pacing at rates faster or slower than the PAT may restore sinus rhythm, presumably by prematurely depolarizing one of the pathways required for continued reentry. In some patients, right atrial pacing may precipitate atrial fibrillation; however, because the latter is generally accompanied by a slower ventricular rate, the patient's clinical status improves.

8. Procainamide (Pronestyl), quinidine, disopyramide (Norpace), or diphenylhydantoin (Dilantin) may be required to terminate PAT in some patients. Unless contraindicated, DC cardioversion should be employed prior to using these agents, which are more often administered to prevent recurrences.

Prevention of recurrences is often more difficult than terminating the acute episode. Precipitating factors such as smoking, alcohol, or excessive fatigue, if identified, should be avoided. Initially, one must decide whether the frequency and severity of the attacks warrant drug phophylaxis. For example, an

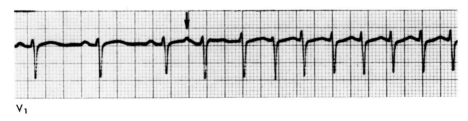

V₁

Fig. 6-25. Paroxysmal supraventricular tachycardia (atrial or junctional). Three sinus beats are interrupted by a premature atrial systole *(arrow)*, which conducts with P-R prolongation and initiates the supraventricular tachycardia.

Rate: Sinus rhythm, 83; paroxysmal supraventricular tachycardia, 190.
Rhythm: Regular during sinus rhythm and during paroxysmal supraventricular tachycardia.
P waves: See in first four beats but not afterward.
P-R interval: Normal during sinus beats (0.16 second), slightly prolonged (0.20 second) during premature atrial systole.
QRS: Normal (0.08 second).
Arrhythmia: Sudden initiation of paroxysmal supraventricular tachycardia by a premature atrial systole that conducts with P-R prolongation.

attempt should probably not be made to supress PAT occurring twice yearly in an otherwise healthy patient.

1. If drug prophylaxis is indicated, digitalis is the initial drug of choice. The speed at which digitalization is achieved is determined by the clinical situation. Using digoxin, rapid oral digitalization can be accomplished in 24 to 36 hours with an initial dose of 1.0 to 1.5 mg, followed by 0.25 to 0.5 mg every 6 hours for a total dose of 2.0 to 3.0 mg. A less rapid oral regimen digitalizes in 2 to 3 days with an initial dose of 0.75 to 1.0 mg, followed by 0.25 to 0.5 mg every 12 hours for a total dose of 2.0 to 3.0 mg. Alternatively, digoxin administered as a maintenance dose of 0.125 to 0.5 mg achieves digitalization in about 1 week. Because of its shorter half-life, digoxin may provide more effective control when administered twice daily. Digitoxin, which has a longer duration of action, may be used instead of digoxin. Oral digitalization with digitoxin may be accomplished in 24 to 36 hours with an initial dose of 0.5 to 0.8 mg, followed by 0.2 mg every 6 to 8 hours until reaching a total dose of 1.2 mg. A slower approach involves administering 0.2 mg three times daily for 2 to 3 days. Complete digitalization can also be accomplished in about 1 month by simply giving a maintenance dose, 0.05 to 0.2 mg daily.

2. If digitalis alone is unsuccessful, one can then add quinidine, 200 to 400 mg every 6 hours, or propranolol (Inderal), 10 to 40 mg every 6 hours.

3. If a combination of digitalis and quinidine or digitalis and propranolol is unsuccessful, concomitant administration of all three drugs, that is, digitalis, quinidine, and propranolol, may be tried. If this regimen also fails, empiric trials with other antiarrhythmic agents such as procainamide, disopyramide, or diphenylhydantoin may be warranted.

4. In particularly resistant cases, sympathectomy, antithyroid measures, permanent pacemaker implantation, and sometimes surgery to interrupt AV conduction may be considered.

Of interest is the recently appreciated fact that as many as 20% to 30% of patients with recurrent PAT or PJT may have an accessory pathway (see preexcitation or Wolff-Parkinson-White syndrome) that conducts only in a retrograde direction. Thus these patients have the two pathways (accessory pathway and normal A-V node) necessary for reentry to occur, but do not exhibit obvious manifestations of having the preexcitation syndrome in the scalar ECG.

ATRIAL FLUTTER (Figs. 6-26 to 6-29)

The atrial rate during atrial flutter is usually 250 to 350 beats per minute; quinidine or procainamide may reduce the rate to 200 beats per minute. In patients with untreated atrial flutter the ventricular rate is usually half the atrial rate, that is, 150 beats per minute. A significantly slower ventricular rate (in the absence of drugs) suggest abnormal A-V conduction. Atrial flutter in children, in patients with the preexcitation syndrome, or occasionally in patients with hyperthyroidism may conduct to the ventricle in a 1:1 fashion, producing a ventricular rate of 300 beats per minute.

The ECG reveals identically recurring, regular, sawtooth-shaped flutter waves and evidence of continual electrical activity (lack of an isoelectric interval between flutter waves), often best visualized in leads II, III, a V_F, or V_1. Commonly, the flutter waves appear inverted in these leads. If the A-V conduction ratio remains constant, the ventricular rhythm will be regular; if the ratio of conducted beats varies (usually the result of a Wenckebach A-V

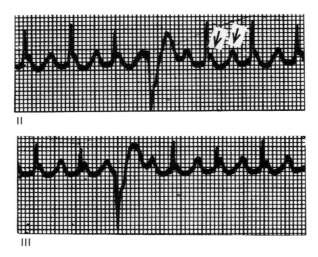

Fig. 6-26. Atrial flutter. Flutter waves indicated by arrows. A single premature ventricular systole occurs in each lead. The conduction ratio is 2:1; that is, flutter waves are conducted alternately to the ventricle.

Rate: Atrial—250 to 350, usually near 300 (280). Digitalis may increase whereas quinidine may slow the flutter rate.
    Ventricular—In untreated atrial flutter, generally one half the atrial rate (140).
Rhythm: Atrial—Regular.
    Ventricular—In untreated atrial flutter, usually regular with 2:1 A-V conduction; in treated atrial flutter, the ventricles respond in an irregular fashion produced by varying degrees of A-V block, for example, 3:2, 3:1, 4:1, or greater (2:1).
P waves: Flutter waves with regular oscillations resembling a sawtooth pattern, best seen in leads II, III, or V_1. Two, three, four, or more flutter waves occur for each QRS complex, depending on the degree of A-V block. Electrical activity appears continuous (lack an isoelectrical interval between flutter waves).
P-R interval: Flutter-R interval may be constant or varying (constant).
QRS: Normal (0.08 second).

block), the ventricular rhythm will be irregular. Impure flutter (flutter-fibrillation), occurring at a faster rate than pure flutter, shows variability in the contour and spacing of the flutter waves and may represent dissimilar atrial rhythms, that is, fibrillation in one atrium and a slower, more regular rhythm in the opposite atrium.

Significance. Atrial flutter is a less common tachyarrhythmia than is atrial fibrillation. Although paroxysmal atrial flutter usually indicates the presence of cardiac disease, it may occur in normal hearts. Uncommonly, it is produced by digitalis excess. Chronic (persistent) atrial flutter rarely occurs in the absence of underlying heart disease. Atrial flutter usually responds to carotid sinus massage with a decrease in ventricular rate in stepwise multiples, returning in a reverse manner to the former ventricular rate at the termination of carotid massage. Very rarely will sinus rhythm follow carotid sinus massage. Exercise, by enhancing sympathetic or lessening parasympathetic tone, may reduce the A-V conduction delay and produce a doubling of the ventricular rate.

Treatment. Treatment for atrial flutter is as follows:

1. Synchronous DC cardioversion is probably the initial treatment of choice for atrial flutter, since it promptly and effectively restores sinus rhythm with energies less that 50 watt-seconds. If DC shock results in atrial fibrillation, a second shock with a higher energy level may be used to restore sinus rhythm or, depending on the clinical circumstance, the atrial fibrillation may be left untreated. The latter will usually revert to atrial flutter or sinus rhythm.

2. If a cardioverter is unavailable or if the atrial flutter recurs at frequent intervals, therapy should be with a short-acting digitalis preparation,

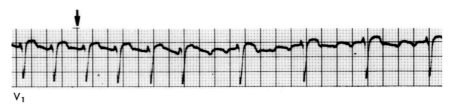

V_1

Fig. 6-27. Atrial flutter. Atrial flutter with a 2:1 ventricular response is present in the left portion of the tracing but cannot be clearly diagnosed from this lead. At the arrow, carotid sinus massage increases the degree of A-V block to 4:1 and clearly exposes the atrial flutter waves.

Rate: Atrial—300.
      Ventricular—150, decreasing to 75.
Rhythm: Atrial—Regular.
      Ventricular—Regular.
P waves: Flutter waves clearly seen after carotid sinus massage *(arrow)* decreases the ventricular response.
P-R interval: Flutter-R interval fairly constant.
QRS: Normal (0.08 second).

such as digoxin or deslanoside. The dose of digitalis necessary to slow the ventricular response varies and at times may result in toxic levels because it is often difficult to slow the ventricular rate during atrial flutter. Frequently, atrial fibrillation develops after digitalization and may revert to normal sinus rhythm on withdrawal of digitalis; occasionally, normal sinus rhythm may occur without intervening atrial fibrillation.

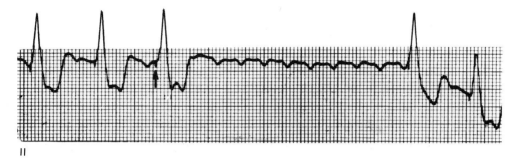

II

Fig. 6-28. Atrial flutter in a patient with complete A-V block. A ventricular pacemaker (pacemaker stimulus indicated by arrow) controls the ventricles and is suddenly turned off in the midportion of the tracing. Atrial flutter waves can be clearly discerned and fail to conduct to the ventricles. In the terminal portion of the tracing the ventricular pacemaker is turned on again.

Rate: Atrial—240.
　　　Ventricular—90 (paced).
Rhythm: Atrial—Regular
　　　　Ventricular—Regular.
P waves: Flutter waves with regular oscillations have no relationship to the ventricular rhythm.
P-R interval: Flutter-R interval varies.
QRS: Ventricular paced beats (0.14 second).

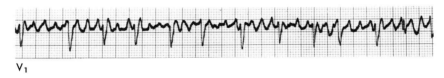

V₁

Fig. 6-29. Impure atrial flutter (coarse atrial flutter or flutter-fibrillation). Impure atrial flutter is characterized by a faster atrial rate than puse atrial flutter and more variability shows in the contour and spacing of the flutter waves.

Rate: Atrial—300 to 500.
　　　Ventricular—72 to 150.
Rhythm: Atrial—Irregular.
　　　　Ventricular—Irregular.
P waves: Variability in the contour and spacing of the flutter-fibrillation waves.
P-R interval: Nonmeasurable.
QRS: Normal (0.09 second).

3. If the atrial flutter persists after digitalization, quinidine, 200 to 400 mg orally every 6 hours, is used to restore sinus rhythm. Large doses of quinidine formerly used to terminate atrial flutter prior to the development of DC cardioversion are no longer warranted. If atrial flutter persists after digitalis and quinidine administration, termination may be attempted with DC cardioversion and the patient maintained on both digitalis and quinidine following reversion to sinus rhythm. Sometimes, treatment of the specific, underlying disorder, for example, thyrotoxicosis, is necessary to effect conversion to sinus rhythm.

4. In certain instances, atrial flutter may continue and if the ventricular rate can be controlled with digitalis, conversion may not be indicated. Quinidine maintenance therapy should be discontinued if flutter remains. It is important to remember that quinidine and procainamide should *not* be used unless the patient is fully digitalized. Both drugs have a vagolytic action and also directly slow the atrial rate. These two effects may facilitate A-V conduction sufficiently to result in a 1:1 ventricular response to the atrial flutter, unless digitalis has been administered previously.

5. Propranolol effectively diminishes the ventricular response to atrial flutter and may be used together with digitalis in patients in whom the ventricular rate is not decreased after digitalization. Propranolol does not appear to affect the atrial rate during atrial flutter.

6. Uncommonly, atrial flutter may be resistant to cardioversion as well as to the A-V blocking effects of digitalis. Rapid atrial pacing, on a temporary or permanent basis, may be used to convert flutter to fibrillation with a decrease in the ventricular rate.

7. Rarely, neostigmine (Prostigmin), 0.25 to 0.5 mg subcutaneously, or edrophonium (Tensilon), 0.25 to 2.0 mg per minute in an IV solution, may be administered over a few days to control the ventricular rate.

Prevention of recurrent atrial flutter is often difficult to achieve but should be approached as outlined for the prevention of PAT. If recurrences cannot be prevented, the aim of therapy is directed toward a controlled ventricular rate when the flutter does recur, with digitalis alone or combined with propranolol.

ATRIAL FIBRILLATION (Figs. 6-30 and 6-31)

Atrial fibrillation is characterized by a total disorganization of atrial activity without effective atrial contraction. The ECG reveals small deflections appearing for the most part as irregular base-line undulations of variable amplitude and contour at a rate of 350 to 600 per minute. The ventricular response is grossly irregular, and, if the patient is untreated, the rate is usually between 100 and 160 beats per minute. Carotid sinus massage slows the ventricular rate, but the rhythm remains grossly irregular. The conversion of atrial flutter to atrial fibrillation is usually accompanied by *slowing* of the ventricular rate because more atrial impulses become blocked at the A-V node. As a result, it is generally easier to slow the ventricular rate with digitalis during atrial fibrillation than during atrial flutter. When the ventricular rhythm becomes regular in patients with atrial fibrillation, four possibilities exist: conversion to sinus rhythm; conversion to atrial flutter; development of atrial tachycardia; or development of an independent junctional or ventricular rhythm (or tachycardia) controlling the ventricles and giving rise to A-V dissociation. In the latter two instances, digitalis intoxication must be suspected.

Significance. Similar to other tachyarrhythmias, atrial fibrillation may be chronic or paroxysmal; the former is almost always associated with underlying heart disease whereas the latter may occur in clinically normal patients. Underlying heart disease is more frequent in patients with atrial fibrillation than in patients with atrial flutter. The arrhythmia is commonly seen in patients with rheumatic mitral stenosis, thyrotoxicosis, cardiomyopathy, hypertensive heart disease, pericarditis, and coronary heart disease.

Approximately 30% of all patients with atrial fibrillation experience systemic or pulmonary emboli. Such a catastrophe is most common is patients with rheumatic mitral valvular disease. Ninety percent of the emboli that occur in patients with mitral stenosis occur in patients who have atrial fibrillation.

Treatment. It is of paramount importance in treating the patient who has atrial fibrillation for the first time to search for a precipitating cause. Thyrotoxicosis, mitral stenosis, acute myocardial infarction, pericarditis, and other known associated causes should be considered.

1. Initial therapy is determined by the patient's clinical status. The primary therapeutic objective is to slow the ventricular rate and, secondarily, to restore atrial systole. Both of these objectives may be accomplished by DC cardioversion. If the sudden onset of atrial fibrillation with a rapid ventricular rate results in acute cardiovascular decompensation, DC cardioversion is the treatment of choice, beginning with 50 to 100 watt-seconds.

2. In the absence of decompensation the patient may be given digitalis to maintain a resting apical rate of 60 to 80 beats per minute, which does not exceed 100 beats per minute after slight exercise. The speed, route, dosage, and type of digitalis preparation administered is determined by

the degree of cardiovascular compensation (see the discussion of the treatment of PAT). The ventricular rate cannot be slowed sufficiently by digitalis administration in some patients and digitalis toxicity may result prior to slowing the ventricular rate. In such cases, complicating factors such as pulmonary emboli, atelectasis, myocarditis, infection, congestive heart failure, and hyperthyroidism should be excluded and treated if found.

3. The combined use of digitalis and propranolol may be used to slow the ventricular rate when digitalis alone fails. Occasionally, conversion of atrial fibrillation to normal sinus rhythm may result from this combination or following the administration of digitalis alone.

4. Most often, however, the use of quinidine together with digitalis administration is necessary to convert the rhythm to a sinus mechanism. Because of the availability and safety of the electric cardioverter, it is preferable not to administer the large doses of quinidine that were used formerly to produce reversion to normal sinus rhythm. Rather, maintenance doses in the range of 1.2 to 2.4 gm per day should be administered for a few days prior to the planned DC cardioversion. During this time, 10% to 15% of patients will establish normal sinus rhythm. If sinus rhythm does not occur, digitalis is withheld for 1 to 2 days (while continuing quinidine) and DC cardioversion is carried out. Pretreatment with quinidine establishes an effective tissue concentration, determines whether the drug will be tolerated, improves chances of maintaining normal sinus rhythm after cardioversion, and reduces the number of shocks and level of energy required to restore normal sinus rhythm. Successful establishment of normal sinus rhythm by electric DC cardioversion occurs in over 90% of patients; with maintenance quinidine therapy, approximately 30% to 50% remain in normal sinus rhythm for 12 months.

Certain patients should not be considered for cardioversion. These include patients who have (1) known sensitivity or intolerance to quinidine or other antiarrhythmic agents (according to some studies, the recurrence rate of atrial fibrillation is higher in the absence of prophylactic quinidine administration), (2) repetitive paroxysmal atrial fibrillation that cannot be prevented by quinidine, (3) digitalis intoxication, (4) numerous conversion procedures without clinical improvement or preservation of sinus rhythm, (5) difficult-to-control atrial tachyarrythmias that finally eventuate into atrial fibrillation, (6) cardiac surgery planned in the near future, (7) a high degree of partial or complete atrioventricular block and thus a slow ventricular response, and (8) sick sinus syndrome.

Many elderly patients in the last two groups tolerate the atrial fibrillation well because the ventricular rate is slow and often do not require treatment with digitalis, unless the ventricular rate increases or congestive heart failure develops. Such patients may demonstrate serious supraventricular and ventricular arrhythmias after cardioversion because concomitant sinus node dis-

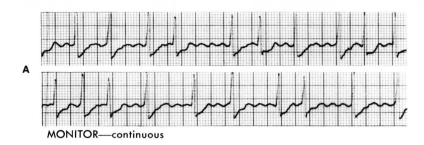

A

MONITOR—continuous

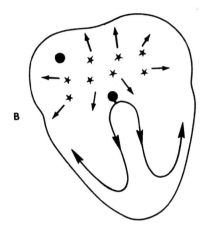

B

Fig. 6-30. **A, Atrial fibrillation.** Atrial activity is present as the undulating, wavy base line. In **B**, schematic is presented.

Rate: Atrial—350 to 600.
       Ventricular—In untreated atrial fibrillation, between 100 and 160 (75 to 160, average 130).
Rhythm: Atrial—Irregularly irregular.
         Ventricular—Irregularly irregular.
P waves: Irregular rapid base-line undulations called fibrillatory (F) waves.
P-R interval: Not measurable.
QRS: Generally normal (0.09 second).

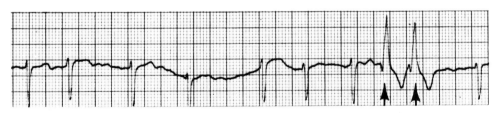

V₁

Fig. 6-31. **Atrial fibrillation.** A long ventricular pause followed by a short ventricular pause precedes the QRS complex with a right bundle branch block contour *(arrow)*; this QRS complex is followed after a short interval by a second QRS complex, also with right bundle branch block *(arrow)*. The aberrant QRS pattern indicates functional right bundle branch block (Ashman phenomenon).

Rate: Atrial—350 to 600.
       Ventricular—65 to 160.
Rhythm: Atrial—Irregularly irregular.
         Ventricular—Irregularly irregular.
P waves: Irregular rapid base-line undulations indicate fibrillatory atrial activity.
P-R interval: Not measurable.
QRS: Generally normal (0.08 second; two complexes indicated by arrows are functional right bundle branch block QRS complexes with a duration of 0.13 second).

ease becomes manifest after cardioversion. A related group of patients may have supraventricular tachycardias that alternate with bradycardias, and represent a subgroup of the sick sinus syndrome called "bradycardia-tachycardia syndrome." Usually, these patients are best treated with a ventricular pacemaker (to correct the slow rates) and digitalis (to control the ventricular rates during the supraventricular tachycardia).

In general, all other patients in whom improved circulatory hemodynamics are desirable may be considered candidates for electrical cardioversion. Failure to maintain normal sinus rhythm after electrical reversion is related to the duration of atrial fibrillation, the functional classification of the patient, and the etiology of the underlying heart disease. The likelihood of establishing and maintaining sinus rhythm should be weighed against the risks of cardioversion or other forms of therapy. The presence of multiple factors that adversely affect maintenance of sinus rhythm militates against cardioversion attempts.

Anticoagulation prior to cardioversion is indicated in patients with a high risk of emboli, that is, those with mitral stenosis and recent onset of atrial fibrillation, recent or recurrent emboli, or enlarged heart. The incidence of embolization during conversion to normal sinus rhythm is 1% to 3%.

ATRIAL TACHYCARDIA WITH A-V BLOCK (Figs. 6-32 and 6-33)

The atrial rate is usually between 150 and 200 beats per minute, with a range, similar to PAT, of 150 to 250 beats per minute. When caused by digitalis excess, the atrial rate is generally less than 200 beats per minute and may be noted to gradually increase as the digitalis is continued. The P-R interval may also gradually lengthen until Wenckebach second-degree A-V block develops. On occasion the degree of A-V block may be more advanced. Frequently, other manifestations of digitalis excess, such as premature ventricular systoles, coexist. In nearly 50% of cases of atrial tachycardia with block the atrial rate is irregular, whereas in paroxysmal atrial tachycardia the atrial rate is generally exceedingly regular. Characteristic isoelectric intervals between P waves, in contrast to atrial flutter, are usually present in all leads. However, at rapid atrial rates the distinction between atrial tachycardia with block and atrial flutter may be quite difficult. As in atrial flutter, carotid sinus massage slows the ventricular rate by increasing the degree of A-V block, but does not terminate the tachycardia.

Significance. Atrial tachycardia with block occurs most commonly in patients who have significant organic heart disease such as coronary artery disease or cor pulmonale. It is associated with digitalis excess in 50% to 75% of such patients.

A different type of atrial tachycardia, multifocal atrial tachycardia, is characterized by atrial rates of 100 to 250 beats per minute and marked variation in P wave morphology and in the P-P interval, is associated with a high mortality, and is rarely produced by digitalis.

Treatment If the ventricular rate is in a normal range and the patient is asymptomatic, often no therapy at all may be necessary.

1. Very slow ventricular rates may respond to atropine (0.5 mg increments IV) or rarely require ventricular pacing.
2. Atrial tachycardia with block in a patient who is not taking digitalis may be treated with digitalis to slow the ventricular rate.
3. If atrial tachycardia with block remains after digitalization, oral quinidine, disopyramide, or procainamide may be added.
4. The rhythm in some patients may resist termination by pharmacologic means, and, if digitalis excess is not the cause, DC cardioversion may be tried.
5. If atrial tachycardia with block appears in a patient receiving digitalis, it should be assumed initially that the digitalis is responsible for the arrhythmia, especially if the patient recently has received diuretics, the serum potassium level is low, the digitalis dose has been increased, or multiple premature ventricular systoles are also present. In such patients, initial therapy includes omission of digitalis and potassium-depleting diuretics and the administration of potassium chloride orally (30 to 45 mEq initially, repeated if necessary in 1 hour) or intravenously (0.5 mEq potassium chloride per minute in 5% dextrose and water during constant electrocardiographic monitoring for a total of 30 to 60 mEq

initially). A gradual slowing of the atrial rate with a decrease in A-V block usually occurs if the arrhythmia is caused by digitalis. In the presence of advanced A-V block, potassium, as well as other antiarrhythmic agents, must be given with great caution and under constant electrocardiographic monitoring. It should be remembered that renal dysfunction, acidosis, and excess digitalis predispose to the development of hyperkalemia and therefore potassium must be administered cautiously, along with frequent ECG, serum potassium, and blood urea nitrogen (BUN) checks.

6. Propranolol, 0.5 to 1 mg per minute IV for a total dose of 0.5 to 3 mg, or diphenylhydantoin, 50 to 100 mg IV every 5 minutes until the tachycardia terminates, the patient develops signs of toxicity such as nystagmus, vertigo, or nausea, or 1 gram is given, may be quite useful for digitalis-induced arrhythmias, including atrial tachycardia with block. The latter agent, since it does not appear to slow A-V conduction, may be particularly useful.

7. If these agents are not effective, further short-acting digitalis preparations may be given cautiously, assuming that the development of atrial tachycardia with block was not caused by digitalis.

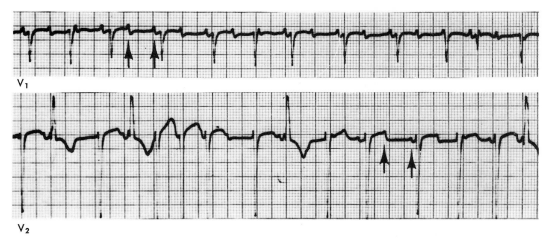

V₁

V₂

Fig. 6-32. Atrial tachycardia with A-V block. In the lower tracing, long-short QRS intervals, which follow longer intervals, set the stage for aberrant ventricular conduction that is manifest as a functional right bundle branch block. Arrows indicate P waves.

Rate: Atrial—150 to 250, generally 150 to 200 (167).
       Ventricular—Varies according to the degree of A-V block (83 to 120).
Rhythm: Atrial—Frequently regular but may be irregular (regular).
          Ventricular—Irregular (2:1, 3:2, and 4.3).
P waves: Contour differs from sinus-initiated P waves.
P-R interval: Wenckebach cycles.
QRS: Generally normal (0.08 second; functional right bundle branch block in lower tracing with a duration of 0.12 second).

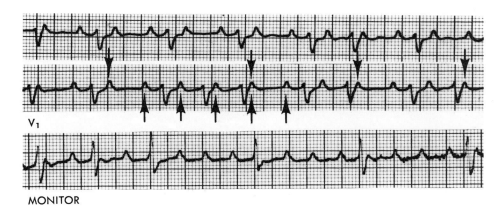

V₁

MONITOR

Fig. 6-33. Atrial tachycardia with A-V block caused by digitalis toxicity. Top two tracings recorded on admission. In the bottom tracing, continued digitalis administration increased the atrial rate to 193 beats per minute and increased the degree of A-V block. Upright arrows indicate P waves; inverted arrows indicate nonconducted P waves.

Rate: Atrial—150, top; 193 bottom.
       Ventricular—83 to 125, top; 50 to 94, bottom.
Rhythm: Atrial—Regular
          Ventricular—Varies (2:1, 3:1, 4:1, 4:3, etc).
P waves: Contour differs from sinus-initiated P waves.
P-R interval: Wenckebach cycles.
QRS: Normal (0.09 second).

PREMATURE A-V JUNCTIONAL SYSTOLES (Fig. 6-34)

Rhythms formerly called nodal, coronary nodal, and coronary sinus are now termed "A-V junctional." the latter term, which includes the A-V nodal–His bundle area, is preferred to terms that imply a more exact site of impulse origin because the exact location at which the impulse originates often cannot be determined from the surface ECG. A premature A-V junctional systole arises in the A-V junction and spreads in an anterograde and retrograde fashion. If unimpeded in its course, the impulse discharges the atrium to produce a premature retrograde P wave and a QRS complex with a supraventricular contour. Retrograde atrial activation generally results in a negative P wave in leads II, III, aV_F, and V_6, with positive P waves in leads I, aV_L, aV_R, and V_1. The retrograde P wave may occur before, be buried in, or less commonly follow the QRS complex. The site at which the impulse originates, as well as the relative speeds of anterograde and retrograde conduction, determines the relationship of the P wave to the QRS complex. A compensatory pause commonly follows a premature A-V junctional systole, but if the atrium and sinus node are discharged retrogradely, a noncompensatory pause results.

Significance and treatment. The significance of premature A-V junctional systoles is discussed under premature ventricular systoles.

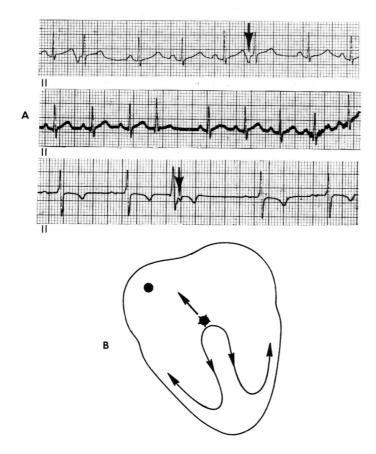

Fig. 6-34. A, Premature A-V junctional systoles. Premature junctional systoles seen in the top, middle, and bottom tracings were formerly called upper, mid, and lower nodal premature systoles, respectively, because the retrograde P wave was inscribed before, during, and after the QRS complex. Since not only the site of origin, but the relative speeds of anterograde and retrograde conduction determine the P-QRS complex relationship during a premature A-V junctional systole, it is best to use the nonspecific term "premature A-V junctional systole" for all three types. Note that the QRS complex maintains an almost identical contour to the normally conducted beats. Slight QRS aberration occurs in the middle recording. Monitor lead from three different patients; arrows-indicate P waves. In **B,** schematic illustration presented.

Rate: Determined by basic rate and number of premature systoles.

Rhythm: Irregular because of premature systoles; may be a regular irregularity as in bigeminy or trigeminy.

P waves: Atria discharged in a retrograde direction, producing negative (inverted) P waves in leads II, III, and aV_R and upright in aV_R. P waves may occur before (top), during (middle), or after (bottom) the QRS complex, depending on the site of origin of the premature systole and the status of anterograde and retrograde conduction.

P-R interval: Less than 0.12 second.

R-P interval: If P wave follows QRS, less than 0.20 second.

QRS: Generally normal, reflecting normal anterograde conduction to the ventricles. Contour may differ slightly from normal (0.08 second).

A-V JUNCTIONAL RHYTHMS (Figs. 6-35 to 6-37)

An A-V junctional escape beat occurs when the rate of impulse formation of the primary pacemaker (usually sinus node) becomes less than that of the A-V junctional region, or when impulses from the primary pacemaker do not penetrate down to the region of the escape focus. The interval from the last normally conducted beat to the escape beat is therefore greater than the normal R-R interval and is a measure of the initial rate of discharge of the A-V junctional focus. The inherent discharge rate of the A-V junctional escape focus (usually 40 to 60 per minute) determines when the junctional escape beat occurs. A continued series of A-V junctional escape beats is called an A-V junctional rhythm. An A-V junctional escape rhythm is usually fairly regular. Intervals between subsequent escape beats after the initial escape beat may gradually shorten as the rate of discharge of the escape focus increases (rhythm of development). The configuration of the QRS complex may differ from the normal sinus-initiated QRS complex; usually, it maintains the same contour as the normally conducted QRS.

The atria may be under retrograde control of the A-V junctional pacemaker or the atria may discharge independently (see discussion of A-V dissociation).

Significance. An A-V junctional escape beat(s) or rhythm may be a normal phenomenon owing to the effects of vagal tone or higher pacemakers or it may occur during pathologic slow sinus discharge and heart block. The escape beat or rhythm serves as a safety mechanism that assumes control of the car-

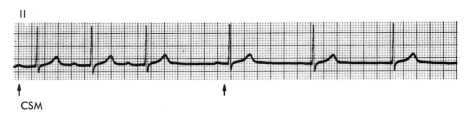

Fig. 6-35. A-V junctional rhythm. Carotid sinus massage (*CSM*, between arrows) produces significant sinus slowing to allow the escape of an A-V junctional rhythm (fourth QRS). Note unchanged QRS complexes and gradual acceleration of the escape rhythm from a rate of 48 beats per minute to 64 beats per minute. Atrial activity to the right of the last arrow is not apparent and may result from A-V junctional rhythm with retrograde capture of the P wave, lost within the QRS complex.

Rate: Atrial—40 to 100; any independent atrial arrhythmia may exist or the atria may be captured retrograde (atrial activity not apparent during the junctional rhythm).
   Ventricular—40 to 60 (48 to 64 during the junctional rhythm).
Rhythm: Ventricular, generally regular.
P waves and P-R interval: Relationship between P and QRS as explained under premature A-V junctional systoles. (P waves not apparent). P-R interval not determinable during junctional rhythm.
QRS: Generally normal (0.08 second); may be conducted with slight aberration.

diac rhythm owing to *default* of the primary pacemaker, so as to prevent the occurrence of complete ventricular asystole.

Treatment. Treatment, if indicated, lies in increasing the discharge rate of higher pacemakers or improving conduction with atropine or isoproterenol. Rarely, pacing may be needed.

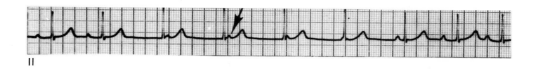

II

Fig. 6-36. A-V junctional rhythm. Transient, spontaneous sinus slowing allows the escape of an A-V junctional rhythm. P waves can be seen to occur just after the onset of the QRS complex *(arrow)* and represent normal sinus-initiated P waves. Gradual acceleration of the sinus rate reestablishes sinus control of the ventricular activity at the end of the tracing and thus terminates the period of A-V dissociation in the midportion of the tracing. The P-R interval is prolonged.

Rate: Atrial—45 to 70.
      Ventricular—58 to 70.
Rhythm: Atrial—Slowing.
      Ventricular—Slowing but fairly regular.
P waves: Normal.
P-R interval: See premature A-V junctional systoles (A-V dissociation in this tracing).
QRS: Normal (0.08 second).

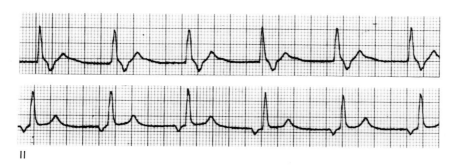

II

Fig. 6-37. A-V junctional rhythm with a changing P-QRS relationship. In the top tracing, retrograde atrial activity follows the QRS complex. In the bottom tracing, retrograde atrial activity precedes the QRS complex. Thus with the same A-V junctional rhythm in the same patient, atrial activity first followed and then preceded the QRS complex.

Rate: Atrial—65.
      Ventricular—65.
Rhythm: Regular.
P waves: Inverted; follow QRS in top tracing; precede QRS in bottom tracing.
P-R interval: 0.12 second, bottom.
R-P interval: 0.12 second, top.
QRS: Generally normal (0.08 second).

NONPAROXYSMAL A-V JUNCTIONAL TACHYCARDIA (Figs. 6-38 and 6-39)

Accepted terminology confers the label of tachycardia to instances when the rate exceeds 100 beats per minute. However, since rates greater than 60 to 70 beats per minute represent, in effect, a tachycardia for the A-V junctional tissue, the term "nonparoxysmal A-V junctional tachycardia" (NPJT), although not entirely correct, has been generally accepted when the rate of junctional discharge exceeds 60 to 70 beats per minute. NPJT usually has a more gradual onset and termination than does PAT or PJT, with a ventricular rate commonly between 70 and 130 beats per minute. The rate sometimes may be slowed by vagal maneuvers, as in sinus tachycardia, and the rhythm may not always be entirely regular. Although retrograde atrial activation may occur more commonly the atria are controlled by an independent sinus or atrial focus resulting in A-V dissociation.

Significance. The distinction between NPJT and PJT is etiologically and therapeutically quite important. NPJT occurs most commonly in patients who have underlying heart disease, such as inferior wall infarction, acute rheumatic myocarditis, and following open heart surgery. Probably the most important cause is excessive digitalis, which only rarely produces PAT or PJT. It is especially important to recognize slowing and regularization of the ventricular rhythm caused by NPJT as an early sign of digitalis intoxication in a patient who has atrial fibrillation.

Treatment. The treatment for NPJT is as follows:

1. If the ventricular rate is rapid, the cardiovascular status compromised, and the patient is not taking digitalis, digitalization should be the first measure.

2. Uncommonly in an emergency situation of if the arrhythmia does not respond to digitalization and is *clearly not induced by digitalis*, electrical DC cardioversion may be employed.

3. However, if the patient tolerates the arrhythmia well, careful monitoring and attention to the underlying heart disease is usually all that is needed. The arrhythmia will usually abate spontaneously.

4. If digitalis toxicity is the causative factor, the drug must be immediately stopped. Potassium may be given (see discussion of treatment of atrial tachycardia with block). The ECG should be monitored, since the blocking effects of potasium administration and digitalis are additive in the A-V junctional tissue and advanced A-V heart block may result. The rate of potassium administration is important, since a rapid infusion of the potassium, especially in a potassium-depleted patient, may result in transient cardiac arrest or depression of A-V conduction.

5. Lidocaine, propranolol, or diphenylhydantoin also may be tried.

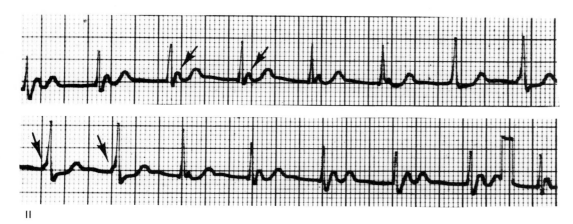

II

Fig. 6-38. Nonparoxysmal A-V junctional tachycardia. Atrial activity *(Arrows)* follows, then slightly precedes, and then once again follows the inscription of the QRS complex. Therefore A-V dissociation is present because of the accelerated A-V junctional discharge. This type of A-V dissociation is called "isorhythmic."

Rate: Atrial—60 to 100; any independent atrial arrhythmia may exist or the atria may be captured retrogradely (100).

    Ventricular—70 to 130; (100).

Rhythm: Atrial—Regular.

    Ventricular—Fairly regular.

P waves: Normal or retrograde capture (normal).

P-R interval: Depends on atrial and ventricular relationships (varying).

QRS: Generally normal (0.08 second); may be slightly aberrant.

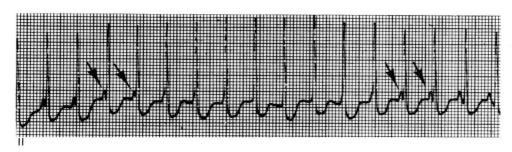

II

Fig. 6-39. Nonparoxysmal A-V junctional tachycardia. Atrial activity *(arrows)* at a very similar rate and rhythm to the QRS can be seen to precede, then occur simultaneously with, and once again precede the onset of the QRS complex. This type of A-V dissociation is called "isorhythmic."

Rate: Atrial—166.

    Ventricular—166.

Rhythm: Atrial—Regular.

    Ventricular—Regular.

P waves: Normal.

P-R interval: Varying.

QRS: 0.06 second.

VENTRICULAR ESCAPE BEATS (Fig. 6-40)

A ventricular escape beat results when the rate of impulse formation of supraventricular pacemakers (sinus node and A-V junctional) becomes less than that of potential ventricular pacemakers or when supraventricular impulses do not penetrate to the region of the escape focus because of S-A or A-V block. The inherent rate of discharge of ventricular escape pacemakers is usually 20 to 40 per minute. A continued series of ventricular escape beats is called a ventricular escape rhythm. The ventricular rhythm is usually fairly regular, although the rhythm may accelerate for a few complexes shortly after its onset (rhythm of development). The duration of the QRS complexes is prolonged to greater than 0.12 second because the origin of ventricular discharge is located in the ventricles. Sometimes the escape focus may shift from one to another portion of ventricle and may generate QRS complexes with a different contour and rate.

Significance. The presence of ventricular escape beats indicates significant slowing of supraventricular pacemakers or a fairly high degree of S-A or A-V block, and would therefore generally be considered abnormal.

Treatment. Depending on the cause, atropine, isoproterenol, or pacing would generally represent the therapeutic approach.

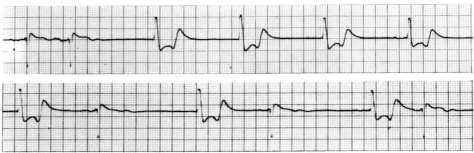

MONITOR—continuous

Fig. 6-40. Ventricular escape beats. Intermittent sinus arrest produced periods of asystole terminated by ventricular escape beats that are characterized by a prolonged, abnormal QRS complex. Intermittent return of sinus node activity establishes periods of supraventricular capture. The reason why A-V junctional escape beats did not terminate the asystolic periods is not known.

Rate: Atrial—40 to 100. Any independent atrial arrhythmia may exist or the atria may be captured retrogradely (intermittent sinus arrest).
  Ventricular—25 to 40 (43).
Rhythm: Atrial—Regular or irregular, depending on atrial rhythm (irregular).
  Ventricular—Generally regular (regular).
P waves: Normal or retrograde capture (normal).
P-R interval: Depends on atrial and ventricular relationships (varying).
QRS (Of ventricular escape rhythm): Prolonged greater than 0.12 second (0.13 second).

PREMATURE VENTRICULAR SYSTOLES (Figs. 6-41 to 6-43, 6-48)

A premature ventricular systole is characterized by the premature occurrence of a QRS complex, initiated in the ventricle, that has a contour different from the normal supraventricular complex and a duration usually greater than 0.12 second. The T wave is generally large and opposite in direction to the major deflection of the QRS. The QRS complex is generally not preceded by a premature P wave, but may be preceded by a sinus P wave occurring at its expected time. One must remember, however, that these criteria may be met by a supraventricular beat or rhythm that conducts aberrantly through the ventricle; in fact, aberrant supraventricular conduction may mimic all the manifestations of ventricular arrhythmia except ventricular fibrillation (see pp. 194 and 223).

Retrograde transmission to the atria from premature ventricular systoles occurs more frequently than stated in the earlier literature, but still probably does not occur commonly. The retrograde P wave produced in this fashion is often obscured by the distorted QRS complex. Usually a fully compensatory pause follows a premature ventricular systole. If the retrograde impulse discharges the sinus node prematurely and resets the basic timing, it may produce a pause that is not fully compensatory. A compensatory pause occurs more commonly with ventricular and A-V junctional premature systoles, but it can be seen that the presence of a compensatory pause is not invariably diagnostic. The normal sinus P wave following a premature ventricular systole may conduct to the ventricles with a long P-R interval, in which case a pause does not follow the premature ventricular systole and the latter is said to be *interpolated*. A *ventricular fusion beat* (the simultaneous activation of one chamber by two foci) represents a blend of the characteristics of the normally conducted beat and the beat originating in the ventricles, indicating that the ventricle has been depolarized from both atrial and ventricular directions. *Atrial fusion beats* may occur during ectopic atrial discharge and represent a blend of the characteristics of the sinus-initiated and ectopic atrial P waves. Whether a compensatory or noncompensatory pause, retrograde atrial excitation, an interpolated systole, a fusion systole or echo beat occurs is merely a function of how well the A-V junction conducts and the timing of the events taking place. The term *"bigeminy"* refers to pairs of beats or two contractions and may be used to indicate couplets of normal and ectopic ventricular systoles. Premature ventricular systoles may have differing contours and are called multifocal. More properly they should be called multiform, since it is not known that there are multiple foci discharging.

Significance. In individuals without organic heart disease, the presence of premature systoles may be manifested by the symptoms of palpitations or discomfort in the chest or neck, because of the greater than normal contractile force of the postectopic beats, or the feeling that the heart has stopped during the long pause after the premature systoles. Long runs of premature systoles in patients who have heart disease may produce angina or hypotension. Frequent interpolated premature systoles actually represent a doubling of the heart rate and may compromise the hemodynamic status. In the absence of underlying heart disease the presence of premature systoles may have no significance and not require suppression. Recently, however, it has been shown that premature ventricular systoles and complex ventricular arrhythmias occurring in asymptomatic middle-aged men are associated with the presence of coronary heart disease and with a greater risk of subsequent death from coronary heart disease.

Most of the drugs used to suppress premature systoles may also produce them on certain occasions. This is especially true of the digitalis preparations. On the other hand, digitalis often is effective in controlling premature atrial and ventricular systoles, especially those related to the presence of congestive heart failure. In patients suffering from acute myocardial infarction, premature ventricular systoles, such as those occurring close to the preceding T wave, greater than five or six per minute, bigeminal, multiformed, or occuring in salvos of two, three, or more, may presage or precipitate ventricular tachycardia or fibrillation.

Treatment. In the patient with an acute myocardial infarction, extremes of heart rate, both fast and slow, may provoke the development of premature ventricular systoles. Frequently, premature systoles accompanying slow ventricular rates caused by sinus bradycardia or A-V block may be abolished by increasing the basic rate with atropine or isoproterenol or by pacing at a faster rate with an artificial pacemaker. If the patient with sinus bradycardia has no hypotension, heart failure, or premature ventricular systoles and can be monitored closely, it appears best not to increase the heart rate. Faster rates increase the oxygen needs of the heart and may increase the degree of ischemia.

1. In the hospitalized patient, lidocaine, 1 to 2 mg per kilogram (50 to 100 mg) given as an IV bolus followed by an IV drip in a dose of 1 to 4 mg per minute, is the initial treatment of choice. A second or third IV injection may be given at approximately 10- to 20-minute intervals after the first dose if necessary, but care should be taken not to exceed 400 to 500 mg per hour. In some instances, lidocaine may be given intramuscularly in a dose of 250 to 300 mg. The onset of action of lidocaine given IV is 45 to 90 seconds and the duration of action is 10 to 20 minutes. Lidocaine produces less hypotension and negative inotropic effects than procainamide or quinidine in doses having equivalent antiarrhythmic effects. It is ideal for use in patients who have renal disease, since less than 10% is excreted unaltered in the kidney and the rest is metabolized by the liver. In patients exhibiting allergic reactions to quinidine or procainamide, lidocaine is useful, since there appears to be no cross-sensitivity.

2. If maximum doses of lidocaine are unsuccessful, then procainamide, administered IV (50 to 100 mg per 1 to 3 minutes until suppression of the premature ventricular systoles occurs, toxic effects such as QRS widening or hypotension result, or 750 to 1000 mg is administered) may be tried. If successful, procainamide may then be given as a continuous IV infusion (2 to 6 mg per minute).

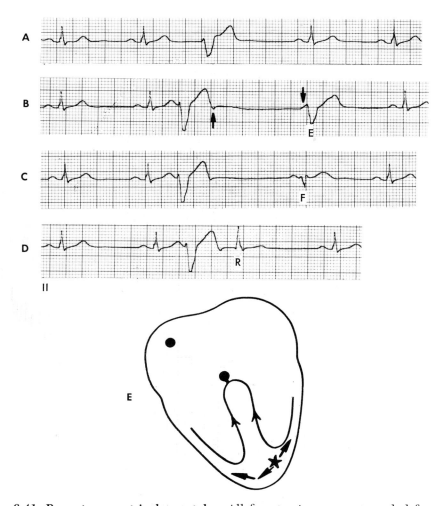

Fig. 6-41. Premature ventricular systoles. All four tracings were recorded from the same patient. In **A,** a relatively late premature ventricular systole is followed by a full compensatory pause. Sinus slowing makes the pause after the ventricular systole minimally greater than compensatory but its characteristics are essentially the same, that is, the interval between the two normal QRS complexes flanking the premature ventricular systole is twice the basic R-R interval. In **B,** an earlier premature ventricular systole in the same patient retrogradely discharges the atria (↑). This resets the sinus node and a ventricular escape beat *(E)* escapes before the next P wave (↓) can conduct to the ventricles. In strip **C,** the squence is the same as in **B,** except that the atrial rate is faster. This permits the P wave, following the premature ventricular systole and retrograde P wave, to partially depolarize the ventricles at the same time the ventricular escape beat occurs, resulting in a fusion beat *(F)*. In **D,** the sequence is the same as in **C,** except that after the impulse from the ventricle retrogradely discharges the atria, it returns to the ventricles to produce a ventricular echo, or reciprocal beat *(R)*. In **E,** a schematic illustration is presented.

Rate: Determined by basic rate and number of ventricular systoles.
Rhythm: Irregular because of premature systoles; may be a regular irregularity as in bigeminy or trigeminy.
P waves: Generally normal; may be captured retrogradely; often lost in QRS or T wave of premature ventricular systole.
P-R interval: Determined by whether P wave is blocked, conducted with a prolonged P-R interval, or retrogradely actived.
QRS: Wide, bizarre, greater than 0.12 second (0.14 second).

PREMATURE VENTRICULAR SYSTOLES (Figs. 6-41 to 6-43, 6-48—cont'd)

3. Oral maintenance therapy can be achieved with procainamide, 375 to 500 mg every 3 to 4 hours to produce therapeutic blood levels of 4 to 8 mg per liter, or with quinidine sulfate, 200 to 400 mg every 6 hours to produce serum levels of 3 to 6 mg per liter.

4. Propranolol or diphenylhydantoin may be tried if lidocaine, quinidine, and procainamide fail (see discussion of treatment of ventricular tachycardia).

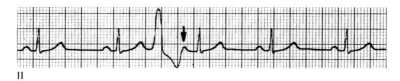

II

Fig. 6-42. Interpolated premature ventricular systole. A sinus-initiated P wave (↓) immediately following the premature ventricular systole conducts to the ventricles with a long P-R interval. Thus the normally expected compensatory pause is not present. The premature ventricular systole does not replace a normally conducted complex (see Fig. 6-41, *A*), but occurs *in addition* to the normally conducted complex. The P-R interval following the premature ventricular systole is prolonged owing to incomplete recovery of the A-V node because of partial retrograde penetration by the interpolated ventricular systole.

Rate, rhthm, and P waves: As in Fig. 6-41.
P-R interval: Prolonged following the interpolated premature ventricular extrasystole (0.20 second).
QRS: Wide, bizarre, greater than 0.12 second (0.14 second).

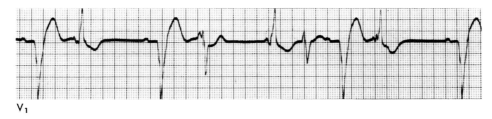

V₁

Fig. 6-43. Multiformed premature ventricular systoles. The normally conducted QRS complexes have a left bundle branch block morphology. The P-R interval is slightly prolonged (0.24 second). Premature QRS complexes with varying contours and coupling intervals are present and called *multiformed* ventricular extrasystoles. It is possible that these arise from different sites within the ventricle, in which case they would be *multifocal* in origin. This cannot be stated with absolute certainty from the surface ECG.

Rate, rhthm, P waves, and P-R interval: As in Fig. 6-41.
QRS: Wide, bizarre, greater than 0.12 second with varying contours and coupling intervals.

VENTRICULAR TACHYCARDIA (Figs. 6-44, 6-45, and 6-47)

Ventricular tachycardia is usually an ominous finding, indicating significant underlying cardiac disease. Although it occurs most commonly in patients with acute myocardial infarction and coronary artery disease, this arrhythmia also has been reported in patients presumed to have clinically normal hearts.

The electrocardiographic diagnosis of ventricular tachycardia is suggested when a series of three or more bizarre, premature ventricular systoles occur that have a duration greater than 0.12 second, with the ST-T vector pointing opposite to the major QRS deflection. The ventricular rate is between 110 and 250 beats per minute and the R-R interval may be exceedingly regular or it may vary. Atrial activity may be independent of ventricular activity (A-V dissociation) or the atria may be depolarized by the ventricles in a retrograde fashion (in which case A-V dissociation is *not* present). A repetitive type of intermittent paroxysmal ventricular tachycardia occurs less commonly and is characterized by bursts of premature ventricular systoles separated by a series of sinus beats.

The distinction between supraventricular and ventricular tachycardia may be difficult at times because the feature of both arrhythmias frequently overlap and under certain circumstances a supraventricular tachycardia can mimic the criteria established for ventricular tachycardia. Ventricular complexes with abnormal configurations only indicate that conduction through the ventricle is not normal; they do not necessarily indicate the origin of impulse formation or the reason for the abnormal conduction (see discussion of supraventricular arrhythmia with abnormal QRS complex).

The presence of fusion and capture beats provides evidence in favor of ventricular tachycardia. Fusion beats indicate simultaneous activation of the ventricles by two separate impulses (inferring that one of the impulses arose in the ventricles) whereas the capture beats signal supraventricular control of the ventricles, generally at a rate faster than the ventricular tachycardia. This proves that normal ventricular conduction can occur at cycle lengths equal to or shorter than the tachycardia in question, again implying that the origin of the wide QRS complexes lies in the ventricles rather than in aberrant supraventricular conduction.

Significance. Symptoms occurring during ventricular tachycardia depend on the ventricular rate, the duration of the tachyarrhythmia, and the severity of the underlying heart disease. The location of impulse formation and therefore the way in which the depolarization wave spreads across the myocardium also may be important. The immediate significance of ventricular tachycardia to the patient relates to the hemodynamic dysfunction it produces and the possible development of ventricular fibrillation.

The importance of a premature ventricular (rarely, atrial) complex initiating ventricular tachycardia or ventricular fibrillation when the premature systole occurs during the vulnerable period of the antecedent T wave must be stressed. The vulnerable period represents an interval of 20 to 40 msec lo-

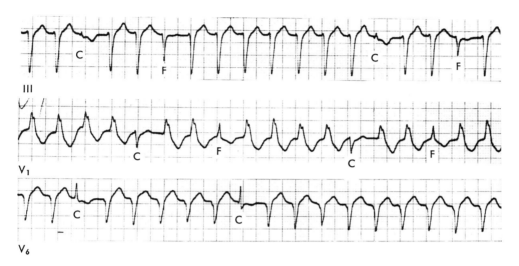

Fig. 6-44. Ventricular tachycardia. QRS complexes with a prolonged duration and a right bundle branch block morphology occur at a regular interval and are occasionally interrupted by QRS complexes with a normal contour (*C*, capture) or QRS complexes with an intermediate contour (*F*, fusion). Atrial activity cannot be seen; most likely, the atria are discharging independently to produce intermittent QRS captures and fusion beats. Therefore the most reasonable diagnosis is a ventricular tachycardia with A-V dissociation.

Rate: Atrial—60 to 100; any independent atrial arrhythmia may exist or the atria may be captured retrogradely (clear P waves not seen).

Ventricular—110 to 250 (150).

Rhythm: Atrial—Regular.

Ventricular—Fairly regular; may be irregular on occasion (regular).

P waves: Often lost in QRS; may be retrograde conduction to atria or atrial activity may be independently under control of sinus node (probably independent).

P-R interval: Generally not measurable.

QRS: Greater than 0.12 second (0.14 second).

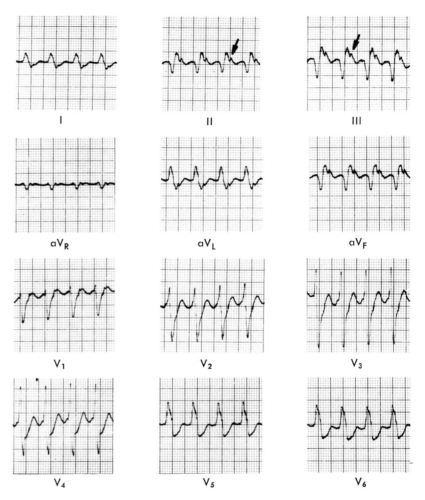

Fig. 6-45. Ventricular tachycardia with retrograde atrial capture. Ventricular tachycardia cannot be diagnosed with certainty from this surface ECG because all the features of this arrhythmia can be mimicked by a supraventricular tachycardia with aberrant ventricular conduction of a left bundle branch block type. His bundle electrocardiography proved that this was a ventricular tachycardia, however. The importance of the illustration lies in demonstrating 1:1 retrograde conduction to the atrium. Retrograde atrial activity indicated by arrows. Thus A-V dissociation is *not* present during this ventricular tachycardia.

Rate: Atrial—150.
      Ventricular—150.
Rhythm: Atrial—Regular.
      Ventricular—Regular.
P waves: Retrograde P waves inverted in 2, 3, and aV$_F$.
R-P interval: 0.16 second.
QRS: 0.12 second.

cated near the apex of the T wave during which the heart, when stimulated, is more prone to developing ventricular tachycardia or fibrillation (see discussion of ventricular fibrillation). The stimulus may be from an intrinsic source such as premature systole or from an extrinsic source such as a pacemaker or DC shock. During the interval of the vulnerable period, maximal electrical nonuniformity in the ventricular muscle is present, that is, ventricular muscle fibers are at varying stages of recovery of excitability. Some fibers have completely repolarized, others only partially repolarized, and still others may be completely refractory. Therefore stimulation during this period establishes nonuniform conduction with some areas of slowed conduction or actual block and sets the stage for repetitive reentrant excitation. Generally this R-on-T phenomenon occurs in patients with organic heart disease such as acute myocardial infarction, which explains the ominous importance of premature systoles in these patients. Slow (and, in some cases, fast) rates, drug toxicity (digitalis, quinidine, procainamide), electrolyte imbalance, and hypoxemia represent other clinical situations in which the R-on-T phenomenon may occur. It cannot be forgotten, however, that ventricular tachycardia or fibrillation may begin without preexisting or precipitating ventricular extrasystoles.

Treatment. The treatment for ventricular tachycardia is as follows:

1. Ventricular tachycardia that does not cause any hemodynamic decompensation may be treated medically by administering lidocaine IV in a bolus of 1 to 2 mg per kilogram body weight. A second or third IV injection of the drug may be given at approximately 10 to 20 minute intervals after the first dose if necessary but care should be taken not to exceed 400 to 500 mg per hour. The dose should probably be reduced in patients who have liver disease, heart failure, or shock. If lidocaine abolishes the ventricular tachycardia, then a continuous IV infusion of 1 to 4 mg per minute should be given to the patient.

2. If maximum doses of lidocaine are unsuccessful, procainamide administered IV (50 to 100 mg per 1 to 3 minutes until termination of the tachycardia occurs, toxic effects such as QRS widening or significant hypotension result, or 750 to 1000 mg is administered) may be tried. If successful, procainamide may then be given as a continuous IV infusion (2 to 6 mg per minute).

3. If the arrhythmia does not respond to medical therapy, cardioversion may be used. However, ventricular tachycardia that precipitates hypotension, shock, angina, or congestive heart failure should be treated *promptly* with DC cardioversion. Very low energies may terminate ventricular tachycardia; we generally begin with a synchronized shock of 10 to 50 watt-seconds (see discussion of Treatment of ventricular fibrillation). Digitalis-induced ventricular tachycardia is best treated medically. After reversion of the arrhythmia to a normal rhythm, it is essential to institute measures to prevent a recurrence (see Chapter 8 for discussion of cardioversion).

4. A search for reversible conditions contributing to the initiation and maintenance of ventricular tachyarrhythmias should be made and the conditions corrected if possible. For example, the ventricular arrhythmia related to hypotension of hypokalemia may at times be terminated by the use of vasopressors or potassium. Slow ventricular rates that are caused by sinus bradycardia or A-V block may permit the occurrence of premature systoles and ventricular tachyarrhythmias that can be corrected by administration of atropine, 0.5 mg IV, temporary isoproterenol administration (1 to 2 μg per minute in an IV drip), or temporary transvenous pacing.

5. Intermittent ventricular tachycardia, interrupted by one or more supraventricular beats, is best treated medically. If lidocaine and procainamide prove unsuccessful, then quinidine (200 to 400 mg orally or intramuscularly every 6 hours), propranolol (0.5 to 3 mg IV, 10 to 60 mg orally every 6 hours), or diphenylhydantoin IV (50 to 100 mg IV every 5 minutes until the tachycardia terminates, 1000 mg is given, or toxic symptoms such as nausea, ataxia, or vertigo result) or orally (250 mg every 6 hours the first day, followed by 100 mg every 6 hours thereafter) may be tried. Maintenance oral therapy with procainamide (375 to 500 mg every 3 to 4 hours) may be useful.

6. Striking the patient's chest may terminate ventricular tachycardia by mechanically inducing a premature ventricular systole that presumably interrupts the reentrant pathway necessary to support the ventricular tachycardia sometimes called ("thumpversion"). Similarly, ventricular pacing may stop a ventricular tachycardia. Stimulation at the time of the vulnerable period during ventricular tachycardia with either method may provoke ventricular fibrillation.

Prevention of recurrences may be difficult at times:

1. Initial preventive drug therapy for recurrent ventricular arrhythmias in the ambulatory patient should be with quinidine or procainamide. Procainamide is given as a loading dose of 0.5 to 1 gm orally, followed by 375 to 500 mg three to six times daily. Because procainamide has a shorter duration of action than quinidine, giving procainamide at 6-hour intervals may fail to provide therapeutic blood levels for the entire 6-hour period. If the arrhythmia fails to respond, procainamide should be administered at 3-hour intervals to ensure adequate therapeutic serum levels in the range of 4 to 8 mg per liter at all times. Hard-to-control arrhythmias may reflect poor absorption of the drug or nontherapeutic blood levels in between too widely spaced doses.

2. Alternatively, quinidine may be tried, administered at a dose of 200 to 400 mg four times daily, to achieve therapeutic blood levels of 3 to 6 mg per liter. Following an initial approach with procainamide or quinidine, diphenylhydantoin or propranolol may be tried.

3. Combinations of drugs with different mechanisms of action may be successful and allow one to use low doses of both agents rather than high or

toxic doses of one drug. For example, propranolol, 40 mg daily, combined with average doses of quinidine or procainamide may be efficacious. Similarly, procainamide or quinidine plus diphenylhydantoin might be effectively combined.

4. Administration of potassium to maintain serum potassium levels in the 5+ range, in addition to antiarrhythmic agents, may be helpful.

5. A trial of ventricular or atrial pacing, combined with antiarrhythmic agents if necessary, may be tried empirically, and if successful, permanent pacing may be instituted.

6. Once contributing factors have been sought and corrected, available antiarrhythmic agents have been tried singly and in combinations using maximally tolerated doses, correlated with blood levels, and administered at sufficiently frequent intervals to provide 24-hour coverage, and a trial of atrial and ventricular pacing has been unsuccessful, therapy begins to take on heroic proportions. Cardiac catheterization and coronary angiograms should be considered in hopes that an arrhythmia-provoking ventricular aneurysm or poorly contracting area may be found and resected, or coronary revascularization procedures may be performed to eliminate the arrhythmia or at least make it more manageable. Creation of hypothyroidism, cardiac sympathectomy, and cardiac surgery to interrupt a reentry pathway have been successful on occasion.

7. A number of new antiarrhythmia agents (see Appendix A) offer promise to control recurrent, life-threatening ventricular tachyarrhythmias.

ACCELERATED IDIOVENTRICULAR RHYTHM (Figs. 6-46 and 6-47)

The ventricular rate, commonly between 50 and 110 beats per minute, usually hovers within 10 beats of the sinus rate so that control of the cardiac rhythm may be passed back and forth between these two competing pacemaker sites. Consequently, long runs of fusion beats often appear at the onset and termination of the arrhythmia as the pacemakers vie for control of ventricular discharge. Because of the slow rates, capture beats are common. The onset of this arrhythmia is generally gradual (nonparoxysmal) and occurs when the rate of ectopic ventricular discharge exceeds the sinus rate because of sinus slowing, S-A or A-V block. The ectopic mechanism may also begin following a premature ventricular complex or the ectopic ventricular rate may simply accelerate sufficiently to overtake the sinus focus. The slow rate and nonparoxysmal onset avoid the problems initiated by excitation during the vulnerable period, and, consequently, precipitation of more rapid ventricular arrhythmias is rarely seen. Termination of the rhythm generally occurs gradually as the dominant sinus rhythm accelerates or the ectopic ventricular rhythm decelerates.

Significance. The arrhythmia occurs as a rule in patients with heart disease such as in the setting of acute myocardial infarction or as an expression of digi-

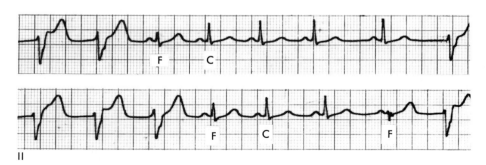

Fig. 6-46. Accelerated idioventricular rhythm. An accelerated idioventricular rhythm is present at the beginning and termination of the top and bottom strips. In the midportion of each tracing, slight sinus node acceleration reestablishes sinus node control by capturing the ventricles (C) and suppresses the accelerated idioventricular rhythm. When the sinus node slows, the accelerated idioventricular rhythm escapes. Fusion beats (F) may occur in the beginning and end of such arrhythmias because sinus and ventricular foci have similar rates.

Rate: Atrial—60 to 100; any independent atrial arrhythmia may exist or the atria may be captured retrogradely (70 to 90).
  Ventricular—50 to 110 (72).
Rhythm: Atrial—Regular.
  Ventricular—Generally regular although may be irregular (regular).
P waves: Often lost in the QRS; may be independent or may be retrogradely depolarized (independent).
P-R interval: Not measurable during accelerated idioventricular rhythm.
QRS: Greater than 0.12 second; fusion beats and capture beats often present (labeled F and C).

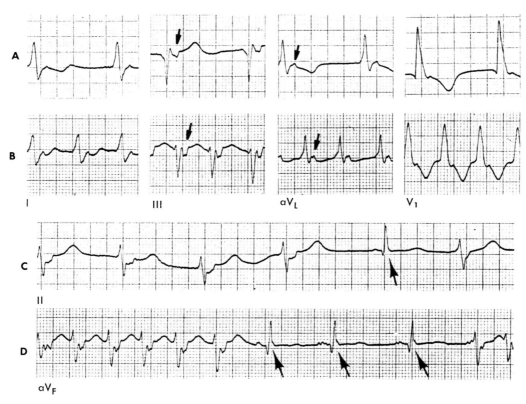

Fig. 6-47. Accelerated idioventricular rhythm and paroxysmal ventricular tachycardia.
An accelerated idioventricular rhythm and a paroxysmal ventricular tachycardia occurred at different times in this patient. **A** illustrates leads, I, III, aV_L V_1, and V_6 during
the accelerated ventricular rhythm, whereas **C** (lead II) illustrates the onset of the
accelerated idioventricular rhythm. **B** illustrates the paroxysmal ventricular tachycardia in leads I, III, aV_L, V_1, and V_6, whereas **D** (aV_F) illustrates the onset and termination
of the ventricular tachycardia. Retrograde atrial capture (↓) occurred during both tachycardias. Normally conducted QRS complexes present in **C** and **D** (↑). Note identical
QRS contours for both tachycardias (aV_L, V_1, and V_6 in **A** were recorded at different
standardization), indicating that they arose at same or similar areas of the ventricle.

Rate: Accelerated idioventricular rhythm (60). Ventricular tachycardia (varying slight, 150).
Rhythm: Accelerated idioventricular rhythm (regular). Paroxysmal ventricular tachycardia (reg-
    ular).
P waves: Retrogradely captured.
P-R interval: 0.14 second.
QRS: 0.14 second.

talis toxicity. It is transient and intermittent, with episodes lasting a few seconds to a minute, and does not appear to seriously affect the course or prognosis of the disease. Suppressive therapy is rarely necessary because the ventricular rate is generally less than 100 beats per minute. Basically, five conditions exist during which therapy may be considered: (1) when A-V dissociation results in loss of sequential atrioventricular contraction and, with it, the hemodynamic benefits of atrial contraction; (2) when accelerated idioventricular rhythm occurs together with paroxysmal ventricular tachycardia; (3) when accelerated idioventricular rhythm begins with a premature ventricular complex that has a short coupling interval that causes discharge in the vulnerable period; (4) when the ventricular rate is too rapid and produces symptoms; and (5) if ventricular fibrillation develops. The latter appears only rarely.

Treatment. Treatment for accelerated idioventricular rhythm is as follows:

1. The best initial therapeutic approach would appear to be close observation, rhythm monitoring, and care for the underlying heart disease.
2. Digitalis administration should be discontinued if the drug is implicated in the genesis of the arrhythmia.
3. Atropine, 0.5 mg IV initially, repeated if necessary to a total dose of 2.0 mg, may be used to speed the sinus rate and capture the ventricles.
4. Lidocaine may be given to suppress the ectopic ventricular focus.

VENTRICULAR FLUTTER AND VENTRICULAR FIBRILLATION (Figs. 6-48 to 6-50)

Ventricular flutter and ventricular fibrillation represent severe derangements of the heartbeat that usually terminate fatally within 3 to 5 minutes unless they are promptly stopped. Ventricular flutter resembles a sine wave in appearance, with regular, large oscillations occurring at a rate between 150 and 300 beats per minute, usually about 200 beats per minute. Ventricular fibrillation is recognized by the presence of irregular undulations of varying contour and amplitude. Distinct QRS complexes, ST segments, and T waves are absent. The difference between rapid ventricular tachycardia and ventricular flutter may be difficult and is usually of academic interest only.

Significance. Ventricular fibrillation occurs in a variety of clinical situations but is most commonly associated with coronary heart disease, acute myocardial infarction, and advanced forms of heart block. The arrhythmia occurs frequently as the terminal event in a variety of disease. It also may be seen during cardiac pacing, cardiac catheterization, operation, anesthesia, drug toxicity (for example, digitalis, quinidine, procainamide), and hypoxia. It may occur after electric shock administered during cardioversion or accidentally by improperly grounded equipment. Premature stimulation during the vulnerable period (R-on-T phenomenon; see discussion of Ventricular tachycardia) may precipitate ventricular tachycardia, flutter, or fibrillation, particularly when the ventricular fibrillation threshold has been lowered by the ischemia of an acute myocardial infarction, after a series of premature ventricular systoles, and during hypoxia and bradycardia.

Ventricular flutter or fibrillation results in faintness followed by loss of consciousness, seizures, apnea, and, if the rhythm continues untreated, death. The blood pressure is unobtainable and heart sounds are usually absent. The atria may continue to beat at an independent rhythm or be retrogradely captured for a time. Eventually, electrical activity of the heart is completely absent.

Treatment. Ventricular flutter and ventricular fibrillation are totally unphysiologic life-threatening arrhythmias for which immediate electrical (nonsynchronized) DC cardioversion, using 200 to 400 watt-seconds, is the only re-

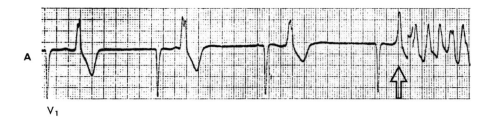

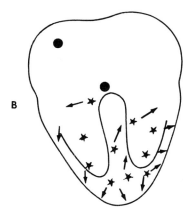

Fig. 6-48. A, Ventricular fibrillation. Premature ventricular systoles occurred in a bigeminal pattern with a decreasing coupling interval. The fourth premature ventricular systole discharged during the vulnerable period of the antecedent T wave and precipitated ventricular fibrillation *(arrow)*. In **B,** schematic illustration presented.

Rate: Atrial—60 to 100; any independent atrial arrhythmia may exist or the atria captured retrogradely.
    Ventricular—400 to 600.
Rhythm: Atrial—Regular; may be irregular if the atria are retrogradely captured.
    Ventricular—Grossly irregular.
P waves: Generally cannot be seen.
P-R interval: Generally not measurable.
QRS: Base-line undulations without distinct QRS contours.

liable treatment. When ventricular tachycardia produces the same hemodynamic response as ventricular flutter or fibrillation, it also must be immediately terminated by DC shock. A sharp blow to the chest may terminate some forms of ventricular tachyarrhythmias ("thumpversion") but time should not be wasted on this procedure if one or two sharp blows fail.

Termination of ventricular flutter or fibrillation within 30 to 45 seconds prevents the biochemical derangements accompanying ventricular fibrillation, eliminates the need for endotracheal intubation, and significantly increases the success rate of such procedures. If necessary, artificial ventilation by means of a tightly fitting rubber face mask and an AMBU bag is quite satisfactory and eliminates the delay attending intubation by inexperienced personnel. *There must be no delay in administering the DC shock.* If the patient is not monitored and it cannot be established whether asystole or ventricular fibrillation has caused the cardiovascular collapse, the electric shock should be administered *without* wasting precious seconds attempting to record the ECG. The DC shock may cause the asystolic heart to begin discharging, as well as terminate ventricular fibrillation if the latter is present. Following a successful cardioversion, measures must be taken to prevent a second episode of ventricular fibrillation, including monitoring of the cardiac rhythm, administration of lidocaine, and so forth.

Ventricular fibrillation is quickly followed by severe metabolic acidosis, and sodium bicarbonate, 1 to 3 ampules containing 44 mEq of sodium bicarbonate per ampule, may be used initially. The exact amount necessary depends on the pH, which in turn is related to the duration of the ventricular fibrillation. An additional ampule is given every 5 to 8 minutes until adequate cardiorespiratory function is achieved. Blood gases and pH should be obtained as soon as possible and further bicarbonate administration adjusted accordingly.

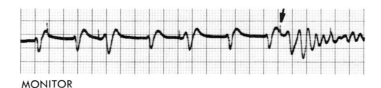

MONITOR

Fig. 6-49. Ventricular fibrillation. Pacemaker spikes *(arrow)* from a malfunctioning pacemaker fall randomly throughout the cardiac cycle at a slightly irregular interval. When the pacemaker spike discharged during the vulnerable period of the antecedent T wave *(arrow)*, it precipitated ventricular fibrillation. Ventricular rhythm preceding onset of ventricular fibrillation is probably slightly irregular, accelerated idioventricular rhythm.

Rate, rhythm, P waves, P-R interval and QRS: As in Fig. 6-48.

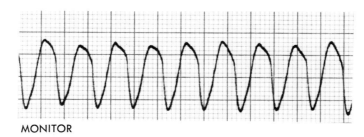

MONITOR

Fig. 6-50. Ventricular flutter. Ventricular flutter presents as a sine wave with regular large oscillations. The QRS complex cannot be definitely distinguished from the S-T segment or T wave.

Rate: Atrial—60 to 100. Any independent atrial arrhythmia may exist or the atria may be captured retrogradely.
　　　Ventricular—150 to 300, usually about 200 (195).
Rhythm: Atrial—Regular; may be irregular if atria are captured retrogradely.
　　　　Ventricular—Usually regular.
P waves: Generally cannot be seen.
P-R interval: Generally not measurable.
QRS: Prolonged to greater than 0.12 second (0.16 second).

FIRST-DEGREE A-V BLOCK (Figs. 6-51 and 6-52)

During first-degree heart block, A-V conduction is abnormally prolonged, manifested by a P-R interval greater than 0.20 second in the adult. P-R intervals as long as 1.0 second have been noted. Every atrial impulse is conducted to the ventricles, producing a regular ventricular rhythm.

Atropine, isoproterenol, and exercise normally shorten the P-R interval as the atrial rate increases; when the atrial rate is increased by atrial pacing, the P-R interval lengthens. Steroids tend to improve A-V conduction, which may lengthen during adrenal insufficiency.

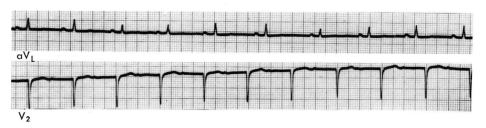

Fig. 6-51. First-degree A-V heart block. Leads aV_L and V_2 were recorded during the course of a 12-lead ECG in this patient. An increase in heart rate probably caused further abnormal lengthening of P-R interval (V_2) in this patient with abnormal A-V conduction.

Rate: Atrial rate and rhythm may vary, depending on whether sinus bradycardia or tachycardia, atrial tachycardia, and so on, is the atrial mechanism; generally normal (62 to 71 in a V_L; 78 in V_2).

Rhythm: Regular.

P waves: Normal contour and precede each QRS complex.

P-R interval: Prolonged to greater than 0.20 second; generally constant interval (0.22 in aV_L; 0.42 in V_2).

QRS: Generally normal (0.08 second).

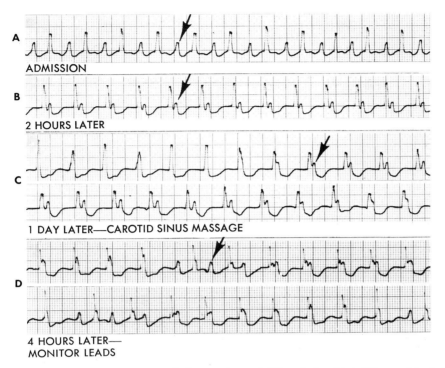

Fig. 6-52. First-degree and second-degree (type I, Wenckebach) A-V heart block in a patient with acute myocardial infarction. P waves indicated by arrows. On admission, **A,** first-degree heart block was present. Two hours later, **B,** the heart rate sped and lengthened the P-R interval. In the tracing recorded the following day, **C,** atrial activity was not apparent. Two possibilities exist: First, an A-V junctional rhythm could be present with retrograde atrial activity hidden within the QRS complex. Second, the patient may have developed a further lengthening of the P-R interval so that the sinus-initiated P wave was hidden within the QRS complex and conducted with a very long P-R interval to the following QRS complex. The P-R interval then would be approximately 0.56 second in duration. Carotid sinus massage, by slowing the sinus rate and the R-R interval as well, proves that the latter possibility is the correct diagnosis. Following release of carotid sinus massage (midportion of the second strip in panel C) the sinus rate speeds back to its previous rate. Four hours later, **D,** A-V conduction has worsened slightly with the development of type I (Wenckebach) second-degree A-V block. Some variations in the QRS complex occur.

Rate: A, 108; **B,** 115; **C,** 105; **D,** atrial rate, 115 to 120.
Rhythm: Regular except for ventricular rhythm in **D.**
P waves: Generally normal (slightly increased in amplitude); precede each QRS.
P-R interval: Prolonged to greater than 0.20 second (varying in the different tracings; **A,** 0.26 second; **B,** 0.42 second; **C,** 0.56 second; **D,** Wenckebach A-V block).
QRS: Normal (0.08 second).

SECOND-DEGREE A-V BLOCK (Figs. 6-53 to 6-57)

Failure of some atrial impulses to conduct to the ventricles at a time when physiologic interference would not be expected constitutes second-degree A-V block. The nonconducted P wave may be intermittent or frequent, occur at regular or irregular intervals, and be preceded by fixed or lengthening P-R intervals. A distinguishing feature is that conducted P waves relate to a QRS complex with recurring P-R intervals, that is, the association of P with QRS is not random. The two types of second-degree A-V block can be distinguished by analysis of the P-R intervals. In type I (Wenckebach) second-degree A-V block a gradual lengthening of the P-R interval occurs because of lengthening A-V conduction time, until an atrial impulse is nonconducted. Then the sequence begins again. The ratio of atrial impulses to ventricular responses is frequently 5:4, 4:3, 3:2, or 3:1. Because the increment in conduction time is greatest in the second beat of the Wenckebach group and then *decreases* progressively over succeeding cycles, the interval between successive R-R

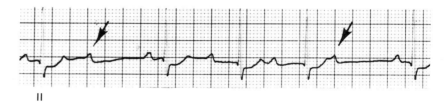

II

Fig. 6-53. Second-degree A-V heart block (type I Wenckebach). A-V Wenckebach is characterized by progressive P-R prolongation preceding the nonconducted P wave. Wenckebach A-V block, in the presence of a normal QRS complex, is virtually always at the level of the A-V node. Conduction ratios are 2:1, 4:3, and 3:2 in this tracing. Because the increment in conduction time is greatest in the second cycle of the Wenckebach group and then decreases progressively over succeeding cycles, the following characteristics are also present: (1) the interval between successive R/R cycles prior to the nonconducted P wave progressively decreases; (2) the duration of the pause produced by the nonconducted P wave is less than twice the shortest cycle, which is generally the cycle immediately preceding the pause; (3) the duration of the R-R cycle following the pause exceeds the duration of the R-R cycle preceding the pause. These features can be seen in the middle 4:3 grouping and should be compared with the P-P intervals in Fig. 6-16. Blocked P waves indicated by arrows.

Rate: Atrial—Atrial rate and rhythm may vary, depending on whether sinus bradycardia or tachycardia, atrial tachycardia, and so forth, is the atrial mechanism; generally normal (83).

Ventricular—Depends on degree of A-V block, which may vary between 2:1, 3:2, 4:3, 5:3, etc.

Rhythm: Atrial—Regular.

Ventricular—Varying, depending on the degree of A-V block.

P waves: More numerous than QRS complexes but are related to ventricular beats in a consistent, repetitive fashion.

P-R interval: Progressive P-R prolongation preceding the nonconducted P wave. Finally, one P wave is blocked and the cycle then repeats.

QRS: Normal; R-R interval gradually shortens until the blocked P wave occurs; the cycle then repeats.

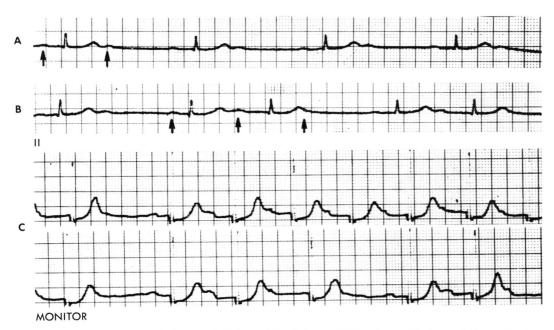

MONITOR

Fig. 6-54. Second-degree A-V heart block (type I Wenckebach). In **A**, 2:1 conduction occurs (arrows indicate P waves). Since 2:1 conduction can occur with either type I or type II second-degree heart block, one sometimes cannot readily distinguish the two. The presence of a normal QRS complex is certainly in favor of this being type I second-degree A-V heart block, however. In **B**, the 2:1 A-V heart block becomes 3:2 and P-R prolongation for the second conducted P wave (second arrow) establishes the diagnosis of type I second-degree A-V heart block. **C** (continuous recording), illustrates the response of Wenckebach A-V block to intravenous atropine. Both the atrial rate and the conduction ratio increase.

Rate: Atrial—(In **A** and **B**, 72; in **C**, 79).
　　　　Ventricular—(In **A**, 36; in **B**, varying; in **C**, varying but increased).
Rhythm: Atrial—Regular.
　　　　　Ventricular—Varying depending on the degree of A-V block.
P waves: Normal.
P-R interval: Progressive increase in P-R interval until one P wave fails to conduct.
QRS: Normal (0.07 second).

SECOND-DEGREE A-V BLOCK (Figs. 6-53 to 6-57—cont'd)

cycles prior to the nonconducted P wave progressively *decreases*, the duration of the pause produced by the nonconducted P wave is less than twice the shortest cycle, and the duration of the R-R cycle following the pause exceeds the R-R cycle preceding the pause.

In type II second-degree A-V block, a P wave is blocked without progressive antecedent P-R prolongation and occurs almost always in the setting of bundle branch block. The P-R interval of the conducted atrial impulses may be prolonged or normal, but usually remains fairly constant. The pause caused by the nonconducted P wave is equal to or may be slightly less than twice the normal R-R interval. Sinus arrhythmia, premature beats, A-V junctional escape beats, or changes in neurogenic influences may disturb the timing of the expected pauses.

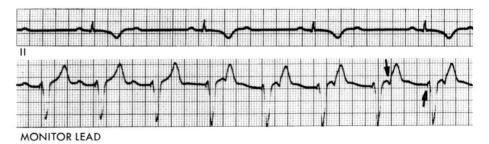

MONITOR LEAD

Fig. 6-55. 2:1 anterograde A-V block and 1:1 retrograde V-A conduction. In the top tracing, alternate P waves conduct to the ventricles. In the lower tracing (same patient), ventricular pacing (upright arrow indicates pacemaker artifact) establishes 1:1 retrograde atrial conduction beginning with the fourth paced QRS complex. Inverted arrow indicates retrograde atrial activation.

Rate: Atrial—Top tracing, 68; bottom tracing, 70.
     Ventricular—Top tracing, 34; bottom tracing, 70.
Rhythm: Atrial—Regular.
     Ventricular—Regular.
P waves: Top tracing, normal; bottom tracing, retrograde.
P-R interval: Top tracing, 0.20 second; conduction of alternate P waves.
R-P interval: Bottom tracing, 0.16 second.
QRS: Top tracing, 0.08 second; bottom tracing, 0.14 second.

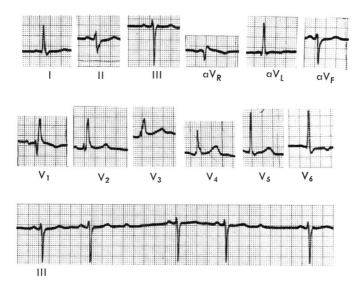

Fig. 6-56. Second-degree A-V heart block, type II. The 12-lead ECG indicates the presence of left anterior fascicular block and right bundle branch block. In the rhythm recording (lead III) sudden failure of A-V conduction results without antecedent P-R prolongation.

Rate: Atrial rhythm and rate may vary, depending on whether sinus bradycardia or tachycardia, atrial tachycardia, and so forth, is the atrial mechanism. Generally, normal sinus rhythm 60 to 100 (62).

Rhythm: Atrial—Regular.

Ventricular—Varying, depending on the degree of A-V block.

P waves: Normal.

P-R interval: Normal, constant (0.14 second) or may be prolonged constant; sudden failure of conduction.

QRS: Prolonged (0.12 second).

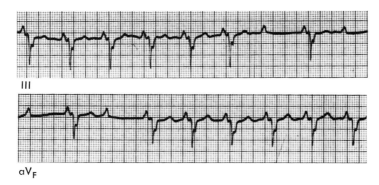

Fig. 6-57. Second-degree A-V heart block, type II. Right bundle branch block (not readily apparent in leads III and aV_F) along with left anterior fascicular block is present in this patient. Sudden failure of A-V conduction results without antecedent P-R prolongation. The P-R interval for the conducted beats is normal, as it often is during type II second-degree A-V heart block.

Rate: 86.

Rhythm: Atrial—Regular.

Ventricular—Varying, depending upon the degree of A-V block.

P waves: Normal.

P-R interval: Normal, constant (0.12 second) or may be prolonged; sudden failure of conduction.

QRS: Prolonged; right bundle branch block and left anterior hemiblock (0.12 second).

COMPLETE A-V BLOCK (Figs. 6-58 and 6-59)

Complete A-V block occurs when no P waves are conducted to the ventricles. The atria and ventricles are controlled by independent pacemakers, and, as such, complete A-V block constitutes one form of complete A-V dissociation. The atrial pacemaker may be sinus of ectopic atial (tachycardia, flutter, or fibrillation). The ventricular focus may be above or below the His bundle bifurcation, depending on the site of the block. In congenital complete A-V block, the block is usually at the level of the A-V node, proximal to the His bundle. The escape focus is supraventricular and, as such, is more stable and faster than that which occurs with distal His block. The rhythm, usually regular, may vary because of premature ventricular beats, a shift in pacemaker site, or an irregularly discharging pacemaker focus. The QRS is normal, and Adam-Stokes syncope occurs less often. In acquired complete A-V block the ventricular rate is 30 to 40 beats per minute because the site of block is distal to the His bundle and consequently the escape focus is in the bundle branch–Purkinje system.

Significance. In the adult, drug toxicity (predominantly digitalis, but other drugs as well) and degenerative disease are the most common causes of acquired A-V heart block. The degenerative process produces partial or complete anatomic or electrical disruption within the A-V nodal region, the A-V bundle, or both bundle branches. Multiple factors may contribute to this degenerative process. They include fibrosclerosis of the cardiac skeleton, fibrosis of the conduction system, coronary artery disease, myocarditis, and cardiomyopathies. Operation is an infrequent but still important cause of heart block. Less commonly, electrolyte disturbances, endocarditis, tumors, Chagas' disease, syphilitic gummas, rheumatoid nodules, myxedema, infiltrative processes such as amyloidosis, sarcoidosis, or scleroderma, and other systemic illnesses may lead to A-V heart block. Calcium deposition in the region of the aortic and mitral valves may extend to involve the conduction pathways. Digitalis excess produces type I, not type II, second-degree A-V block.

A-V heart block occurring during a myocardial infarction may be divided into two groups: that which occurs during an anterior or anteroseptal infarction and that which occurs during a diaphragmatic (inferior) infarction. When an anterior wall infarction produces A-V block, it is usually the result of extensive necrosis of the summit of the interventricular septum, which spares the A-V node and His bundle but inflicts severe damage to the bundle branches. Consequently, the block is apt to be distal to the His Bundle (type II) and associated with right bundle branch block and a form of fascicular block. Complete A-V block may develop, during which the ventricular rate is less than 40 beats per minute, asystole and syncope occur more commonly, and the mortality rate is 75% or higher. Death results from pump failure or shock, owing to the large size of the infarction.

When A-V block results from diaphragmatic infarction, the block, type I, usually occurs in the region of the A-V node, owing to inflammation or edema that results from ischemia or infarction of neighboring myocardium. The ventricular pacemaker is faster and more stable, located in the region of the A-V node or His bundle, and the block is usually transient, without residua. Advanced block and syncope are uncommon, and the mortality in patients without associated heart failure does not appear to be increased. Some overlap occurs between these two divisions.

Symptoms during second-degree A-V block are infrequent unless long periods of A-V block occur. The slow ventricular rate during complete heart block may not maintain circulation effectively and may result in angina, congestive heart failure, or syncope. Ventricular asystole may occur or the slow rate may initiate ventricular premature systoles or tachyarrhythmias.

Treatment

First-degree A-V block. Generally no therapy is required. If digitalis,

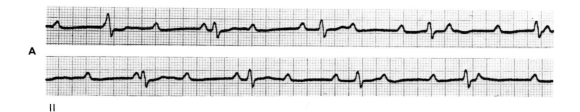

A

II

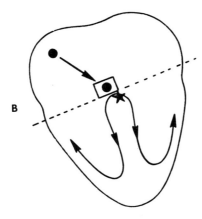

B

Fig. 6-58. A, Third-degree (complete) A-V heart block. Complete A-V dissociation is present *resulting from* complete heart block. The abnormal QRS complexes (prolonged duration) indicate a ventricular origin for the escape rhythm. In **B,** schematic illustration is presented.

Rate: Atrial—Any independent arrhythmia may exist or the atrial may be captured retrogradely. Generally, sinus rhythm 60 to 100 (85).

Ventricular—Less than 40 (38).

Rhythm: Atrial—Regular.

Ventricular—Regular.

P waves: Normal.

P-R interval: Completely variable.

QRS: Prolonged (0.12 second).

quinidine, or procainamide is implicated, the offending drug must be stopped or its dosage reduced.

Second-degree A-V block

TYPE I. Generally no therapy is required. Treatment may be necessary for patients who are symptomatic with very slow ventricular rates. Atropine, 0.5 mg increments IV or isoproterenol, 1 to 2 μg per minute, may be tried initially. If there is no response or if the block remains for prolonged periods, pacemaker therapy may be used. Digitalis, if implicated, must be stopped.

TYPE II. If type II block develops in the setting of an acute myocardial infarction, temporary transvenous pacing is necessary because this form of block presages the occurrence of sudden complete A-V block with ventricular asystole and Adams-Stokes syncope. Prior to pacemaker insertion, isoproterenol may be used temporarily. Atropine, by increasing the atrial rate without decreasing the A-V block, may cause more P waves to block and reduce the ventricular rate.

Third-degree (complete) A-V block.

If third degree, or complete, A-V block develops in the setting of an acute myocardial infarction, temporary transvenous pacing is necessary; isoproterenol may be used initially if necessary. Patients with chronic stable complete A-V block who are asymptomatic may need no specific therapy. For those patients with symptoms of congestive heart failure or Adams-Stokes syncope caused by ventricular asystole, severe ventricular bradycardia, or ventricular tachyarrhythmias occurring as a result of the A-V block, long-term drug therapy is generally unreliable and permanent pacemaker implantation is indicated.

BUNDLE BRANCH BLOCK

Anatomic or functional discontinuity in one of the bundle branches may prevent or slow conduction so that the ventricle on the affected side becomes activated late, because this ventricle, normally supplied by the blocked bundle branch, must be activated by impulses traveling through the ventricular wall and interventricular septum from the unaffected side. Conduction along this circuitous route proceeds more slowly and therefore the QRS complex becomes widened to 0.10 to 0.12 second (incomplete) or more than 0.12 second (complete right or left bundle branch block). Transient bundle branch block may occur as a result of tachycardia, pulmonary embolism, anemia, infection, myocardial infarction, congestive heart failure, metabolic derangements, or hypoxia.

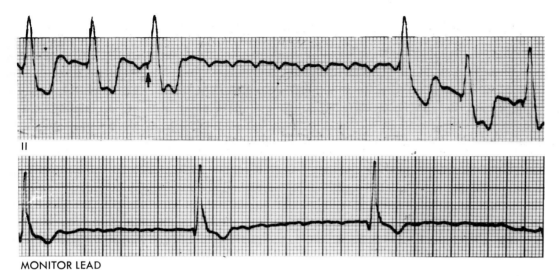

II

MONITOR LEAD

Fig. 6-59. Complete (third-degree) A-V heart block during atrial flutter and atrial fibrillation. In the top tracing a ventricular pacemaker controls ventricular activity (arrow indicates pacemaker artifact). In the midportion of the tracing the ventricular pacing was temporarily discontinued and one can easily see the atrial flutter waves that fail to conduct to the ventricle. In the terminal portion of the tracing the ventricular pacemaker was turned on once again. In the bottom tracing the undulating baseline indicates the presence of atrial fibrillation. The regular ventricular rhythm establishes that none of the atrial fibrillatory impulses conduct to the ventricles; thus complete A-V block is present during atrial fibrillation.

Rate: Atrial—Top tracing, 250; bottom tracing, 400 to 600.

  Ventricular—Top tracing, 100; bottom tracing, 32.

Rhythm: Atrial—Top tracing, regular; bottom tracing, irregular.

  Ventricular—Top tracing, regular; bottom tracing, regular.

P waves: Top tracing, atrial flutter; bottom tracing, atrial fibrillation.

P-R interval. Totally variable or nonmeasurable.

QRS: Top tracing, ventricular paced beats (0.16 second); bottom tracing, 0.14 second.

LEFT BUNDLE BRANCH BLOCK (Fig. 6-60)

In complete left bundle branch block (LBBB) the QRS complex becomes prolonged more than 0.12 second, with the major slowing occurring in the mid and terminal forces. The initial forces are deformed and prevent the development of the normal septal Q wave in I or V_6. Initial R waves in V_1 to V_3 are small or absent, followed by deep, large, slurred S waves, and large, prolonged R waves in V_5 and V_6. Significant mean axis deviation is usually absent. The ST segment and T wave shift are characteristically 180 degrees opposite the major QRS deflection.

Significance. LBBB is often associated with serious heart disease such as coronary artery disease, valvular heart disease, and hypertension. Although both RBBB and LBBB can occur in patients without apparent heart disease, LBBB correlates significantly with cardiomegaly and suggests a more serious prognosis. The conduction defect caused by LBBB alters the initial QRS vector, often obscuring the Normal ECG signs of an acute myocardial infarction.

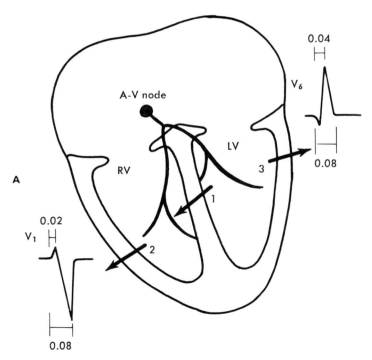

Fig. 6-60. A, Normal intraventricular conduction. Intrinisicoid deflection (interval from onset of QRS complex to peak of R wave, upper brackets) is usually about 0.02 second in right precordial leads and 0.03 to 0.04 second in left precordial leads. The intrinisicoid deflection prolongs during bundle branch block. **B,** Twelve-lead ECG illustrating left bundle branch block. The axis is −30 degrees. **C,** Schematic illustration is presented.

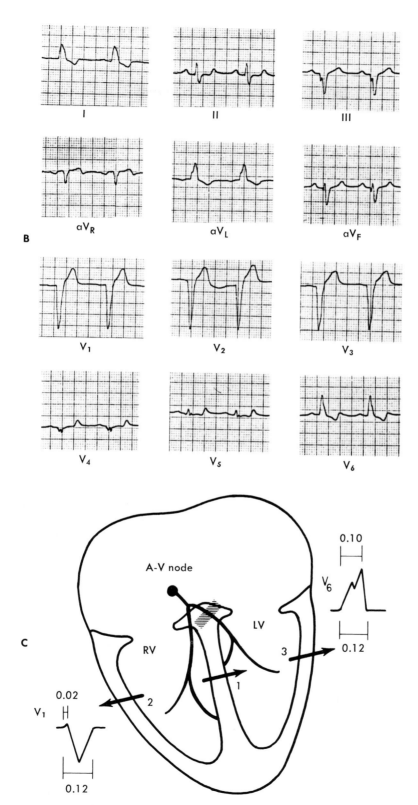

Fig. 6-60, cont'd. For legend see opposite page.

RIGHT BUNDLE BRANCH BLOCK (Fig. 6-61)

In uncomplicated complete right bundle branch block (RBBB) the QRS complex is 0.11 second or wider. The initial and mid forces of the vector loop are in a normal direction, and the terminal force is directed to the right and anteriorly. These changes produce large S waves in I, II, V_5, and V_6, often a terminal R wave in III, and R' in V_1 and V_2. Incomplete RBBB is associated with the same electrocardiographic pattern, but the QRS complex is 0.10 second or less.

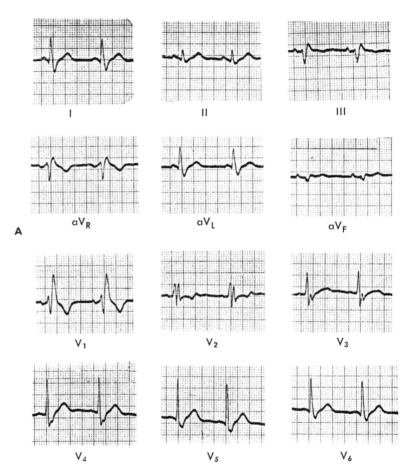

Fig. 6-61. A, Twelve-lead ECG illustrating right bundle branch block. In **B,** schematic illustration is presented.

Significance. In a young individual, right ventricular hypertrophy may produce RBBB; in an older patient, coronary artery disease is a more likely cause. Early supraventricular complexes that are conducted aberrantly through the ventricle are more likely to develop an RBBB than LBBB because the right bundle branch takes longer to repolarize than does the left bundle branch. The initial forces in RBBB are not altered and therefore the ECG signs of myocardial infarction are not obscured.

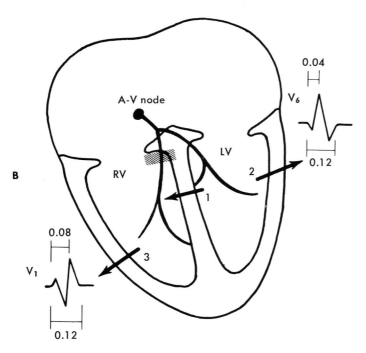

Fig. 6-61, cont'd. For legend see opposite page.

FASCICULAR BLOCKS (Figs. 6-62 and 6-63)

According to recent concepts, the left bundle branch divides into anterior and posterior divisions or fascicles. Block may occur in one or the other division (hemiblock) and give rise primarily to a shift in the frontal plane QRS axis without significant QRS prolongation. *Left anterior fascicular block* results in a QRS angle in the frontal plane of about −60 degrees, an initial Q wave in lead I, a terminal S wave in lead III, and a normal or slightly prolonged QRS duration. *Left posterior fascicular block* produces a QRS angle in the frontal plane of about +120 degrees, an initial Q wave in lead III, and a terminal S wave in lead I; forces of the first half of the QRS complex are also directed toward +120 degrees. Right ventricular hypertrophy and a vertical heart must be excluded. Fascicular blocks may combine with RBBB, thus representing examples of bilateral bundle branch block.

Significance. Fascicular blocks may result from coronary artery disease, particularly in the setting of an acute anteroseptal myocardial infarction that simultaneously involves the right bundle branch and one of the divisions of the left bundle branch. Another large group of patients develop ventricular conduction disorders owing to a sclerodegenerative process limited to the conduction system (Lenegre's disease) fibrosclerosis of structures adjacent to the conduction system (Lev's disease). Patients with Lenegre's disease appear to be younger than those with Lev's disease and more prone to developing A-V block.

If left anterior of left posterior fascicular block is present with RBBB, it must be remembered that the unblocked fascicle constitutes the only conduction pathway from the His bundle to the ventricle. The posterior division of the left bundle branch seems to be the least vulnerable segment of the specialized ventricular conduction system and, therefore, left posterior fascicular block, with or without RBBB, occurs least often. When lesions are sufficiently extensive to involve the posterior fascicle, they often involve the anterior fascicle and right bundle branch as well. Left posterior fascicular block carries a worse prognosis than does left anterior fascicular block, with increased likelihood to progress to more advanced stages of A-V block.

Treatment. In the presence of an acute myocardial infarction, the development of RBBB with left anterior or posterior fascicular block generally requires prophylactic temporary transvenous pacemaker insertion because more advanced A-V block may follow. Pacemaker implantation may not be necessary for the asymptomatic patient without acute myocardial infarction who develops one of the chronic forms of bilateral bundle branch block as a result of degenerative cardiac changes. (See discussion of therapy under A-V block.)

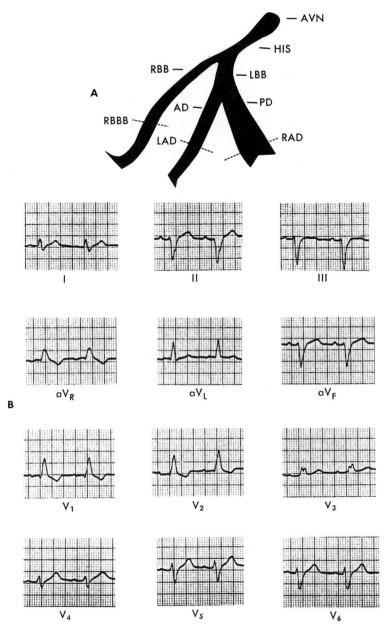

Fig. 6-62. A, Schematic illustration of the trifascicular nature of ventricular conduction. *AVN,* Atrioventricular node; *His,* bundle of His; *RBB,* right bundle branch; *LBB,* main portion of left bundle branch; *AD,* anterior division (fascicle) of left bundle branch; *PD,* posterior division (fascicle) of left bundle branch. Interrupted lines indicate block or delay in conduction, with resultant right bundle branch block *(RBBB),* left axis deviation *(LAD),* right axis deviation *(RAD).* LAD and RAD, in this context, are called left anterior fascicular and left posterior fascicular block, respectively. **B.,** Twelve-lead ECG illustrating right bundle branch block and left anterior fascicular block. See also Figs. 6-56 and 6-57.

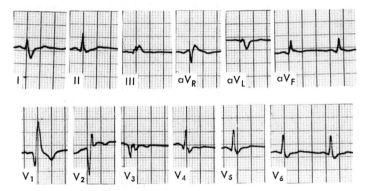

Fig. 6-63. Twelve-lead ECG illustrating right bundle branch block and left posterior fascicular block. The abnormal Q waves in leads V_1 to V_4 indicate the presence of an anteroseptal myocardial infarction.

PARASYSTOLE (Fig. 6-64)

Premature systoles that lack a fixed relationship to the preceding complex (varying coupling intervals) may result from a parasystole. A parasystolic focus is a protected pacemaker focus that discharges at a fixed rate. It becomes manifest when the site in which the parasystolic focus originates has recovered excitability. The parasystolic focus then may depolarize the atrium or ventricle to produce a premature systole. The resulting P wave or QRS complex has a configuration different from that of the dominant rhythm, depending on the site of origin. Although the dominant rhythm may be discharged by the parasystolic focus, the dominant rhythm does not depolarize the parasystolic focus because the latter is protected by unidirectional entrance block, that is, impulses may exit from the parasystolic focus to discharge the surrounding myocardium but no impulse may enter the parasystolic focus and discharge it. The manifest parasystolic rate may be much less than the actual rate because of exit block from the parasystolic

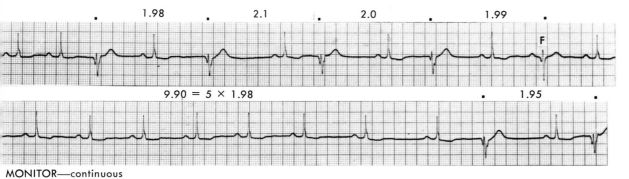

MONITOR—continuous

Fig. 6-64. Ventricular parasystole. The interval between ectopic ventricular systoles ranges between 1.98 and 2.1 seconds. The coupling interval varies. A ventricular fusion beat is labeled *F*. Ventricular refractoriness prevents the emergence of the ventricular parasystole during the long interval in which it is absent. This interectopic interval equals 9.90 seconds and is five times the normal interectopic interval. The dark circles above the tracing indicate the parasystolic ventricular systoles.

Rate: Atrial—Atrial rhythm and rate may vary, depending on whether sinus bradycardia or tachycardia, atrial tachycardia, and so forth, is the atrial mechanism. Generally, normal (approximately 60).
    Ventricular parasystole—(30).
Rhythm: Atrial—Regular.
    Ventricular parasystole—Regular; may be interrupted by exit block or ventricular refractoriness.
P waves: Normal.
P-R interval: During normally conducted beats, normal.
QRS (of ventricular parasystole): Prolonged (0.13 second).

focus. Exit block from the parasystolic focus may produce irregular spacing of the interectopic intervals. However, because the rate of discharge of the parasystolic focus is constant, the interectopic intervals between parasystolic impulses reduce to a common denominator. A continuously discharging atrial or ventricular artificial pacemaker serves as a good example of (artificial) parasystole. Premature systoles that are caused by a parasystolic focus ordinarily have no fixed relationship to the basic rhythm and often result in the production of fusion beats.

Significance. Atrial and junctional parasystole may occur in patients without clinical evidence of heart disease. Ventricular parasystole generally manifests in patients with heart disease; it is rarely, if ever, caused by digitalis excess.

Treatment. The therapeutic approach is basically the same as that discussed under atrial, junctional, and ventricular premature systoles.

PREEXCITATION (WOLFF-PARKINSON-WHITE) SYNDROME (Figs. 6-65 to 6-69)

Preexcitation exists when the atrial impulse activates the whole or some part of ventricular muscle earlier than would be expected if the atrial impulse reached the ventricles by way of the normal specific conduction system only. Four basic features typify the usual ECG of a patient with the preexcitation syndrome: (1) P-R interval less than 0.12 second during sinus rhythm, (2) QRS complex duration greater than 0.12 second with a slurred, slow rising onset of the R wave upstroke in some leads (delta wave) and usually normal terminal QRS portion, (3) secondary ST-T wave changes that are usually directed opposite the major delta and QRS vectors, and (4) paroxysmal tachyarrhythmias in 40% to 80% of patients. The explanation for those findings is the presence of a rapidly conductive accessory pathway, which bypasses the A-V node by communicating directly from atrium to ventricle. Other patients may possess variants of the preexcitation syndrome; one variant is characterized by a short P-R interval (less than 0.12 second) and normal QRS complex. Supraventricular tachycardia may also occur in this group (Lown-Ganong-Levine syndrome).

Patients with the preexcitation syndrome may be divided in two broad types, depending on the form of QRS in the leads recorded from the right precordium, particularly V_1 and V_2. In type A the R wave is the sole or largest deflection in V_1 and V_2 and the bypass is located between the left atrium and the left ventricle. In type B the S or QS deflection is largest in V_1 and V_2 and the bypass is located between the right atrium and the right ventricle. Some patients may have septal bypasses.

Significance. The reported incidence of the preexcitation syndrome averages about 1.5 per 1000. It occurs in all age groups and more often (60% to 70%) in males. Two thirds of patients with the short P-R interval and normal QRS complex are females. Patients may seek help because of recurrent supraventricular tachycardia, atrial fibrillation with a rapid ventricular response, heart failure, syncope, or symptoms related to associated cardiac anomalies, or they may be discovered during examination for noncardiac-related reasons. Sixty to seventy percent of adults with preexcitation syndrome have normal hearts; a higher proportion of children have heart disease. A variety of acquired and congenital cardiac defects have been reported in patients with the preexcitation syndrome, including Ebstein's anomaly, idiopathic hypertrophic subaortic stenosis, septal defects, and tetralogy of Fallot.

Forty to eighty percent of patients with the preexcitation syndrome experience recurrent tachyarrhythmias; paroxysmal atrial tachycardia occurs most often (80%), followed by atrial fibrillation (15%), and atrial flutter (5%). Ventricular tachycardia rarely occurs, and most reports have misdiagnosed as ventricular tachycardia the aberrant QRS complexes caused by anomalous conduction. Recognition of the preexcitation syndrome is clinically important, since the tachyarrhythmias at times do not respond to conventional therapy and may be associated with very rapid ventricular rates. The anomalous complexes may mask or mimic myocardial infarction, bundle branch block, or ven-

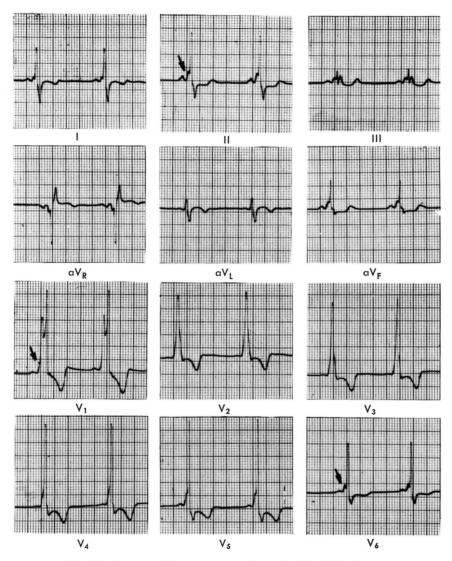

Fig. 6-65. Twelve-lead ECG illustrating preexcitation (Wolff-Parkinson-White) syndrome, type A indicated by positive delta wave and QRS complex in V_1 and V_6. Arrows indicate delta waves. The short P-R interval is apparent.

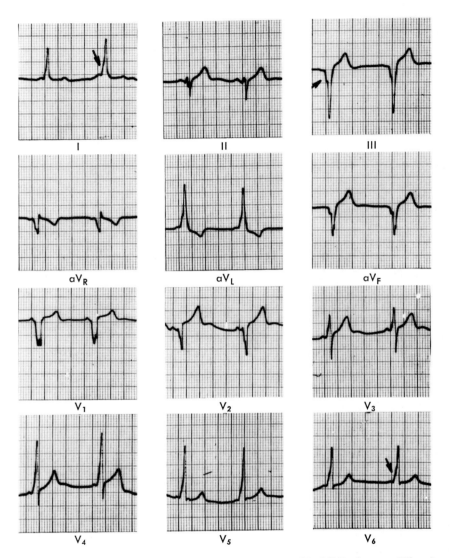

Fig. 6-66. Twelve-lead ECG illustrating preexcitation (Wolff-Parkinson-White) syndrome, type B indicated by negative delta wave and QRS complex in V_1 and positive delta wave and QRS complex in V_6. Arrows indicate delta waves. The short P-R interval is apparent.

tricular hypertrophy, and the presence of the preexcitation syndrome may call attention to an associated cardiac defect.

The prognosis is excellent in patients without tachycardia or associated cardiac anomaly. In patients with recurrent tachycardia the prognosis is good in most, but sudden unexpected death occurs, especially when the ventricular rate during tachycardia is rapid or associated congenital defects are present. Ventricular fibrillation has been documented in man and dog and is probably caused by extremely rapid ventricular rates, permitted by the bypass during atrial flutter or fibrillation, that exceed the ability of the ventricle to follow in an organized fashion. Consequently, fragmented, disorganized ventricular activation results and leads to fibrillation. Alternatively, supraventricular discharge, bypassing the A-V nodal delay, may activate the ventricle during the vulnerable period of the antecedent T wave and precipitate fibrillation.

Treatment. The tachycardia in patients with the Wolff-Parkinson-White syndrome may not respond to conventional therapy and may be associated with very rapid ventricular rates. Many patients with the preexcitation syndrome have rare or infrequent bouts of tachycardia that are not incapacitating and subside spontaneously or with vagal maneuvers. Some patients are moderately or severely incapacitated by recurrent tachyarrhythmias that require suppressive therapy. In this category are patients with frequent attacks of tachycardia, patients with very fast heart rates during attacks, and patients experiencing severe hypotension, heart failure, or syncope during attacks. In addition, prophylactic suppressive therapy may be considered in those pa-

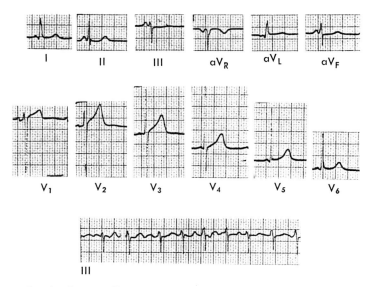

Fig. 6-67. Twelve-lead ECG illustrating a short P-R interval and normal QRS complex, perhaps resulting from the Lown-Ganong-Levine (LGL) syndrome. Lead III (below) illustrates a supraventricular tachycardia in this patient.

tients whose accessory pathway has a short refractory period (established by atrial pacing) and who therefore might develop a very rapid ventricular response to atrial flutter or fibrillation.

PAT that exhibits normal QRS complexes can be approached as ordinary PAT, as if it were unassociated with the preexcitation syndrome. Therefore agents that slow A-V nodal conduction and prolong A-V nodal refractory period, like cholinergic drugs, digitalis, reflexly induced vagal stimulation, propranolol, or any other agent that depresses A-V nodal conductivity, may terminate the PAT; digitalis, quinidine, and propranolol may be used prophylactically (see discussion of therapy PAT). When PAT is characterized by widened QRS complexes of Wolff-Parkinson-White contour, digitalis alone is usually contraindicated and quinidine or other drugs that depress conduction in the accessory pathway may be required.

For atrial flutter or fibrillation, atrial impulses are not obligated to travel the normal A-V node–His bundle route, but can reach the ventricles via the bypass. Drugs possessing a vagal action (like digitalis) may actually *speed* the ventricular rate, since these drugs improve conduction in atrial *muscle* (which may compose the bypass). Quinidine, procainamide, and certain antihis-

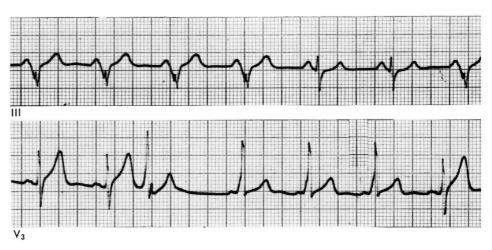

Fig. 6-68. Preexcitation (Wolff-Parkinson-White) syndrome, type B. Spontaneous onset and termination of preexcitation conduction account for the variable QRS conduction in lead III and V_3. In lead V_3 the onset of anomalous conduction follows a premature atrial systole (third QRS) with a Wolff-Parkinson-White pattern. This patient was erroneously admitted to the coronary care unit because of the Q waves in lead III, which were misinterpreted as indicating an inferior myocardial infarction.

Rate: 78.
Rhythm: Regular.
P waves: Normal.
P-R interval: Varies between 0.10 and 0.13 second.
QRS: Normal (0.08 second) during conduction over the A-V node with a normal P-R interval; abnormal (0.12 second) during conduction over the bypass tract with a short P-R interval.

tamines prolong atrial muscle refractory period and are useful in treating atrial flutter and fibrillation. Frequently the combination of digitalis and quinidine to slow conduction in both the normal and the accessory pathways may be effective. Lidocaine depresses conduction in the accessory pathway and may be useful acutely to slow the ventricular rate during atrial flutter or atrial fibrillation. Some patients who have PAT may also intermittently develop atrial fibrillation. In these patients, digitalis alone should not be used, but can be combined with quinidine, for example.

If the ventricular rate is exceedingly rapid, in the range of 250 beats per minute, the development of ventricular fibrillation is possible and DC shock should be considered the initial treatment of choice.

For patients who are symptomatic owing to drug-refractory, recurrent tachycardia, surgery to interrupt the accessory pathway has been extremely useful.

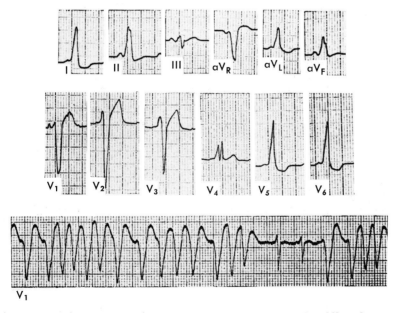

Fig. 6-69. Twelve-lead ECG illustrating the preexcitation (Wolff-Parkinson-White) syndrome, type B. The lower recording (V₁ half standard) demonstrates an extremely rapid ventricular rate during atrial fibrillation in this same patient. The grossly irregular ventricular rhythm, extremely rapid rate, and gradations in QRS contour from normal to prolonged (as conduction changes from the normal A-V nodal pathway to the anomalous route) help differentiate this arrhythmia from ventricular tachycardia. Bypass of the safety valve features provided by normal A-V nodal delay accounts for the rapid ventricular rate that, less commonly, may actually cause the ventricles to fibrillate and result in sudden death.

A-V DISSOCIATION

As the words imply, A-V dissociation means that atria and ventricles are dissociated; they are controlled by separate pacemakers for one or more beats. The term used generically tells nothing regarding the nature of atrial or ventricular activity, except that these chambers are beating independently for a period of time. It is as if the term described a "symptom" without indicating what caused it. The atria may be fibrillating, fluttering, or responding to an ectopic tachycardia or sinus impulses; the ventricles may be controlled by A-V junctional or ectopic ventricular beating. The only fact conveyed is that whatever controls one chamber does not also control the other during the period of A-V dissociation.

A-V dissociation is *never* a primary disturbance of rhythm but rather a consequence of a more basic disorder; for the term to be used properly, the cause(s) producing A-V dissociation must also be described. These are as follows:

1. Slowing of the primary pacemaker to allow the escape of a subsidiary (latent) focus. In Fig. 6-12, sinus slowing allows two ventricular beats to escape under the control of a separate focus while the sinus node still controls the atria. During these two beats, A-V dissociation exists. Fig. 6-36 presents a similar example.

2. Accelerated discharge of subsidiary focus. In Fig. 6-38, accelerated A-V junctional discharge results in a nonparoxysmal A-V junctional (nodal) tachycardia without retrograde atrial capture. Since the atria remain under sinus domination, separate pacemakers control atria and ventricles, resulting in A-V dissociation. Fig. 6-39 presents a similar example, called "isorhythmic" A-V dissociation because atria and ventricles maintain similar rates and rhythms. A-V dissociation may also occur during ventricular tachycardia if retrograde atrial capture does not ensue (see Figs. 6-44 to 6-47).

3. A-V block. In Fig. 6-58, A-V block reduces the number of effective (conducted) atrial impulses; this allows the escape of a subsidiary focus to produce A-V dissociation. When A-V block results in A-V dissociation, the atrial rate generally exceeds the ventricular rate (see Fig. 6-59).

4. Combinations of 1, 2, or 3 may initiate A-V dissociation, as, for example, when digitalis causes both first-degree (or Wenckebach) A-V block and NPJT.

In all these examples, but for diverse reasons, the ventricular rate either exceeds or becomes equal or nearly equal to the effective (conducted) atrial rate. It is this fact that allows A-V dissociation to occur.

The preceding discussion makes it apparent that the presence or absence of A-V dissociation depends on the rate and temporal relationships of the two pacemakers and the intactness of A-V and V-A conduction. Should the atrial pacemaker capture control of the ventricle, or vice versa, A-V dissociation would be terminated during that period of capture (incomplete A-V dissociation).

SUPRAVENTRICULAR ARRHYTHMIA WITH ABNORMAL QRS COMPLEXES (Figs. 6-70 to 6-72)

Wide, bizarre QRS complexes may accompany isolated supraventricular beats or sustained supraventricular rhythms. The term "aberrant ventricular conduction" is commonly applied to such complexes. Thus QRS contours that display prolonged abnormal configuration indicate that conduction through the ventricle is abnormal; they do not necessarily mean that the impulse *originated* in the ventricles. The presence of fusion and capture complexes strongly supports the diagnosis of ventricular tachycardia or accelerated ventricular rhythm. However, the electrocardiographic manifestations of ventricular tachycardia, including the presence or absence of A-V dissociation, and complexes that appear to represent capture or fusion beats, may be mimicked, under certain circumstances, by supraventricular arrhythmias.

Intraventricular conduction defects, bundle branch blocks, and anomalous pathway conduction may all initiate abnormal ventricular excitation with

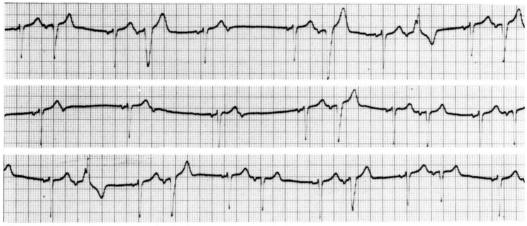

V₁—continuous

Fig. 6-70. Functional right and left bundle branch block following atrial premature systoles. Premature atrial systoles occur at varying coupling intervals. When they occur with a very short R-P interval, they fail to reach the ventricle and are therefore non-conducted atrial systoles. At slightly longer R-P intervals, they conduct with both functional right and functional left bundle branch block. Differences in the duration of the preceding long cycle and in the duration of the short cycle account for whether functional right or left bundle branch block results.

Rate: Determined by the number of premature atrial systoles.

Rhythm: Irregular because of premature atrial systoles.

P waves: Both sinus-initiated and premature atrial systolic P waves are abnormal.

P-R interval: Normal (0.12 second) for the sinus-initiated P waves; prolonged following the premature atrial systoles. Some premature atrial systoles failed to conduct to the ventricle.

QRS: Normal, following the sinus initiated P waves; functional left bundle and functional right bundle branch block following the premature atrial systoles.

widened QRS complexes. Also, premature supraventricular stimulation may conduct to the ventricles before ventricular repolarization has been completed, causing the impulse to conduct aberrantly. The resulting widened QRS complex may display characteristic features that distinguish it from those beats arising in the ventricles during a true ventricular tachycardia. The following analysis may be helpful in differentiating aberrant ventricular conduction initiated by a supraventricular impulse from ventricular tachycardia.

Identification of atrial activity. During sinus rhythm or an ectopic supraventricular rhythm, identification of distinct atrial activity initiating ventricular depolarization, regardless of how deformed the QRS complex may appear, establishes the diagnosis of supraventricular rhythm with QRS abberrancy. A cause-and-effect relationship between the P and QRS complexes may be demonstrated in one or more of the following ways, depending on the nature of the supraventricular rhythms:

1. P waves with a normal contour precede and bear a constant relationship to each QRS complex during sinus rhythms.
2. Interventions that alter the sinus rate, such as carotid sinus massage or exercise, secondarily alter the ventricular rate in exactly the same manner and maintain the same, or nearly so, P-R interval. This indicates that ventricular activation follows as a consequence of atrial discharge. Atrial pacing has been employed to alter the atrial rate during a tachycardia characterized by wide QRS complexes, and a diagnosis of ventricular tachycardia was considered likely when fusion and capture complexes resulted.
3. When atrial flutter, atrial fibrillation, or atrial tachycardia exists, carotid sinus massage, digitalis, or edrophonium chloride (Tensilon) administration produces characteristic slowing of the ventricular response (at times also normalizing the QRS complex); during paroxysmal atrial tachycardia, the rhythm may remain unchanged or terminate and allow sinus rhythm to resume.
4. Atrial and ventricular rhythms may be so related as to suggest dependency of the latter on the former, for example, during typical A-V Wenckebach cycles.
5. When atria and ventricles are dissociated, finding ventricular captures that have the same contour as the QRS of the tachyarrhythmia indicates a supraventricular rhythm.
6. Bursts of an intermittent tachycardia that are always initiated by a premature or ectopic atrial complex provide indirect evidence supporting a supraventricular diagnosis.
7. During retrograde atrial capture the R-P interval is of too short duration to be explained by retrograde conduction from a ventricular focus (about 0.10 second or less).
8. If the rate and rhythm of abnormal QRS complexes are the same as the rate and rhythm of a known supraventricular tachycardia, this provides some support in favor of aberration.

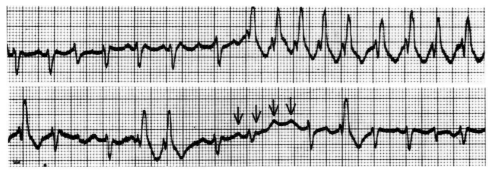

V₁—continuous

Fig. 6-71. Functional right bundle branch block. At first glance the tracing appears to be sinus rhythm interrupted by a burst of ventricular tachycardia and intermittent premature ventricular systoles. Closer inspection reveals flutter waves *(arrows)* when the ventricular rate slows slightly and suggests that the widened QRS complexes may be aberrantly conducted supraventricular beats. These beats conform in all respects to criteria established to differentiate supraventricular aberration from ventricular tachycardia. (See text.) The patient requires digitalis to slow the ventricular rate rather than lidocaine to suppress ectopic ventricular discharge.

Rate: Atrial—280.
    Ventricular—90 to 200.
Rhythm: Atrial—Regular.
    Ventricular—Irregularly irregular.
P waves: Flutter waves *(arrows)* can be seen when the ventricular rate slows and can be marched out with regularity.
P-R interval: Flutter-R interval varies.
QRS: Varying contour between normal and functional right bundle branch block.

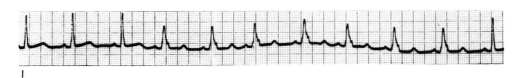

I

Fig. 6-72. Rate-dependent aberrancy of the left bundle branch block type. Gradual acceleration of the sinus rate results in a functional left bundle branch block that remains until the sinus rate slows sufficiently at the end of the tracing. This type of abberancy is much more commonly of the left bundle rather than the right bundle branch block type and is more apt to be associated with cardiac disease than is functional right bundle branch block.

Rate: 60-78.
Rhythm: Slightly irregular.
P waves: Normal.
P-R interval: Normal and constant (0.14 second).
QRS: Varies between normal and functional left bundle branch block.

Analysis of QRS contours and intervals. The following clues suggest aberrant ventricular conduction initiated by a supraventricular impulse:

1. The contour of the QRS is a triphasic rsR' in V_1. RBBB patterns occur more frequently than LBBB patterns because, at a slower heart rate, the right bundle branch requires more time to repolarize than the left. Therefore premature discharge is more likely to encounter a refractory right bundle branch and produce right bundle branch block.

2. Faster rates speed repolarization, whereas slower rates retard it; the refractory period is proportional to the preceding cycle length. Therefore the heart takes longer to repolarize following a long cycle than it does after a short cycle. Because of this, when an early beat succeeds a long cycle, the early beat may encounter refractory tissue and conduct aberrantly. A comparison of such long-short cycle sequences aids in determining aberrant conduction. Uncommonly, aberrancy may occur at slow ventricular rates.

3. Aberrantly conducted beats tend to persist in runs rather than maintain a bigeminal pattern and lack a compensatory pause.

4. The initial vectors of aberrant and normal beats are similar, since RBBB preserves the normal initial forces.

5. Aberrantly conducted supraventricular QRS complexes are not wildly bizarre or lengthened, most of the QRS prolongation occurring in the latter portion of the beat.

6. A fixed coupling interval between the normal and aberrant beat is absent during atrial flutter or atrial fibrillation. Conversely, fixed coupling favors ventricular ectopy.

7. The aberrant beats are not excessively premature.

8. The QRS configuration appears the same as that resulting from known supraventricular conduction at similar rates. Conversely, if the QRS contour is the same as that resulting from known ventricular conduction, the tachycardia is probably ventricular in origin.

9. Vagal maneuvers remain the most important differentiating point, since vagal discharge does not usually affect ventricular tachycardia, whereas it slows the ventricular rate in most supraventricular mechanisms. However, ventricular tachycardia terminated by vagal discharge has been reported recently.

ELECTROLYTE DISTURBANCES

Potassium (Figs. 6-73 and 6-74). During induced hyperkalemia in animals, the ECG correlates closely with the potassium blood level: The T wave peaks when potassium concentration reaches about 5.5 mEq per liter; the corrected Q-T interval is normal or shortens initially but may prolong as the QRS complex widens. The QRS complex may widen when the external potassium concentration exceeds 6.5 mEq per liter; above 7.0 mEq per liter, P wave

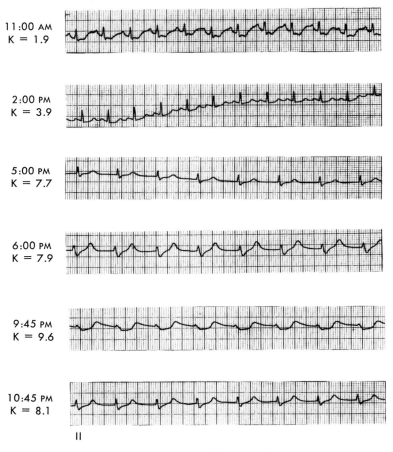

Fig. 6-73. Serial ECG tracings in a patient with marked changes in serum potassium level. In the 11:00 A.M. tracing the depressed S-T segment and low amplitude T wave blending into a probable U wave (this cannot be seen with clarity because of the superimposed P waves) indicate the presence of hypokalemia. Following the administration of potassium the 2:00 P.M. tracing becomes relatively normal. Continued potassium administration results in hyperkalemia with the disappearance of atrial activity on the ECG and some prolongation of the QRS complex. By 7:00 P.M. the QRS complex is more prolonged, and by 9:45 P.M. the QRS complex is greatly prolonged. Secondary ST-T wave changes are present. Improvement follows the administration of bicarbonate, glucose, and insulin at 10:45 P.M. with reduction in serum potassium level; improvement in the ECG results.

amplitude diminishes, and P wave and P-R interval duration are prolonged. Above 8.0 to 9.0 mEq per liter, the P wave frequently disappears. Sometimes S-T segment deviation, both elevated and depressed, occurs and simulates an injury pattern. Clinically occurring potassium alterations do not correlate as well as during these experimental changes; less than 25% of patients with hyperkalemia may develop the characteristic tall, peaked T waves. It is believed that external potassium concentration accounts for the ECG patterns rather than changes in total body potassium or internal potassium concentration.

During hypokalemic states the S-T segment becomes depressed, the U wave is exaggerated, and the T wave amplitude is decreased without changing the actual duration of Q-T or Q-U interval (as long as it can be measured accurately). The P and QRS amplitude and duration may increase and the P-R interval may be prolonged. Clinical hypokalemia does not normally slow A-V conduction significantly. However, isolated cases have been reported demonstrating varying degrees of P-R prolongation. Intraventricular conduction in adults seldom lengthens by more than 20 msec, but may be more prolonged in children.

Spontaneous hyperkalemia rarely, if ever, produces more advanced A-V block than simple P-R prolongation; large doses of potassium administered rapidly may produce further advanced forms of A-V block, however. Often the P wave disappears, which precludes the diagnosis of A-V block. As the plasma potassium level continues to rise above 6.5 and 7.0 mEq per liter, slowed intraventricular conduction results, manifested by uniform widening of the QRS complex. Areas of intraventricular block may occur and lead to ventricular fibrillation.

Potassium may potentiate the slowing effects of digitalis on A-V conduction, particularly if plasma potassium level rises rapidly. However, if A-V conduction is also hampered by a rapid atrial rate, slowing the atrial rate with potassium actually may improve A-V conduction and offset any direct depressing effects of potassium. Fortunately, potassium administration to patients with digitalis-induced arrhythmias suppresses ectopic discharge at a much lower blood potassium level than that which further depresses A-V conduction.

Low blood potassium levels encourage spontaneous ectopic pacemaker discharge, presumably by enhancing automaticity and also possibly by slowing dominant pacemakers or producing conduction defects. Low potassium levels may initiate ventricular fibrillation in man. Reduced potassium concentration may precipitate arrhythmias in animals and humans receiving digitalis at plasma potassium levels that ordinarily do not produce ectopic beating in the absence of digitalis. Possibly the synergistic effects of digitalis and reduced potassium on automaticity and conduction make animals and humans receiving digitalis particularly prone to arrhythmias precipitated by hypokalemia.

The antiarrhythmic effects of potassium administration may suppress varied rhythms, regardless of cause and whether or not hypokalemia exists. Digitalis-induced ectopic discharge generally responds to potassium therapy at sufficiently low doses to avoid further A-V conduction delay. Many believe that potassium remains the drug of choice for ectopic rhythms produced by excessive digitalis. Animals and humans with elevated potassium levels may tolerate large doses of digitalis without developing ectopic arrhythmias, whereas reduced potassium level predisposes to ectopic activity in digitalized animals or patients. Also, a low level of potassium may worsen the depression of A-V conduction produced by digitalis.

Sodium. In general the magnitude of sodium change necessary to produce ECG alterations is not compatible with life, making clinical electrocardiographic manifestations of sodium derangements rarely seen, if ever.

Calcium (Fig. 6-75). In the ECG, low calcium level prolongs the duration of the S-T segment and Q-T interval without prolonging the duration of the T wave, although the T wave may reverse polarity. Elevated calcium level shortens the S-T segment and Q-T interval; the QRS duration may be pro-

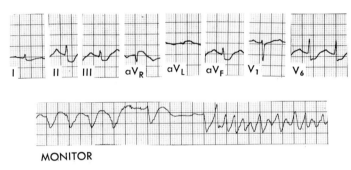

MONITOR

Fig. 6-74. Hypokalemia-induced ventricular tachycardia and fibrillation. The ECG demonstrates the characteristic changes of hypokalemia: depressed S-T segment, low amplitude T wave, and large U wave, blending into the following P wave. In the monitor lead a ventricular tachycardia briefly stops and then degenerates into ventricular fibrillation that was reversed with DC shock.

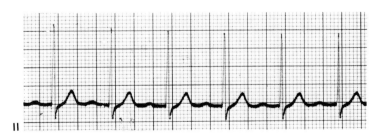

Fig. 6-75. The effects of hypercalcemia on the ECG. Serum calcium level, 14.0/100 ml. The S-T segment and Q-T interval are shortened and the P-R interval is slightly prolonged (0.22 second).

longed during severe hypercalcemia, and A-V block may develop. High calcium level opposes the effects of high level potassium, whereas low calcium level opposes the effects of low potassium. If the calcium level varies in a direction opposite that of potassium level, the effects of the latter are enhanced.

HIS BUNDLE ELECTROCARDIOGRAPHY (Fig. 6-1)

The technique of His bundle electrocardiography involves passing an electrode catheter that is introduced percutaneously into the femoral vein, in a cephalad direction up the inferior vena cava and positioning the catheter tip near the septal leaflet of the tricuspid valve. The His potential (H) appears as a well-defined, most often bipolar spike between the low right atrial (A) and ventricular (V) electrograms. The interval between the earliest onset of the surface P wave or a high right atrial deflection (P) and the low right atrial deflection (P-A interval) is a measure of intra-atrial conduction. The A-H interval is a measurement of the conduction across the A-V node and varies in duration from 50 to 120 msec, depending on the cycle length and autonomic influences. The interval from H to V (H-V interval) is determined by the interval between the His deflection and the earliest ventricular activity recorded in any lead. The H-V interval is a measure of conduction through the His bundle distal to the recording electrode, the bundle branches, and the Purkinje system up to the point of ventricular activation. In contrast to a relatively wide range of values for the A-H interval, the H-V interval is fairly constant, measuring 30 to 55 msec, with an average value of 45 msec. In some patients, discharge of the right bundle branch may be recorded.

The ability to separate A-V nodal and His-Purkinje conduction has enhanced our understanding of normal and abnormal atrioventricular (A-V) conduction. Abnormal A-V conduction may be caused by prolongation of P-A, A-H, or H-V intervals or all three. In addition, intra-His block has been demonstrated. During type I(Wenckebach) A-V block in a patient with a normal QRS complex the conduction disturbance occurs at the A-V node, proximal to the His bundle. Type II A-V block in a patient with a bundle branch block virtually always results distal to the His bundle. Thus in type I A-V block the blocked P wave is not followed by a His spike, whereas in type II A-V block, the blocked P wave is followed by a His spike.

His bundle electrocardiography has been useful in differentiating ventricular tachycardia from aberrant ventricular conduction, in understanding the nature of many supraventricular and ventricular tachycardias and other arrhythmias, in evaluating patients with the preexcitation syndrome or A-V block, and in other areas as well. Further discussion is beyond the scope of this text, and the reader is referred to the many papers written on this subject. The utility of His bundle electrocardiography as a routine clinical tool necessary to the care of patients with heart disease is not yet completely defined. Clearly, however, in most instances a carefully analyzed surface ECG provides the necessary information required to make clinical therapeutic decisions.

ARTIFACTS (Figs. 6-76 and 6-77)

Electronic instrumentation has provided vast dividends to the care of patients with heart disease. However, because we now rely so heavily on various types of monitoring devices, one must constantly be alert and recognize artifacts that mimic arrhythmias. A tracing that resembles ventricular fibrillation *must* be artifactual if the patient is found sitting up in bed in no distress, reading his newspaper!

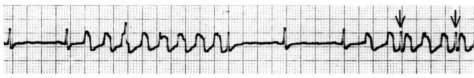

MONITOR

Fig. 6-76. Artifact. Regularly moving a loose electrode creates an artifact that mimicks ventricular tachycardia. However, careful scrutiny uncovers the fairly regularly occurring normal QRS complexes *(arrows)*, each preceded by a P wave. The question of ventricular tachycardia may be eliminated and the diagnosis of artifact established by observing that the QRS complexes continue uninterrupted and unaffected by the "apparent" ventricular tachycardia.

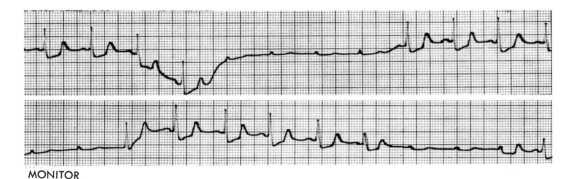

MONITOR

Fig. 6-77. Artifact simulating A-V block. These tracings were recorded in a patient who presented with an acute anteroseptal myocardial infarction and 1 day later developed left anterior fascicular block. The monitored recording was interpreted as illustrating the development of advanced A-V block with sequentially blocked P waves. Temporary transvenous pacemaker insertion was deemed immediately necessary. However, careful observation of the tracing reveals that the nonconducted P waves are artifactual in origin. In reality the "nonconducted P waves" are QRS complexes with a grossly diminished amplitude because of intermittent poor ECG lead contact. The diagnosis is established by noting QRS complexes with intermediate amplitudes, by noting T waves that follow the diminutive QRS complexes and by "marching out" the QRS complexes and finding that they occur at the same time as the apparent P waves.

REFERENCES

Azevedo, I. M., Watanabe, Y., and Dreifus, L. S.: Reassessment of A-V junctional rhythms, Heart Lung 1:626, Sept.-Oct., 1972.

Constant, J.: Learning electrocardiography, Boston, 1973, Little, Brown and Co..

DeJoseph, R. L., and Zipes, D. P.: His bundle electrocardiography—its clinical value. In Controversy in cardiology, New York, 1975, Springer-Verlag New York Inc.

Dubin, D.: Rapid interpretation of electrocardiograms, Tampa, Fla., Cover Publishing Co..

Goldman, M. J.: Principles of clinical electrocardiography, ed. 9, Los Altos, Calif., 1976, Lange Medical Publications

Hurst, J. W., and Logue, R. B.: The heart, arteries, and veins, ed. 4, New York, 1978, McGraw-Hill Book Co.

Katz, L., and Pick, A.: Clinical electrocardiography. I. The arrhythmias, Philadelphia, 1956, Lea & Febiger.

Lindsay, A. E., and Budkin, A., The cardiac arrhythmias, ed. 2, Chicago, 1975, Year Book Medical Publishers, Inc.

Marriott, H. J. L.: Practical electrocardiography, ed. 5, Baltimore, 1972, The Williams & Wilkins Co.

Miller, R. R., Amsterdam, E. A., Massumi, R. A., Zelis, R., and Mason, D. T.: Procainamide: reappraisal of an old anti-arrhythmic drug, Heart Lung 2:277, March-April, 1973.

Noble, R. J., Dickerson, L. S., and Fisch, C.: The use and abuse of digitalis in acute myocardial infarction, Heart Lung 1:762, Nov.-Dec., 1972.

Pick, A.: A-V dissociation. A proposal for a comprehensive classification and consistent terminology, Am. Heart J. 66:147, 1963.

Pick, A., and Dominguez, P.: Nonparoxysmal A-V nodal tachycardia, Circulation 16:1022, 1957.

Rosenbaum, M. B.: The hemiblocks: diagnostic criteria and clinical significance, Mod. Conc. Cardiovasc. Dis. 39:141, 1970.

Selzer, A.: The use and abuse of quinidine. Heart Lung 1:755, Nov.-Dec., 1972.

Zipes, D. P., and McIntosh, H. D.: Cardiac arrhythmias. In Conn, H., and Horwitz, O., editors: Cardiac and vascular diseases, Philadelphia, 1971, Lea & Febiger.

Zipes, D. P., Watanabe, A. M., & Besch, H. R.: Clinical electrophysiology and electrocardiography. In Wilkerson, J. T., and Sanders C. A., editors: The science and practice of clinical medicine, New York, 1977, Grune & Stratton, Inc.

Zipes, D. P.: Tachycardia. In Conn, H. F., editor: Current therapy, Philadelphia, 1975, W. B. Saunders Co.

Zipes, D. P.: Cardiac arrythmias. In Conn, H. F., editor: Current diagnosis, Philadelphia, 1977, W. B. Saunders Co.

Arrhythmia test section

It is suggested that the reader use this section to test his knowledge of arrhythmias. Cover the interpretations on the right side of each legend and calculate intervals and irregularites as previously discussed, providing the information called for. Consider also the significance of each arrhythmia and what form of treatment would most likely be employed. There may be disagreements in interpretation of rhythm strips, but the essential point is to make your diagnosis by using the analytic method described in this chapter. This approach offers a justification for your interpretation.

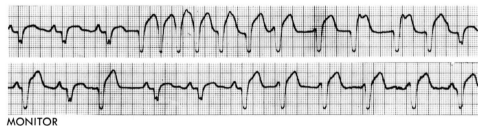

MONITOR

Fig. 6-78

Rate:	Atrial	78.
	Ventricular	Varies between 78 and 180.
Rhythm:	Atrial	Regular.
	Ventricular	Varying.
P waves:		Normal when visible.
P-R interval:		0.16 second preceding the normally conducted QRS complexes. Not measurable in front of the ventricular ectopy.
QRS:		Normal for the sinus-conducted beats (0.09 second); prolonged for the ventricular ectopy (0.14 second).
Arrhythmia:		Paroxysmal ventricular tachycardia coexisting with an accelerated idioventricular rhythm.

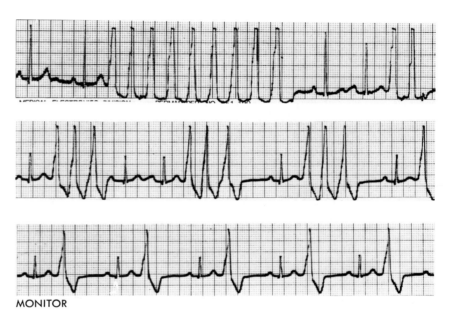

MONITOR

Fig. 6-79

Rate:	Atrial	60 to 75.
	Ventricular	170 to 210.
Rhythm:	Atrial	Slightly irregular.
	Ventricular	Irregular because of bursts of ventricular ectopy.
P waves:		Normal for the sinus-initiated QRS complexes.
P-R interval:		Normal for the sinus-initiated QRS complexes, 0.16 second.
QRS:		Normal for the sinus-initiated complexes; wide, bizarre, prolonged (0.12 second) for the ventricular ectopy.
Arrhythmia:		Paroxysmal ventricular tachycardia gradually decreasing in frequency to bigeminy and then complete disappearance. This result followed administration of lidocaine, 50 mg IV in a patient with an acute myocardial infarction.

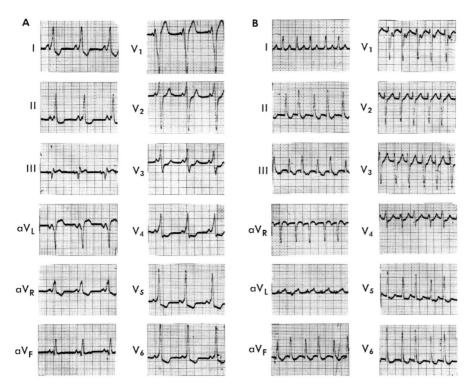

Fig. 6-80

Rate:	**A,** 82 beats per minute; **B,** varying between 150 and 180.
Rhythm:	**A,** regular; **B,** slight variation in R-R intervals with long cycles alternating with short cycles.
P waves:	**A,** normal; **B,** retrograde; see V_1.
P-R interval:	**A,** 0.08 second; **B,** R-P interval 0.12 second.
QRS:	**A,** prolonged 0.12 second; **B,** normal 0.08 second.
Arrhythmia:	**A,** normal sinus rhythm during preexcitation syndrome, type B; **B,** paroxysmal supraventricular tachycardia in the same patient.

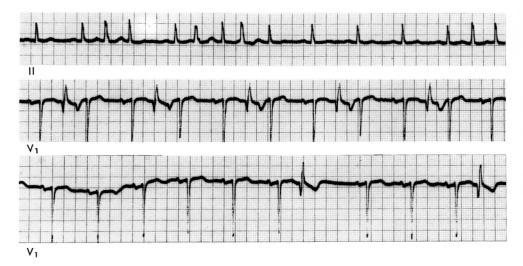

II

V₁

V₁

Fig. 6-81

Rate:	75, with premature systoles.
Rhythm:	Irregular because of premature systoles.
P waves:	Normal and precede each of the normal QRS complexes.
P-R interval:	Prolonged following the premature systoles.
QRS:	Normal for the sinus-initiated systoles; prolonged to almost 0.12 second for the premature systoles.
Arrhythmia:	Interpolated premature ventricular systoles in the top and middle tracings. In the bottom tracing, premature ventricular systoles produce a compensatory pause and are therefore no longer interpolated.

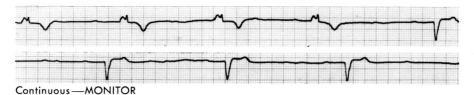

Continuous—MONITOR

Fig. 6-82

Rate:	Atrial	86.
	Ventricular	Upright complexes 38; negative complexes 28.
Rhythm:	Atrial	Regular.
	Ventricular	Fairly regular.
P waves:		Normal and have no relationship to the QRS complexes. Clear P waves cannot be seen throughout the entire tracing.
P-R interval:		Not measurable.
QRS:		Abnormal; upright complexes 0.14 second, negative complexes 0.12 second.
Arrhythmia:		Complete A-V block with a ventricular escape rhythm. The simultaneous change in ventricular contour and rate probably indicates a shift in the ventricular escape focus site.

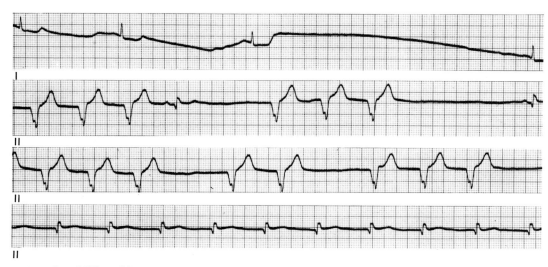

Atropine, 0.75 mg IV

Fig. 6-83

Rate:	Top tracing, slow with periods of asystole. Second and third strips (75) with periods of asystole. Bottom tracing (65).
Rhythm:	Top three tracings, irregular; bottom tracing, regular.
P waves:	Normal contour, preceding the sinus-initiated QRS complexes in lead II but are hard to see in lead I.
P-R interval:	Normal for the sinus-initiated P waves, not present for the other QRS complexes. In the bottom tracing, no P wave or P-R interval is apparent.
QRS:	Normal for the sinus-initiated QRS complexes, prolonged (0.13 second) for the ventricular ectopic beats.
Arrhythmia:	Various arrhythmias recorded in a patient with an acute inferior myocardial infarction. Top tracing, marked sinus bradycardia and periods of sinus arrest. Middle two tracings, an accelerated idioventricular rhythm, slightly irregular. The duration of the pauses in the third strip appears to be a multiple of the basic idioventricular cycle length, thus suggesting the possible presence of an intermittent exit block. Bottom tracing, a junctional rhythm following atropine administration, suppresses the ventricular ectopy.

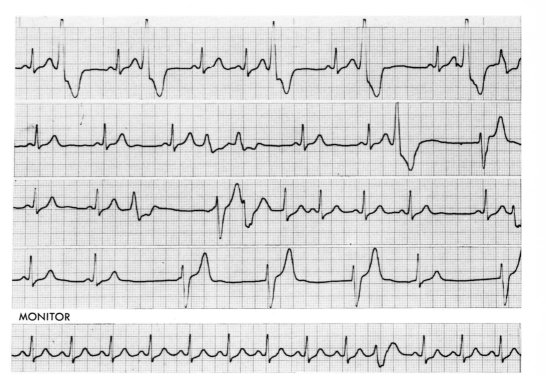

MONITOR

Atropine, 0.5 mg IV—MONITOR

Fig. 6-84

Rate:	45 to 125.
Rhythm:	Irregular.
P waves:	Normal and present before each of the sinus-initiated QRS complexes. Intermittent sinus slowing occurs.
P-R interval:	Normal and constant before each of the sinus-initiated QRS complexes (0.14 second).
QRS:	Normal for the sinus-initiated QRS complexes, prolonged (0.14 second) for the ventricular systoles.
Arrhythmia:	Frequent multiformed ventricular systoles occurring singly and in pairs in a patient with an acute myocardial infarction. Sinus bradycardia results in the emergence of a slow idioventricular rhythm (fourth strip). Atropine (bottom tracing) produced a sinus rhythm and suppressed the ventricular ectopy.

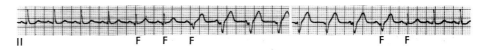

II   F   F   F   F   F

Fig. 6-85

Rate:	94 to 105.
Rhythm:	Fairly regular.
P waves:	Normal and precede each of the sinus-initiated QRS complexes. They do not precede the ventricular ectopic systoles.
P-R interval:	Normal for the sinus-initiated P waves.
QRS:	Normal for the sinus-initiated P waves; prolonged (0.14 second) for the abnormal QRS complexes. Fusion beats labeled *F*.
Arrhythmia:	Accelerated idioventricular rhythm that becomes manifest because of gradual sinus slowing.

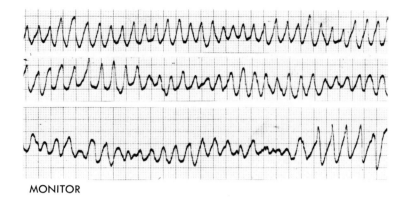

MONITOR

Fig. 6-86

Rate:	300 to 500.
Rhythm:	Grossly irregular.
P waves:	None seen.
P-R interval:	Not measurable.
QRS:	Wide, bizarre, irregular.
Arrhythmia:	Ventricular flutter that becomes ventricular fibrillation in the bottom tracing. The ventricular fibrillation then seems to organize and merge into ventricular flutter or possibly ventricular tachycardia in the terminal portion of the tracing.

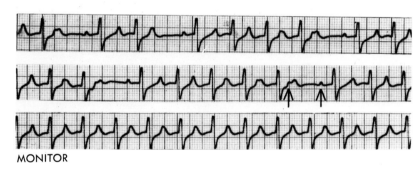

MONITOR

Fig. 6-87

Rate:	Atrial	115.
	Ventricular	Varying, depending on the degree of block.
Rhythm:	Atrial	Regular.
	Ventricular	Irregular.
P waves:		Precede each of the QRS complexes (arrows).
P-R interval:		Progressively lengthens until one P wave fails to conduct (Wenckebach A-V block).
QRS:		Normal (0.08 second).
Arrhythmia:		Atrial tachycardia with varying block. Note the varying T wave contour as P waves fall during different portions of the antecedent T wave. In the bottom tracing, 1:1 A-V conduction occurs.

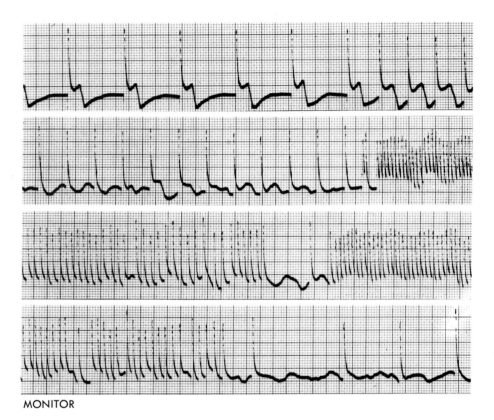

MONITOR

Fig. 6-88

Rate:	Ventricular	74 to very rapid rates.
Rhythm:	Ventricular	Periods of regularity replaced by gross irregularity.
P waves:		None seen.
P-R interval:		Not measurable.
QRS:		Wide, distorted, initiated by pacemaker spikes.
Arrhythmia:		Runaway pacemaker discharging at irregular and, at times, extremely rapid rates and finally initiating ventricular fibrillation. The pacemaker rate sped from 71 beats per minute to approximately 145 beats per minute and then greater than 1000 stimuli per minute.

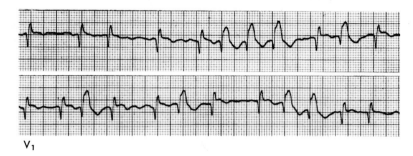

V_1

Fig. 6-89

Rate:	Ventricular	73 to 180.
Rhythm:	Ventricular	Grossly irregular.
P waves:		None seen.
P-R interval:		Not measurable.
QRS:		Normal (0.08 second) and abnormal (0.12 second) with a right bundle branch block contour.
Arrhythmia:		Atrial fibrillation with a rapid ventricular response. QRS complexes, which demonstrate a right bundle branch block, terminate a short cycle (or a series of short cycles) that follows a long preceding cycle. The development of functional right bundle branch block caused by cycle length changes in this fashion is called the "Ashman phenomenon."

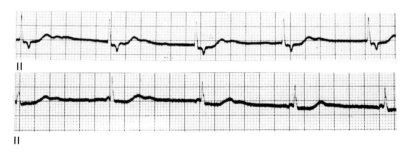

II

II

Fig. 6-90

Rate:	Top, 52; bottom, 48.
Rhythm:	Regular.
P waves:	Retrograde.
P-R interval:	Bottom, 0.06 second.
R-P interval:	Top. 0.08 second.
QRS:	Normal (0.06 second).
Arrhythmia:	A-V junctional rhythm recorded on two occasions in the same patient. In the top tracing, retrograde P waves followed the QRS complex; in the bottom tracing, retrograde P waves preceded the QRS complex.

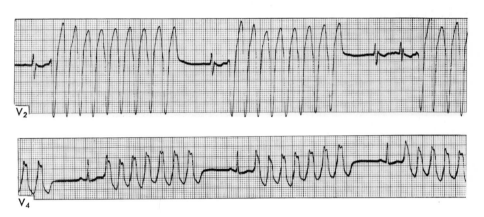

Fig. 6-91

Rate:	Ventricular	250.
Rhythm:	Ventricular	Regular in a recurrent paroxysmal fashion.
P waves:		Precede the normally conducted QRS complexes.
P-R interval:		Normal for the normally conducted QRS complexes.
QRS:		Normal for the sinus-initiated QRS complexes. QRS prolonged for the ventricular ectopic systoles (0.14 second).
Arrhythmia:		Repetitive intermittent paroxysmal ventricular tachycardia. The lack of fusion or capture beats and precise determination of atrial activity during the tachycardia prevent an unequivocal diagnosis of ventricular tachycardia from this tracing, although the diagnosis is highly suggestive.

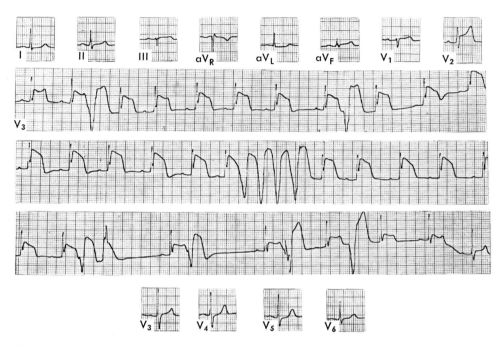

Fig. 6-92

Rate:	During V_3, approximately 75, interrupted by ventricular ectopy.
Rhythm:	Fairly regular except when interrupted by ventricular ectopy.
P waves:	Normal and precede each of the normally conducted QRS complexes.
P-R interval:	Normal (0.16 second) and constant.
QRS:	Note abrupt S-T segment elevation between V_1 and V_2 and during the V_3 rhythm strip. Then V_3 at the bottom shows a normal S-T segment. Abnormal complexes have a QRS duration greater than 0.12 second.
Arrhythmia:	Atypical (Prinzmetal) angina pectoris characterized by S-T segment *elevation.* Premature ventricular systoles trigger a short run of ventricular tachycardia in the midportion of the tracing. S-T segments return to the base line as the chest pain abates and the ectopic ventricular activity ceases.

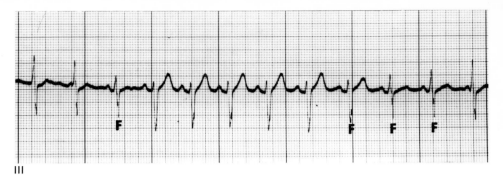

III

Fig. 6-93

Rate:	107.
Rhythm:	Regular.
P waves:	Normal and precede each of the QRS complexes in the midportion of the tracing.
P-R interval:	Constant (0.16 second) for the QRS complexes in the midportion of the tracing.
QRS:	Normal duration (0.08 second) for both types of QRS complexes, Fusion QRS complexes indicated by *F*.
Arrhythmia:	Nonparoxysmal A-V junctional tachycardia at beginning and end of tracing, which generates QRS complexes with a slightly different contour than during sinus tachycardia that occurs in the midportion of the tracing. The supraventricular origin of the tachycardia is suggested by the QRS duration (<0.12 second). However, recent data suggest that such a tachycardia actually may be ventricular, originating in the upper portions of the fascicular system and generating a QRS complex with a duration *less* than 0.12 second. The presence of fusion beats (*F*) supports this conclusion. In any event, during the tachycardia at the beginning and end of the ECG, QRS complexes are not related to atrial activity. Thus A-V dissociation is present because of nonparoxysmal A-V junctional (or ventricular) tachycardia. In the midportion of the tracing, slight acceleration of the sinus rate allows the sinus node to regain capture of the ventricles, suppress the nonparoxysmal A-V junctional tachycardia, and eliminate the periods of A-V dissociation.

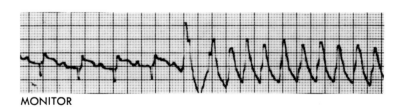

MONITOR

Fig. 6-94

Rate:	Atrial	110.
	Ventricular	230.
Rhythm:		Regular.
P waves:		Precede the normal QRS complexes but not seen during the tachycardia to the right.
P-R interval:		0.24 second, preceding the normal QRS complexes; not measurable during the tachycardia.
QRS:		Normal (0.07 second) for the sinus-initiated QRS complexes; prolonged (0.14 second) during the tachycardia.
Arrhythmia:		Ventricular tachycardia that began, in this patient who experienced an acute myocardial infarction, *without* preexisting or precipitating ventricular extrasystoles. Although it is possible that the P wave preceding the widened QRS complex initiates a supraventricular tachycardia with aberration, it is unlikely.

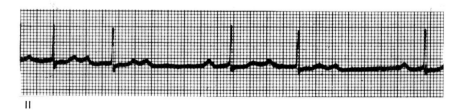

II

Fig. 6-95

Rate:	Atrial	75.
	Ventricular	3:2 conduction, average 50.
Rhythm:	Atrial	Regular.
	Ventricular	Irregular.
P waves:		Normal and precede each QRS complex.
P-R interval:		Progressively lengthens prior to the nonconducted P wave.
QRS:		Normal (0.06 second).
Arrhythmia:		Second-degree A-V block, type I (Wenckebach).

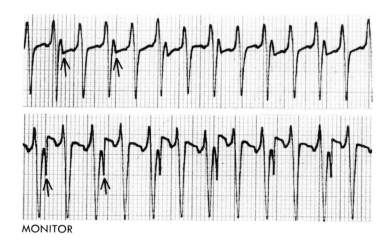

MONITOR

Fig. 6-96

Rate:	Atrial	120.
	Ventricular	240.
Rhythm:		Regular.
P waves:		Follow alternate QRS complexes.
P-R interval:		0.08 second.
QRS:		Normal (0.10).
Arrhythmia:		Nonparoxysmal A-V junctional tachycardia with 2:1 retrograde block to the atrium. Arrows indicate P waves. Top tracing, monitor lead; bottom tracing, intracavitary right atrial lead.

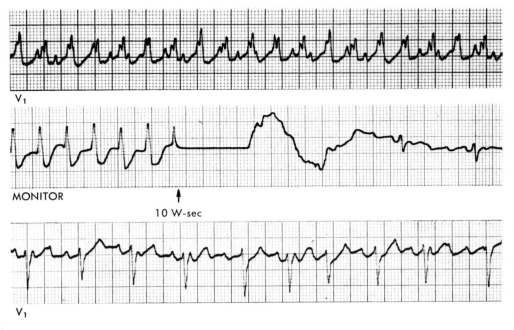

Fig. 6-97

Rate:	Atrial	300 (top panel).
	Ventricular	200 (top panel).
Rhythm:	Atrial	Regular.
	Ventricular	Regular.
P waves:		Atrial flutter.
P-R interval:		Completely variable.
QRS:		Wide, prolonged (0.12 second).
Arrhythmia:		Atrial flutter and ventricular tachycardia in top tracing. Thus complete A-V dissociation is present. In the monitor recording (middle tracing) the left portion reflects the same activity seen in V₁ above. However, the particular monitor lead fails to reveal the atrial flutter waves. Direct current cardioversion (*arrow*, 10 watt-seconds) terminates the ventricular tachycardia but allows the atrial flutter to persist, seen more clearly in V₁ below. The atrial flutter at this point is not as precisely regular at it was prior to the cardioversion.

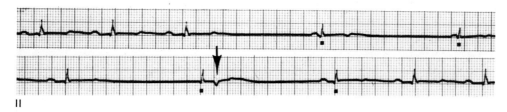

II

Fig. 6-98

Rate:	30 to 50.
Rhythm:	Fairly irregular.
P waves:	Precede and conduct to the QRS complexes that do not have dots beneath them. Those with dots beneath them are junctional escape beats.
P-R interval:	Prolonged (0.26 second) and constant for the QRS complexes that do not have a dot beneath them.
QRS:	Normal duration and contour (0.08 second). Dots indicate A-V junctional escape beats. The third A-V junctional escape beat (lower tracing) retrogradely activates the atrium *(arrow)*.
Arrhythmia:	Sinus bradycardia with intermittent sinus arrest and A-V junctional escape beats, the "sick sinus syndrome."

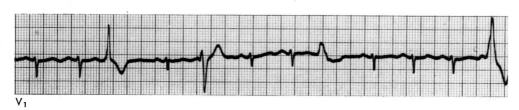

V₁

Fig. 6-99

Rate:	98.
Rhythm:	Irregular because of premature ventricular systoles.
P waves:	Normal and precede each sinus-initiated QRS complex.
P-R interval:	Normal for the sinus-initiated QRS complexes (0.14 second).
QRS:	Normal for the sinus-initiated QRS complexes (0.08 second). Premature systoles are characterized by varied contour and a duration greater than 0.12 second.
Arrhythmia:	Multiformed premature ventricular systoles with four different contours.

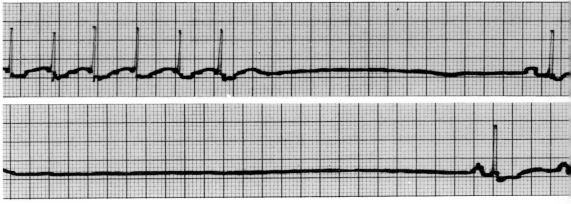

MONITOR

Fig. 6-100

Rate:	140, abruptly slowing following carotid sinus massage. Two periods of asystole are finally terminated by sinus rhythm.
Rhythm:	Regular, followed by asystole, an atrial escape beat, and then sinus rhythm.
P waves:	Can be seen when tachycardia terminates.
P-R interval:	Normal (0.18 sec) in those beats preceded by P waves.
QRS:	Normal.
Arrhythmia:	Abrupt termination of paroxysmal supraventricular tachycardia by carotid sinus massage (at beginning of recording). A lengthy period of asystole results when the tachycardia stops, before sinus rhythm resumes.

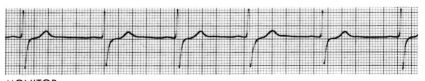

MONITOR

Fig. 6-101

Rate:	56.
Rhythm:	Regular.
P waves:	Normal and precede each QRS complex.
P-R interval:	Normal, constant (0.18 second).
QRS:	Normal (0.10 second).
Arrhythmia:	Sinus bradycardia.

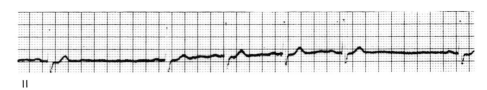

II

Fig. 6-102

Rate:	33 to 66.
Rhythm:	Irregular.
P waves:	Normal contour. Long P-P cycles are exactly twice the short P-P cycles.
P-R interval:	Normal (0.20 second).
QRS:	Normal (0.08 second).
Arrhythmia:	2:1 sinus exit block.

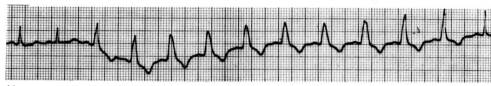

V₆

Fig. 6-103

Rate:	Gradually accelerates from 105 to 115.
Rhythm:	Fairly regular.
P waves:	Normal and precede each QRS complex.
P-R interval:	Normal (0.14 second) and constant.
QRS:	Normal at the slower rates; left bundle branch block (0.12 second) at the faster rates.
Arrhythmia:	Rate-dependent aberration with functional left bundle branch block.

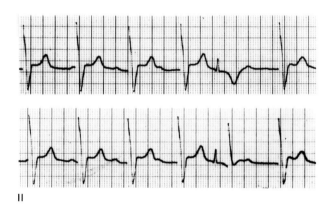

II

Fig. 6-104

Rate:	68.
Rhythm:	Fairly regular.
P waves:	Normal contour but have no consistent relationship to ventricular depolarization.
P-R interval:	Completely variable.
QRS:	All but the fifth QRS complex in each panel are initiated by a pacemaker spike and have a duration of 0.16 second. The fifth QRS complexes represent supravricular captures with a duration of 0.07 second.
Arrhythmia:	Left panel, ventricular inhibited pacemaker; right panel, conversion of ventricular inhibited pacemaker to a continuously discharging, asynchronous pacemaker by holding a magnet over the pacemaker. Note that the fifth QRS complex in right panel no longer suppresses pacemaker discharge. The ventricles are still refractor at the time of pacemaker discharge, and no QRS complex is generated.

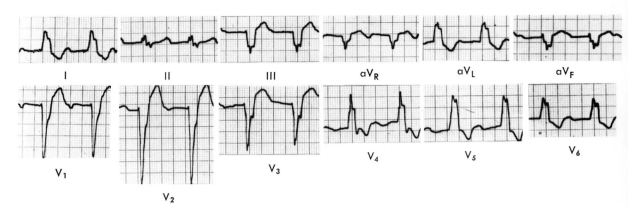

Fig. 6-105

Rate:	72.
Rhythm:	Regular.
P waves:	Hidden within the preceding T waves.
P-R interval:	Prolonged (0.4 second).
QRS:	Wide (0.16 second).
Arrhythmia:	Normal sinus rhythm with left bundle branch block and first-degree A-V block.

Electrocardiogram test section

This section provides a series of ECG tracings of various conditions that have been previously discussed. It is suggested that you cover the interpretations at the end of each legend and attempt to identify the abnormal patterns in each electrocardiogram.

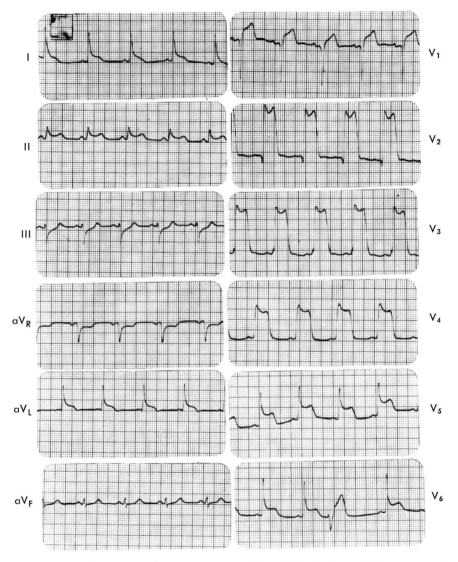

Fig. 6-106. Normal sinus rhythm. Q waves in V_1 and V_2. Marked S-T segment elevation in leads I, II, a V_L, and V_1 through V_6. T waves have not yet inverted.

Electrocardiogram: *Hyperacute anterolateral, possibly apical, myocardial infarction.*

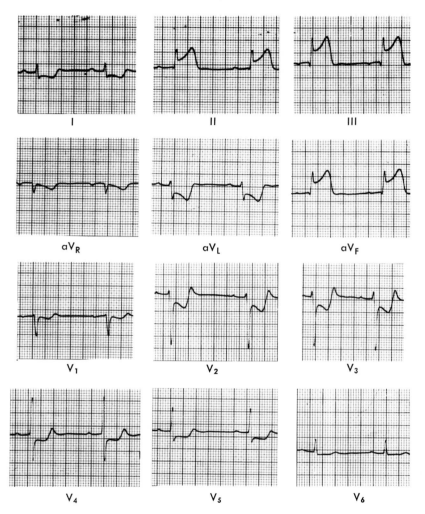

Fig. 6-107. Normal sinus rhythm. No pathologic Q waves have developed. Marked S-T segment elevation in leads II, III, and aV$_F$ with reciprocal depression in leads I, aV$_L$ and the anterior precordium. T waves are still upright.

Electrocardiogram: *Hyperacute inferior (diaphragmatic) myocardial infarction.*

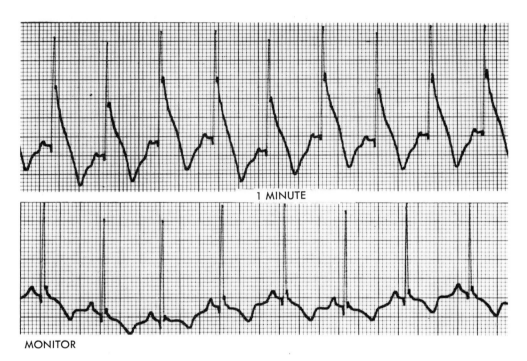

1 MINUTE

MONITOR

Fig. 6-108. Top tracing demonstrates marked S-T segment elevation and T wave inversion. One minute later (bottom tracing) the S-T segments have returned to base line. The T waves are still inverted.

Electrocardiogram: *The rapid S-T changes from elevation to normal are characteristic of atypical (Prinzmetal) angina pectoris.*

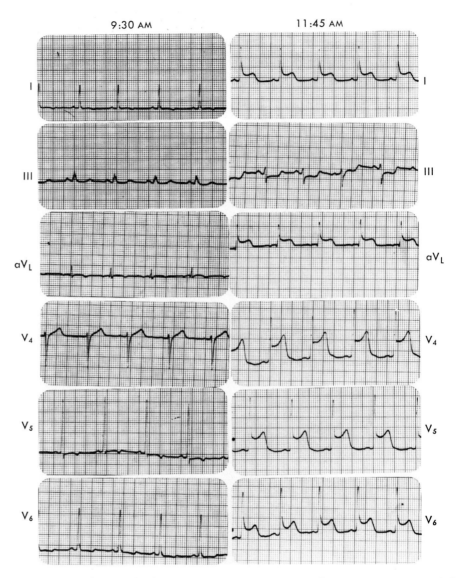

Fig. 6-109. Normal sinus rhythm. Tracing at 9:30 AM, normal; tracing at 11:45 AM (after the patient developed more chest pain) demonstrates S-T segment elevation in leads I, aV_L, and V_4 through V_6. The T waves are still upright and no pathologic Q waves have developed.

Electrocardiogram: *Hyperacute lateral myocardial infarction.*

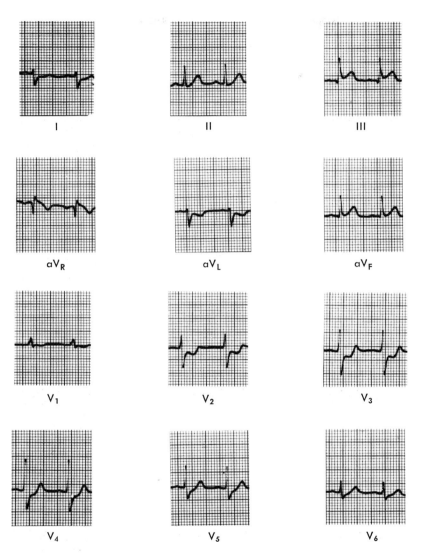

Fig. 6-110. Normal sinus rhythm. Right axis deviation suggesting left posterior hemi-block. S-T segment elevation in lead III and slight S-T segment elevation in lead aV_F. Large R wave in V_1 with slight S-T segment depression in V_1, more marked in V_2 and V_3. T waves are still upright except for diphasic T waves in leads V_1 and V_2.

Electrocardiogram: *Acute posteroinferior myocardial infarction.*

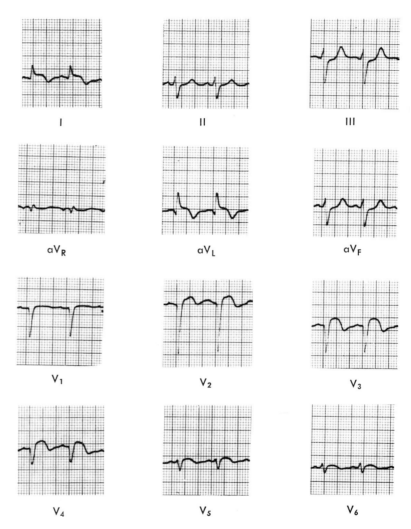

I II III

aV_R aV_L aV_F

V_1 V_2 V_3

V_4 V_5 V_6

Fig. 6-111. Normal sinus rhythm. Left axis deviation characteristic of left anterior hemiblock. S-T segment elevation in leads I, aV_L, and V_2 through V_6. Abnormal Q wave in V_1 through V_4 with small R waves in V_5 and V_6. T wave inversion in leads I and aV_L and terminal T wave inversion in V_2 through V_5.

Impression: *Acute anterolateral myocardial infarction and left anterior hemiblock.*

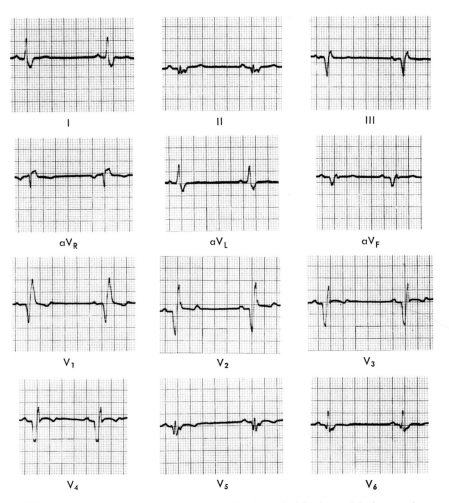

Fig. 6-112. Normal sinus rhythm, right bundle branch block, and left axis deviation characterisic of left anterior hemiblock. S-T segments are normal. There are nonspecific T wave changes. A pathologic Q wave is present in leads II, III, aV$_F$, and V$_1$ through V$_4$, and makes the diagnosis of left anterior hemiblock difficult.

Electrocardiogram: *Right bundle branch block, possible left anterior hemiblock, and anteroinferior myocarcial infarction, probably old.*

CHAPTER SEVEN

ARTIFICIAL CARDIAC PACEMAKERS

A pacemaker is an electronic device (also called a pulse generator) that delivers an electrical stimulus to the heart through electrodes sewn directly on the epicardium or placed in contact with the endocardium. The stimulus lasts from 0.08 to 2 msec and has a milliampere amplitude that depends on the resistance of the electrode circuit and the voltage output of the pacemaker.

Electrical stimuli applied in such a manner repetitively depolarize the ventricles (or the atria) to increase the heart rate by a controlled amount. These devices were originally developed to increase heart rate in patients with complete heart block. However, today they find a wider diagnostic as well as therapeutic use in patients with cardiac disorders. Approximately 300,000 patients have been treated with pacemakers.

Indications for pacemaker insertion
TEMPORARY PACING—THERAPEUTIC USES

Temporary transvenous pacing is generally indicated as follows:
1. Prior to replacing the pulse generator or initially inserting a permanent pacemaker
2. Prophylactically in patients who have complete A-V block and are undergoing surgical procedures requiring general anesthesia
3. Prophylactically after open heart surgery (wires may be inserted into the atrial and ventricular wall at the time of surgery and removed when the patient's condition has stabilized)
4. On a trial basis to control drug-refractory tachyarrhythmias
5. To treat congestive heart failure in patients with medically unresponsive, slow ventricular rates
6. In general, to treat any situation that is thought to be transient and reversible (outlined under indications for permanent pacemaker implantation)

For patients developing A-V block *during* the course of acute myocardial infarction, controversy exists regarding the indications for pacemaker insertion. Reasons for this controversy are the following: Catheter insertion, even by skilled personnel, during an acute myocardial infarction may be dangerous. Although A-V block develops in 7% to 10% of the patients with diaphragmatic myocardial infarction, it is generally transient and usually does not progress past the Wenckebach grade. If necessary, medical therapy with atropine or isoproterenol usually reverses the block or speeds the ventricular rate to acceptable levels, thus preventing the need for pacemaker insertion. Mortality in patients with this type of block in the absence of heart failure or shock is no greater than in patients without Weckebach block. A-V block has an incidence of 1% to 3% in patients with anterior myocardial infarction. However, type (Mobitz) II A-V block or other forms of bilateral (bifascicular) bundle branch block more commonly develop in patients with anteroseptal myocardial infarction; this block may suddenly progress to complete A-V block with an inadequate spontaneous escape pacemaker. It is recommended that a prophylactic pacing catheter be inserted only in patients with bifascicular block complicating acute anteroseptal infarction, especially if this is associated with a prolonged AV conduction. Temporary pacing may not be necessary in patients with bifascicular block of less than 6 hours' duration or of onset more than 24 hours after the onset of the infarction. Unfortunately, prophylactic pacemaker insertion has not significantly altered the 60% to 80% mortality seen in this group of patients with complete A-V block, since pump failure frequently complicates the course of their disease.

Most physicians would agree on inserting a pacemaker catheter in any patient symptomatic from a slow ventricular rate that does not speed up after atropine or isoproterenol administration. Pacing also may be useful to suppress ventricular ectopic arrhythmias that are difficult to control medically or are related to slow heart rates.

TEMPORARY PACING—DIAGNOSTIC USES

Temporary transvenous pacing, usually of the right atrium, is being used with increasing frequency as part of a diagnostic evaluation in the following situations:

1. Atrial pacing may be performed to increase heart rate and thereby provide a stress that may provoke electrocardiographic, biochemical, or hemodynamic signs of ischemia in patients with coronary artery disease.
2. Atrial pacing is usually performed during electrophysiologic studies involving His bundle recordings to assess the effect of changes in heart rate on atrioventricular conduction. In addition, sudden cessation of rapid atrial pacing allows assessment of intrinsic S-A node pacemaking function.
3. Premature stimuli may be delivered to induce and terminate various tachyarrhythmias such as paroxysmal atrial or ventricular tachycardia and thus provide evidence supporting reentry versus automaticity as a cause of the specific arrhythmia.

PERMANENT PACING

All permanent pacing is done for therapeutic reasons. The most common instance is complete heart block, which may be constant or intermittent but is not likely to result from a reversible process. Patients with complete A-V block usually have symptoms caused by low cardiac output (fatigue), congestive heart failure (dyspnea, edema), syncope (Adams-Stokes attacks), or myocardial ischemia (angina). Adams-Stokes attacks are "spells" characterized by sudden syncope or seizures that result from a sudden cardiac arrhythmia, that is, ventricular standstill or ventricular fibrillation. However, many studies suggest that even asymptomatic patients with complete heart block distal to the bundle of His (characterized by widened QRS complexes) should have a permanent pacemaker implantation because such patients have a higher mortality without permanent pacemaker implantation. The 12 month survival rate for unpaced patients with complete A-V block is 30% to 40%; for paced patients with complete A-V block, approximately 80%.

Other indications for permanent pacing include the presence of symptomatic sinus bradycardia ("sick sinus syndrome"), hypersensitive carotid sinus syndrome, and some forms of tachyarrhythmias, like paroxysmal atrial tachycardia (PAT), that cannot be controlled with drug therapy and have been demonstrated in the laboratory to terminate with pacing. In this circumstance, PAT is thought to be terminated by an atrial or ventricular stimulus that, delivered at an appropriate time, interrupts the tachycardia.

The right ventricle remains the pacing site for most instances of permanent

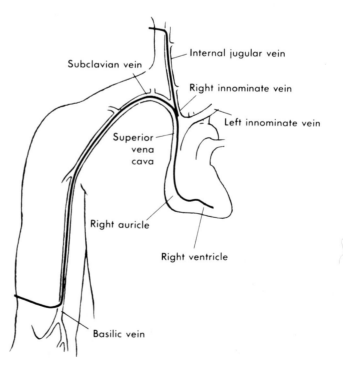

Fig. 7-1. Two venous pathways commonly used to insert a transvenous pacing catheter into the right ventricle.

and temporary pacing. However, as will be discussed later, atrial pacing sites may be utilized under certain circumstances. Demand pacemakers generally are preferred for permanent pacing to avoid competition with other intrinsic spontaneous ventricular rhythms such as ventricular ectopy or the return of A-V conduction in patients with intermittent A-V block. In many patients who develop complete A-V block after an acute myocardial infarction and who survive, A-V conduction may return to normal. If A-V block remains, permanent pacing may be needed. Permanent pacing for the group in whom bifascicular block developed at the time of infarction and remained is controversial. Some studies have shown a high incidence of sudden death in this group after discharge, creating the opinion that these patients should have a permanent pacemaker implanted prophylactically. Further follow-up data are required to resolve the question of whether permanent prophylactic pacemaker implantation is indicated in patients with residual bifascicular block following acute myocardial infarction.

Methods of pacemaker electrode insertion

Temporary pacing employs a catheter with electrodes on its tip, inserted percutaneously or by a small cutdown, into a peripheral vein. The basilic (median antecubital), femoral, external jugular, internal jugular, or subclavian veins may be used. The femoral approach may offer some advantages if permanent implantation subsequently becomes necessary because the neck veins may then be used without increased risk of infection.

The catheter is advanced under fluoroscopic or electrocardiographic* control (or both) to the desired position in the right atrium or ventricle (Fig. 7-1). Stable placement of the catheter tip in the right atrium is difficult to achieve but may be accomplished by manipulating the catheter into the atrial appendage or coronary sinus. For ventricular pacing the catheter is wedged

---

*Connecting the V lead of the ECG machine to the catheter electrode allows the latter to be used as an exploring, intracavity lead. When the catheter is in the atrium the P wave is large; as it passes into the right ventricle, the amplitude of the P wave becomes reduced while that of the QRS complex becomes large (Fig. 7-2).

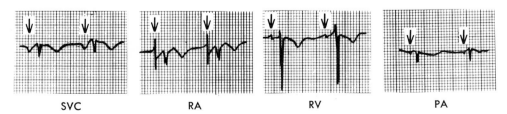

Fig. 7-2. Tracings that demonstrate the characteristic P and QRS contours, recorded from within the superior vena cava *(SVC)*, right atrium *(RA)*, right ventricle *(RV)*, and pulmonary artery *(PA)*. Arrows indicate P waves.

beneath trabeculae in the apex of the right ventricle; less commonly, the outflow tract of the right ventricle may be paced.

If the electrode is adequately positioned very close to or directly touching the endocardium, the amount of electrical energy necessary to depolarize the heart (pacing or excitability threshold) becomes less than 1.5 milliamperes. The setting for energy delivered by the pulse generator should be at least twice this threshold. A stable pacing position with a low threshold is confirmed after having the patient breathe deeply, cough, and shift about slightly.

Extreme emergencies may not allow sufficient time to move the patient to a fluoroscopic unit and to mobilize the skilled help necessary for this type of pacemaker catheter insertion. Alternative approaches are available, although generally they are not as successful. A flexible, lightweight catheter may be directed by the flow of venous blood returning to the right heart to the desired atrial or ventricular position. The "floating" of such a catheter into the right ventricle is made easier by the presence of an inflatable balloon near the end of the catheter. This is accomplished at the bedside, using electrocardiographic monitoring. A second emergency method involves passing a long needle, such as a No. 20 spinal needle with stylet in place, percutaneously through the left chest directly into the right or left ventricle. The stylet is removed and is replaced by a pacing catheter that is advanced until endocardial contact is made. The needle is then withdrawn, leaving the pacing catheter secured in place (Fig. 7-3). Coronary artery trauma, pericardial tamponade, or arrhythmias are risks incurred by this approach.

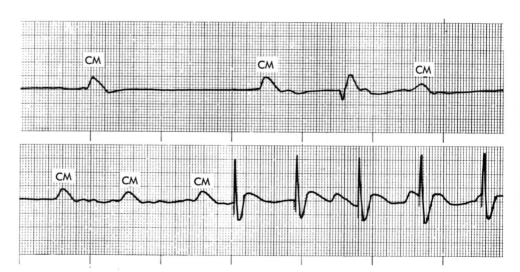

Fig. 7-3. Continuous tracing. This was recorded during resuscitation attempts performed on a patient with cardiac arrest. A thin unipolar catheter electrode, inserted through a needle that penetrated the chest wall into the ventricle, initiated ventricular depolarization at the end of the recording. Deflections labeled *CM* indicate external cardiac massage.

In all these methods of temporary pacing the electrodes are connected to an external pulse generator that may be part of a monitoring unit or may be an independent self-contained battery unit. The latter is preferable to reduce the risks of improperly grounded equipment that may induce ventricular fibrillation.

Depending on the method of temporary pacing, a unipolar (one-electrode) or bipolar (two-electrode) catheter may be used. The unipolar catheter must be connected to an indifferent electrode elsewhere. This is accomplished by inserting a small metal needle into the skin and connecting the negative terminal of the pulse generator to the catheter electrode and the positive terminal to the needle. The patient should be warned that a tingling sensation at the needle site may occur. The bipolar catheter may be more advantageous becuase it does not need a skin electrode, and if one electrode fails, the bipolar catheter sometimes may be used as a unipolar one after a skin electrode is added.

Permanent pacing utilizes one of three approaches:

1. The *transvenous* is the most common technique and the simplest (Fig. 7-4). Under local anesthesia, a small incision is made just above the clavicle on the right side of the neck. The catheter is threaded into the external jugular vein, advanced to the apex of the right ventricle, and secured to the vein by ligature. A loop is fashioned and the proximal end of the catheter is directed downward through a subcutaneous tun-

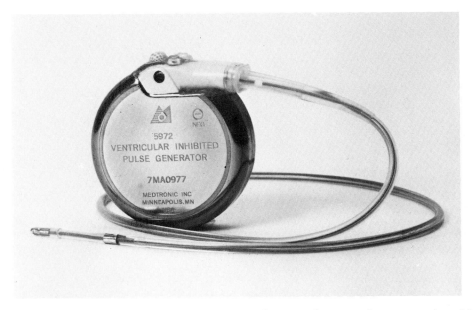

Fig. 7-4 Photograph of one of many types of pacemakers, Medtronic implantable pacemaker, with a transvenous catheter. (Courtesy Medtronic, Inc., Minneapolis, Minn.)

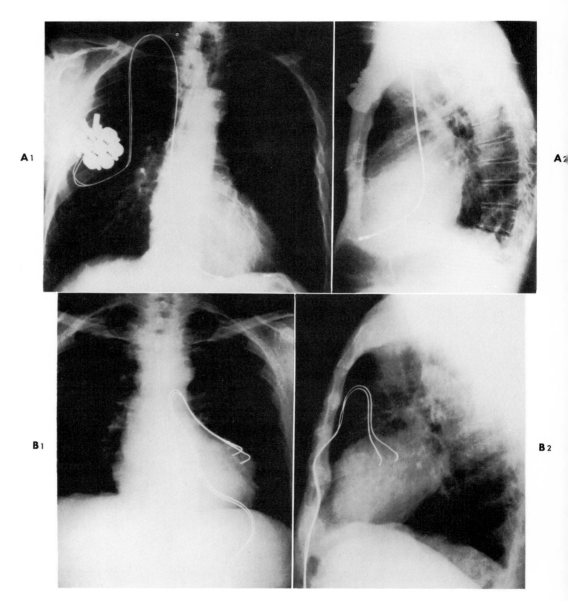

Fig. 7-5. A, Photographs of x-ray films that show a transvenous pacing catheter inserted to the apex of the right ventricle, with the pulse generator implanted beneath the right clavicle. **1.** Posteroanterior view; **2**, lateral view. **B,** Pacemaker electrodes that were sewn on the myocardium at the time of thoracotomy, with the pulse generator implanted in the the abdominal wall (not seen). **1,** Posteroanterior view; **2,** lateral view. (Courtesy Medtronic, Inc., Minneapolis, Minn.)

nel and joined to the battery-powered pulse generator that is placed in a pocket beneath the skin in the right anterior chest area below the clavicle. This same approach may be performed on the left side or using the internal jugular vein. With the transvenous approach, hospitalization time is short and morbidity is low. However, a relatively high incidence of electrode displacement in inexperienced hands results in loss of capture in the early postimplantation period. If careful attention is paid to pacing and sensing thresholds, electrode position, and surgical technique, the percentage of displacement does not exceed 10% for experienced surgeons.

2. With the *transthoracic* approach the chest is opened so that the epicardial pacing electrodes may be sutured directly to the myocardium. The electrode is then directed through a subcutaneous tunnel to the abdominal wall. There it is connected to the pulse generator and placed subcutaneously (Fig. 7-5). The epicardial approach via thoracotomy may offer greater reliability of pacing. Also, it is usually necessary to use this approach when synchronous atrial pacing is desired. Furthermore, pacemaker implantation by thoracotomy may be indicated for young people who have not attained full growth. The fixed length of the electrode used in transvenous implantation does not adjust to vertical growth of the chest, whereas an additional length of electrode may be inserted at the time of thoracotomy.

3. The *transmediastinal* approach is an adaptation of the transthoracic approach and involves opening the chest in the midline. In this situation the pleural cavity is not entered. Consequently, the patient does not need chest tubes and postoperative recovery is expedited. The electrodes are attached to the right ventricular epicardium, and hence this technique offers stable epicardial pacing without the need for thoracotomy. Electrodes shaped like screws may be screwed into the myocardium, thus facilitating the transmediastinal approach.

Electrocardiogram

The electrical stimulus (pacemaker artifact, spike) delivered by a pacemaker produces a sharp narrow deflection (Fig. 7-6). Unipolar pacemakers generate larger spikes than bipolar pacemakers; these spikes may significantly distort the ECG. The pacemaker artifact immediately precedes the P wave when the atrium is paced or the QRS complex when the ventricle is paced. The contour of the pacemaker-induced P wave or QRS complex generally differs significantly from the spontaneous beat. The exact rhythm produced by artificial pacing depends on whether atrium or ventricle is paced, the type of spontaneous cardiac rhythm, if any, and the type of pacemaker used. In addition, the site of ventricular pacing may be predicted from the ECG. Transvenous endocardial pacing of the right ventricle results in a LBBB pattern in the ECG; epicardial transthoracic pacing of the left ventricle results in an RBBB pattern.

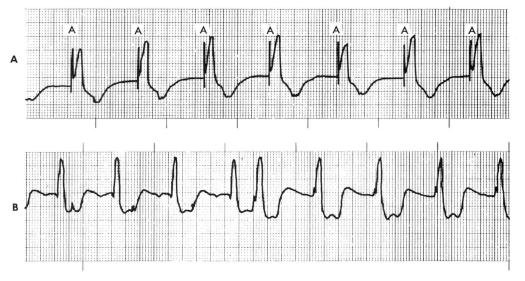

Fig. 7-6. A, Continuously discharging ventricular pacemaker. The pacemaker stimulates each ventricular contraction in this tracing. Atrial activity is not readily apparent. Pacemaker artifacts are labeled **A. B,** Unlike the previous figure, spontaneous ventricular activity competes with the pacemaker for control of the cardiac rhythm. A poorly defined P wave precedes the first four QRS complexes, indicating spontaneous sinus rhythm. Pacemaker spikes "march through" these first four beats but remain completely uninfluenced by spontaneous activity. Finally, the ventricles are in a nonrefractory state in time to be discharged by the fourth pacemaker spike. The last five QRS complexes are each initiated by a small spike and represent pacemaker-driven beats. Both conducted and pacemaker-induced QRS complexes have similar contours because the patient has intrinsic left bundle branch block that is mimicked by pacing the right ventricle.

Types of pacemakers

The different types of pacemakers are as follows:
1. Continuously discharging with fixed or adjustable rates
   a. Atrial
   b. Ventricular
2. Synchronous
   a. Atrial
   b. Ventricular
3. Demand
   a. Atrial
   b. Ventricular

Continuously discharging (fixed rate, asynchronous) *pacemakers* duplicate the ECG features of parasystole, that is, the rate and rhythm of pacemaker discharge remain unaffected by spontaneous beats, and paced beats maintain a constant interectopic interval. This means that the interval between two

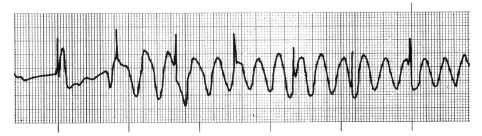

Fig. 7-7. Continuously discharging ventricular pacemaker. The initial pacemaker-stimulated QRS complex is followed by a spontaneous premature ventricular contraction. The next pacemaker discharge occurs during the vulnerable period of this beat and precipitates ventricular tachycardia-fibrillation.

successively paced beats becomes a multiple of the basic pacing rate, regardless of the number of intervening nonpaced beats (Figs. 7-6 and 7-7). The discharge rate in many models may be *adjusted* to suit the clinical situation. The term *"fixed rate"* derives from the fact that, once the rate is set, it remains fixed and continuously discharging, uninfluenced by spontaneous cardiac rhythm.

The fixed-rate, asynchronous method of ventricular pacing in patients with complete A-V block may initiate competition if normal A-V conduction returns, as it may in 25% to 30% of patients, or if premature ventricular complexes occur. The resulting competition between paced and spontaneous beats ordinarily does not produce any problems even though pacemaker stimuli may discharge during the *vulnerable period* of a preceding T wave (a period of 20 to 40 msec located near the apex of the T wave). A fivefold to tenfold safety factor existing between the electrical energy provided by a pacing stimulus and the energy necessary to precipitate ventricular fibrillation protects against pacemaker-precipitated ventricular tachyarrhythmias. However, under conditions that lower the amount of energy necessary to produce ventricular fibrillation—for example, during acute myocardial infarction, electrolyte imbalance, frequent premature systoles, during use of sympathomimetic agents, or immediately after pacemaker insertion when the amount of energy delivered by the pulse generator has not yet become attenuated by the developement of fibrosis at electrode sites—a stimulus delivered to the ventricles during the vulnerable period may initiate ventricular tachycardia or fibrillation (R on T phenomenon) (See Figs. 6-49 and 7-7.)

This mode of pacing does not enable the pacemaker rate to change in response to physiologic demands such as fever or increased physical activity. Also, ventricular pacing eliminates sequential atrioventricular contraction, and the effectiveness of the atrium as a booster pump is lost. Particularly in patients with reduced cardiovascular function, properly timed atrial contraction contributes significantly to maintaining an adequate cardiac output.

Atrial pacing, reserved for the patient with intact A-V conduction and without persistent atrial flutter or fibrillation, provides the electrical and hemodynamic benefits of normal atrioventricular contraction. Atrial pacing also reduces the dangers of ventricular competition (Fig. 7-8).

Since the electronic circuitry is relatively simple and therefore quite reliable, continuously discharging ventricular pacemakers are still useful for patients with stable unvarying complete A-V heart block. Both atrial and ventricular pacing have helped control certain medically refractory arrhythmias and have been useful in terminating various arrhythmias such as atrial flutter and paroxysmal atrial tachycardia.

Synchronous atrial pacing employs an atrial sensing circuit and a ventricular stimulating circuit provided by separate atrial and ventricular electrodes. The pacemaker "senses" or is activated by spontaneous atrial depolarization through the atrial electrodes. After waiting a preset delay interval, it discharges the ventricles through the ventricular electrodes in response to the sensed P wave. The period of delay between the sensed P wave and ventricular stimulation duplicates the normal P-R interval (Fig. 7-9). The pacemaker unit also serves as an electronic A-V node–His bundle by discharging the ventricles at a fixed rate in the event of atrial asystole and by inducing 2:1 or greater block between sensed P waves and ventricular stimulation if the atrial rate becomes excessively rapid.

The advantages of synchronous atrial pacing are to enable the atria to vary the ventricular rate according to physiologic demands, to reduce competition, and to preserve sequential atrioventricular contraction. Complex circuitry,

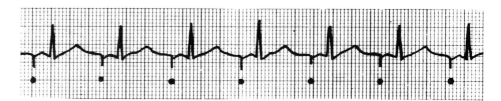

Fig. 7-8. Continuously discharging atrial pacemaker. The pacemaker initiates each atrial depolarization, indicated by pacemaker spikes (dots) preceding each P wave.

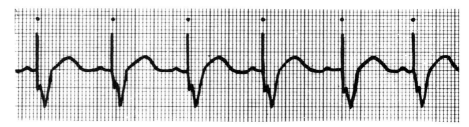

Fig. 7-9. Synchronous atrial pacing. Each sensed P wave is followed by a delay of 0.16 second; at that time the pacemaker discharges to produce ventricular depolarization. Dots indicate pacemaker discharge.

frequent need for thoracotomy to achieve stable sensing and pacing, short battery life, and the precipitation of other arrhythmias have limited the clinical use of this type of pacemaker.

Synchronous ventricular (ventricular triggered) pacing is simply another type of demand ventricular pacing. A ventricular pacemaker electrode serves to both sense and stimulate ventricular depolarization. Spontaneous ventricular beats activate the pacemaker to discharge harmlessly during the absolute refractory period of the sensed beat (about 0.02 second after the onset of the spontaneous QRS complex). In the event of a decrease in ventricular rate below the escape rate of the pacemaker, this pacemaker depolarizes the ventricle at a fixed continuous rate.

Synchronous atrial and ventricular pacemakers have a "refractory period" of about 0.4 to 0.5 second after discharge, during when they fail to sense spontaneous cardiac activity (Fig. 7-10). Because of this, these pacemakers potentially may stimulate during the T wave of a nonsensed ventricular beat. Another disadvantage of the ventricular synchronous pacemakers is that the firing of the pacemaker into a conducted QRS may distort the QRS, and make electrocardiographic interpretation of the ECG more difficult. In addition, the current drain on the pacemaker while the patient is in sinus rhythm may be relatively large. For these reasons, the ventricular synchronous pacemaker is less commonly used.

A *demand atrial* or *ventricular* (atrial or ventricular inhibited, stimulus-

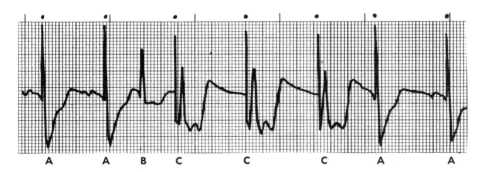

Fig. 7-10. Synchronous ventricular pacing. This seeminly complex tracing is easily explained when the type of pacemaker is known and careful attention is given to the initial portion of each beat. Three different QRS contours are apparent: *A, B,* and *C.* Beats *A* begin with a small Q wave and are preceded by a P wave with a constant P-R interval; 0.02 second *after* the onset of the QRS, the pacemaker discharges and distorts the inscription of the remainder of the QRS complex with its large spike. These represent normally conducted beats that stimulate the pacemaker to discharge during the ventricular refractory period. Beat *B,* a premature atrial contraction, occurs during the refractory period of the pacemaker and is too early to be sensed. Beat *A* would resemble beat *B* (the initial portions are the same) if not altered by the pacemaker spike. Because beat *B* is not sensed, the pacemaker is able to escape and initiates beats *C,* which *begin* with a pacemaker spike, until the sinus node again resumes control. Pacemaker spikes are indicated by dots. The pacemaker is functioning normally and the rhythm produced is not unusual.

blocking, standby) pacemaker discharges when the sensed rate of spontaneous cardiac beating decreases below a preset minimum value of the pacemaker. In other words, the pacemaker behaves as an escape focus: When the spontaneous heart rate decreases below the pacemaker escape rate, the pacemaker fires. The pacemaker is equipped with a sensing circuit, which registers the P wave or QRS complex, and an electrical blocking circuit, which prevents pacemaker discharge as long as the spontaneous rate exceeds the minimum set escape rate of the pacemaker (Fig. 7-11). Escape intervals may not have the same duration as that occurring between repetitive discharges.

The demand mode of pacing effectively eliminates competition, but at times a spontaneous beat occurs too late to prevent pacemaker discharge and results in a fusion beat (Fig. 7-12). Demand pacemakers have a shorter "refractory period" than ventricular synchronous pacemakers and are able to sense electrical activity 150 to 150 msec after pacemaker discharge. Because A-V block may be intermittent or may disappear completely for long periods of time in some patients, this mode of pacing is employed routinely in many centers to eliminate the dangers of competition, as mentioned previously. Ventricular demand pacing is the most common type of permanent pacing currently in use.

A new generation of pacemakers that have more flexibility is being tested;

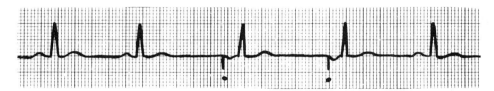

Fig. 7-11. Demand atrial pacing. Sudden sinus slowing after the second P wave allows escape of a demand pacemaker, which then initiates atrial depolarization until the atrial rate increases. Pacemaker spikes indicated by dots.

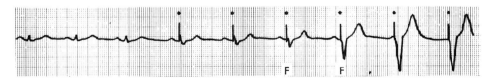

Fig. 7-12. Demand ventricular pacing. A decrease in the ventricular rate, in this case produced by carotid sinus massage that gradually slows the sinus rate, permits the pacemaker to escape. The first two pacemaker discharges merely distort the inscription of the QRS complex; the second two discharges produce fusion beats *(F)* with the sinus-conducted impulse, and the last two discharges solely initiate ventricular beating. Pacemaker artifacts indicated by dots.

some of these will provide for dual chamber (atria and ventricles) sensing and pacing. Most of the pacemaker's parameters, such as discharge rate, voltage output, and level of sensitivity, can be altered externally.

External (temporary) pacemakers may be set either in demand or fixed-rate modes and have an output in milliamperes that is adjustable, as well as an adjustable rate and sensitivity (demand mode). Most *implantable* pacemakers have a fixed output and rate, which are set during manufacture. Some, however, allow adjustment of rate and output subsequent to implantation, either percutaneously with a needle or transcutaneously with a battery-operated programming device.

PACEMAKER POWER SOURCES

All pacemakers contain batteries that provide a power source for the circuits that are responsible for the frequency of discharge and the waveform of the pulse delivered. The common pacemaker power source in the past has been the zinc–mercuric oxide battery cell. In most pacemakers, four to five of these cells have been placed in series to provide a total voltage output of around 6 volts. Most pacemakers will function for 2 to 3 years with this type of cell. Newer developments include improved zinc–mercuric oxide cells, lithium iodide battery power, nuclear-powered pacemakers, and pacemakers that have batteries that are rechargeable transcutaneously by induction coils and an external power source. Pacemakers with a life expectancy of greater than 5 years with a high degree of dependability are now feasible.

Complications
PACEMAKER FAILURE

Life expectancy of the pacemaker varies, as discussed previously. Battery failure accounts for 90% of pacemaker failures and may occur prematurely. Mercury batteries lose their voltage charge precipitously at the time of failure. Battery failure in almost all pacemakers now available is indicated by decrease (greater than 5 beats per minute) in pacing rate. Lithium iodide batteries display a linear decrease in voltage throughout their life span up to the point of battery depletion. This results in a gradual drop in paced rate in most pacemakers utilizing these batteries. Decreased amplitude or otherwise altered pacing stimulus on the ECG and absent stimulus at a time when pacemaker discharge is expected may also occur, as well as failure of a stimulus to cause a ventricular depolarization.

Units that sense as well as pace may lose their sensing ability and discharge continuously. Patients may notice signs of battery failure themselves and complain of palpitations, weakness, or decrease in heart rate. Components of the pulse generator can fail, which may result in changes of rate, no pacing, or, rarely, "runaway" firing when the pacemaker discharges 200 to 1000 times per minute, sometimes inducing ventricular fibrillation. (See Fig. 6-88.) The electrodes take a tortuous course to the heart and may fracture from recurrent stress. A fractured electrode eliminates or otherwise alters the stimulus registered by the ECG, and the heart fails to pace. Fibrosis developing at the electrode tip may insulate the heart from the stimulus and prevent pacing. Despite these problesm, the overall success of pacemakers has been remarkably advanced, and the life expectancy of patients with heart block can be restored to essentially normal in the absence of other cardiac disease.

The most common problems with temporary pacemakers relate to catheter positioning. Inadequate or excessive stimulation of the heart or inadequate sensing of spontaneous heart activity can occur if the catheter is not positioned properly.

OTHER COMPLICATIONS

Other complications generally relate to the method of pacemaker insertion. With temporary pacemakers, cellulitis around the insertion site may occur. Localized phlebitis may also occur. Peripheral veins may thrombose if the catheter remains in place for as long as a week, and if this occurs the catheter may have to be removed.

With the transvenous approach, catheter dislodgment, right ventricular perforation, diaphragmatic stimulation, and, rarely, pulmonary embolism may occur. The occurrence of an air embolism at the time of catheter insertion has been reported. Fortunately, ventricular perforation caused by a pacing catheter gradually penetrating the right ventricular wall occurs uncommonly and does not often produce pericardial tamponade. Thoracotomy implantation incurs the risks of major surgery in an elderly population and carries significant morbidity and mortality. Epicardial electrodes may be dislodged, but much less commonly than endocardial electrodes. Problems common to both systems include infection, pericardial inflammation, and pressure necrosis of the skin overlying the pulse generator, causing it to erode through the skin. The problems produced by competing spontaneous and pacemaker-induced rhythms have been discussed.

Care of the patient with a temporary pacemaker

A. Preoperative care
  1. Provide explanations about the procedure to the patient and family. Be certain that someone has signed an operative permit.
  2. Provide *sedation* if the patient needs it.
  3. Be prepared for *emergency measures*. Establish an IV and have emergency equipment available. In addition, prepare a syringe with lidocaine, as ventricular premature beats may develop with catheter insertion. Isoproterenol and atropine should be available also.
  4. *Monitor* the cardiac rhythm. Place the electrodes on the extremities prior to catheter insertion.
  5. Connect the ECG machine and monitor to a *common ground*. Disconnect the patient from other electrical equipment.

B. Postoperative care
   1. Following pacemaker insertion *record* the *date* and *time* of insertion, the mode of pacing employed, the pulse amplitude necessary to pace, and the set rate (if a fixed rate pacemaker is used).
   2. If the procedure has been done at the bedside, obtain a *chest x-ray film*, and 12-lead ECG to ascertain the electrode position.

   3. *Prevent catheter displacement* by securely fastening the catheter to the skin and minimizing motion of the extremity or torso at the site of catheter insertion. Slight tension on, or movement of, the catheter may alter its position in the heart. An Ace bandage wrapped around the catheter and its connection to the power source facilitates immobilization. Periodically check the ECG and compare it with the tracing taken at the time of insertion. A change in the threshold or vector of the pacemaker stimulus artifact or a change in the pacemaker-initiated QRS complex indicates change in position of the catheter. This may not be serious but becomes significant if the pacemaker then fails to capture.

   4. *Prevent infection* by maintaining absolute sterile technique. Cleanse the area of catheter insertion daily with hydrogen peroxide or a similar agent, and follow with application of a topical antibiotic and sterile dressing. A bland lubricating cream or oil lightly rubbed into the surrounding skin, with padding beneath the catheter wire, helps to prevent ulceration of the underlying tissue.

      Check the patient's temperature immediately after insertion of the pacing catheter and then routinely four times daily. Temperature elevation may indicate infection or inflammation and should be reported to the physician. A sterile, as well as an infected, thrombophlebitis may occur after the catheter has been in place for a few days. Culturing the electrode tip at the time of removal may provide clues to an underlying infection.

   5. *Provide an electrically safe environment* by properly grounding all equipment in the room. This is particularly important when externally powered pulse generators are employed. A self-contained battery pacemaker reduces these hazards and is generally preferable to externally powered units. The exposed terminals at the end of the catheter electrode may be safely insulated at their junction with the pulse generator by a rubber glove that covers the entire connection. Anyone connecting or disconnecting the pacemaker or adjusting the terminals at the end of the pacing catheter should wear rubber gloves. The patient should not be connected to two pieces of electrical equipment unless both pieces of equipment are connected to a common ground before they are attached to the patient. (See electrical safety section in Chapter 8 for further precautions.)

   6. *Observe for rhythm disturbance* and monitor cardiac rhythm constantly to ensure proper pacemaker function. Periodically, rhythm

strips should be obtained and evaluated. Since the type of rhythm produced depends on the method of pacing, be certain of the pacing mode used and the nature of the ECG rhythm to be expected.

Competing rhythms should be observed closely. If possible, demand pacing is used to avoid competition, particularly in patients with an acute myocardial infarction. Periodically, demand pacemakers should be switched to discharge continuously so that pacemaker function, including pacing stimulation thresholds, can be adequately evaluated.

Check the threshold at least every 8 hours. The amplitude of the pacemaker stimulus is set at two to three times the diastolic threshhold, that is, two to three times the amount of current necessary to produce depolarization during diastole. The monitor lead should display clearly the pacemaker stimulus; however, the pacemaker artifact should not be so large that it distorts the ECG recording or is registered by the monitor as a QRS complex and prevents monitor recognition of significant bradycardia or asystole and the sounding of an alarm. Some monitors equipped with special filters sense only contours similar to a QRS complex and therefore remain unaffected by pacemaker stimuli.

7. *Observe the patient for electrolyte changes* that may alter the susceptibility of the myocardium to excitation or conduction.
8. After removal, sterilize the temporary pacing catheter by placing it in a bacteriocidal solution or by gas sterilizing. Autoclaving should not be used.

Care of patient with a permanent pacemaker

A. Preoperative care
1. Preoperative preparation of the patient for implantation of a permanent pacemaker incorporates the details mentioned previously as well as routine preparations for any surgical procedure. Explanations are particularly important at this time. Preparing the patient's family with appropriate information and reassurance will greatly enhance the rehabilitation process.
2. In addition to the routine preoperative care, ask the patient to practice the arm range of motion exercises required postoperatively.

B. Postoperative care
The approach used for implantation of the pacemaker—thoracotomy or transvenous—determines the emphasis of patient care. Obviously the patient who has general anesthesia and a thoracotomy procedure for pacemaker insertion will need a great deal more attention to physical needs during the postoperative period. However, both surgical procedures necessitate similar patient observations.
1. Following pacemaker implantation and prior to patient discharge from the hospital, obtain and record *baseline values* of pacemaker function, including the different parameters in which the pacemaker may

discharge. These include the escape interval, continuously discharging interval (both spontaneous and magnet induced), refractory period, sensed P to QRS stimulus interval (synchronous atrial pacing), sensed QRS complex (demand ventricular pacemakers), current or voltage delivered by the pacemaker, 12-lead ECG artifact size, stimulation thresholds, and posteroanterior and lateral chest x-ray films. Most of this information (as well as date of pacemaker insertion, name, address, and phone number of the responsible physician) should be preserved in the patient's chart but should also be given in a permanent form to the patient to carry at all times.

When the patient's spontaneous rate is rapid and prevents demand or synchronous ventricular pacemakers from discharging, vagal stimulation may be used to slow the spontaneous sinus rate or induce A-V block to allow testing. Also, a magnet placed on the skin overlying the pulse generator of demand and synchronous ventricular pacemakers actuates a switch that causes the pacemaker to revert to a coninuously discharging mode. These methods permit evaluation of pacemaker stimulation.

2. *Prevent catheter displacement.* To reduce the risk of catheter dislodgment, restrict activity for the first few days in patients with transvenous catheter placement.

3. *Prevent infection.* Antibiotics may be prescribed for the initial 5 to 7 days. Sterile dressings cover the operative site. After 7 to 10 days the sutures are removed.

4. *Prevent postoperative complications.* Administer postoperative care according to the patient's needs from the type of insertion procedure. Implement passive range of motion exercises to the arm on the side of the operation to prevent "frozen shoulder." Inspect the operative site daily to detect any abnormalities, such as hematoma formation.

5. *Monitor cardiac rhythm.* As discussed previously, sinus rhythm and premature ventricular depolarizations may compete with the fixed rate pacemaker. When a permanent pacemaker is implanted, the pulse generator initially delivers a large amount of energy to the myocardium. This is necessary because some fibrosis around the electrodes will eventually occur and dissipate this energy to a degree. If the pacing stimulus should discharge during the vulnerable period of the cardiac cycle, ventricular tachycardia or ventricular fibrillation may ensue. After a permanent pacemaker is implanted, a week or more is required for adequate fibrosis to develop. Also the new, stiff, catheter stimulating the myocardium produces a certain amount of injury that may result in premature ventricular systoles. Consequently, this is a critical period, and premature ventricular systoles during this time must be vigorously suppressed. This problem is relieved by routine use of demand pacemakers, where competition is not a problem.

Rehabilitation
PSYCHOLOGIC FACTORS

Most patients appear to make positive adjustments to pacemaker insertion. The extent of the patient's adjustment seems to correlate with general health, the function of the pacemaker, and especially the patient's relationship with the physician.

It is important to assess the patient's attitude about the pacemaker. Although the cardiac rhythm disability is potentially cured by the pacemaker, the patient may experience many kinds of fears associated with the need to have a pacemaker. Fear of sudden death as a result of pacemaker failure, fear of a "fragile" heart and subsequent physical exertion or exercise, and concern about being dependent for life on this object are concerns voiced by patients having pacemakers. They cannot help at times being preoccupied with the pacemaker's function.

These fears must be recognized and handled appropriately in the rehabilitation process. It may be useful for the patient to talk with others who have pacemakers and have successfully adjusted to them. A specialized pacemaker clinic may be useful in this regard. The patient's family also will have many concerns about the pacemaker, and they, too, need to be informed about its function and limitations.

PATIENT TEACHING

Instruction should be geared to the patient's interest level and intellectual capabilities. The family is included in the teaching program. This is particularly important if the patient is unreliable.

Instruction given to the patient must include information about cardiac physiology, pacemaker function, and the patient's particular condition and therapeutic program. Initially, assessment is made of the patient's level of knowledge regarding this information. Subsequently, a teaching program can be formulated and incorporated into the patient care plan.

Cardiac physiology. The patient needs some understanding of normal heart function, including the concepts of the heart as a pump and the impulse formation and conduction that influence atrial and ventricular contraction.

Pacemaker function. Since there are a variety of pacemakers manufactured, it is important that patients understand the particular function of their own pacemaker. To enhance this learning a battery and pacing catheter may be shown. The location of the components and how the pacemaker stimulates the heart are explained. This inculdes the type of pacemaker that the patient has: fixed rate, demand, or synchronous.

Periodic checking of pacemaker function is essential and may be accomplished several ways: (1) patients counting their own pulses, (2) telephone transmission of ECG, and/or (3) periodic ECGs in the physician's office. Most patients are instructed to count their pulse for a full minute daily and report any changes. Certain manufacturers provide a device that is sold with the pacemaker for purposes of counting the rate. Recently, equipment has been developed and is available in certain centers for telephone transmission of the ECG. With this system the patient is given a transmitting device. This device can convert electrical potential changes associated with pacemaker discharge and cardiac depolarization into sounds that may be transmitted via telephone lines to a central receiving station with special equipment. These sounds are demodulated back to electrical signals. The physician then can analyze the pacemaker and accordingly monitor its function. This system, where available, affords numerous advantages to the patient and physician. Patients "telephone" their ECGs periodically, thus saving the cost and inconvenience of office visits and travel while enabling frequent checks of pacemaker function.

In addition to checking the rate, patients should be instructed to report immediately any rate change or symptoms that may represent pacemaker malfunction. These may include syncope or dizziness, palpitations, hiccoughs (diaphragmatic stimulation), chest pain, low cardiac output, or congestive heart failure symptoms. Patients should be alerted to signs of infection, that is, inflammation, discoloration, or drainage around the battery insertion site.

An understanding that prophylactic pacemaker replacement may be necessary at the estimated end of battery life to prevent pacemaker failure is also important. There are varying opinions as to when replacement is necessary. The pacemaker manufacturer indicates the expected battery life. Prophylactic replacement near the end of this period may depend on numerous factors such as the type of monitoring or follow-up checks available to the patient, the costs of replacement versus frequent checks, and the patient's own concerns regarding pacemaker failure. For example, a patient may be planning a trip some distance from clinical resources around the time that battery life is expected to end. In this situation, prophylactic replacement may be appropriate to prevent failure and allay the patient's concerns.

Pacemaker replacement is a simple procedure necessitating a very brief hospital stay. Under local anesthesia the pulse generator is replaced with a new one. It is a common misconception of patients that only the batteries will be replaced. An entire new power unit replaces the old unit when needed. The patient's cardiac rhythm is observed for a few days to ensure proper pacemaker function.

Some people may be very concerned about the cosmetic effect of the surgical procedure. Initially, the suture line and insertion site of the pulse generator appear bruised and traumatized. The pulse generator does protrude, causing a bulge in the skin. All of this may be startling. Reassurance that the discoloration is temporary and a part of the healing process and some guidance in selecting comfortable undergarments and clothing may be helpful. Generally, undergarments that bind the site of the pulse generator will be uncomfortable.

Therapeutic program. Although the patient's symptoms may be "cured" by the pacemaker, the underlying pathologic condition is *not* cured.

Medications may be an important part of the patient's treatment program.

Diuretics to help regulate blood volume, digitalis, or other cardiac drugs may be necessary. The patient should understand the purpose of these drugs and the specifics of how to take them.

Any changes or additions in *diet* should be emphasized. A high-protein and high-vitamin diet is recommended to enhance postoperative recovery. Patients who require digitalis and diuretics should be encouraged to eat foods high in potassium (Appendix A).

Patients need a clear understanding of *activities* they may resume. After surgery, most patients are encouraged to return to the way of life they enjoyed previously. Limitations, if any, must be specifically defined. In addition, a well-defined exercise program should be implemented.

The patient may have questions about using electrical equipment. Most electrical appliances may be used safely. Improperly grounded appliances, however, and certain electrical sources with high-frequency signals, as used in diathermy or electrocautery, may interfere with the pacemaker's normal function. This equipment may produce current within the body that can suppress the activity of a demand pacemaker. Most pacemakers currently manufactured revert to a fixed rate mode when sensing alternating current. This helps to reduce the hazard of cessation of pacing in these circumstances. However, patients should be instructed to inform doctors or dentists that they have a pacemaker so that such equipment will not be used. Adequate information about the characteristics of their own particular unit and the appropriate precautions minimize these hazards. The importance of radiant electrical signals has been minimized by the shielding of most modern pacemakers.

FOLLOW-UP-CARE

Follow-up visits are a necessary part of care for patients with permanent pacemakers. Periodic ECGs, physical checks, and x-ray studies are necessary. Specialized pacemaker clinics are extremely beneficial; they also provide the patient opportunities to meet others who have pacemakers and who have successfully adjusted to normal life. The frequency of visits has to be individualized, both with respect to the type of pacemaker implanted and the time of implantation. Patients should be instructed also in counting their own pulse rate on a regular basis, since a decrease in heart rate frequently precedes and warns of pacemaker failure resulting from battery depletion. The recent development of equipment for telephone transmission of ECGs has simplified the follow-up of patients with cardiac pacemakers. In addition, public health consultation may be useful. In one way or another, reassurance must be readily available to the patient and family. In this way the pacemaker can be a positive addition to health and happiness.

REFERENCES

Amikam, S., et al.: Long-term survival of elderly patients after pacemaker implantation, Am. Heart J. **9**:445-449, 1976.

Barold, S. S., and Winner, J. A.: Techniques and significance of threshold measurement for cardiac pacing. Relationship to output circuit of cardiac pacemakers, Chest **70**:760-766, 1976.

Brenner, A. S., et al.: Transvenous, transmediastinal, and transthoracic ventricular pacing: a comparison after complete two-year follow-up, Circulation **49**:407-414, 1974.

Escher, D. J. W.: Medical aspects of artificial pacing of the heart, Cardiovasc. Nurs. **8**:1-5, 1972.

Escher, D. J. W.: Types of pacemakers and their complications, Circulation **68**:1119-1131, 1973.

Fisher, J. D., et al: Cardiac pacing and pacemakers. II. Serial electrophysiologic-pharmacologic testing for control of recurrent tachyarrhythmias, Am. Heart J. **93**:658-668, 1977.

Furnam, S.: Cardiac pacing and pacemakers. I. Indications for pacing bradyarrhythmias, Am. Heart J. **93**:523-530, 1977.

Furman, S., and Escher, D. J. W.: Principles and techniques of cardiac pacing, New York, 1970, Harper & Row, Publishers.

Furman, S. and Fisher, J. D.: Cardiac pacing and pacemakers. V. Technical aspects of implantation and equipment, Am. Heart J. **94**:250-259, 1977.

Furman, S., Hurzeler, P., and DeCaprio, V.: Cardiac pacing amd pacemakers. III. Sensing the cardiac electrogram, Am. Heart J. **93**:794-801, 1977.

Furman, S., Hurseler, P., and Mehra, R.: Cardiac pacing and pacemakers. IV. Threshold of cardiac stimulation, Am. Heart J. **94**:115-124, 1977.

Goldreyer, B. N.: Intracardiac electrocardiography in the analysis and understanding of cardiac arrhythmias, Ann. Intern. Med. **77**:117-136, 1972.

Greene, W. A. and Moss, A. J.: Psychosocial factors in the adjustment of patients with permanently implanted cardiac pacemaker, Ann. Intern. Med. **70**:897, 1969.

Hunn, V. K.: Cardiac pacemakers, Am. J. Nurs. **69**:479, 1969.

Jenkins, A. C.: Patients with pacers, Nurs. Clin. North Am. **4**:605, 1969.

Kahn, A., Morris, J. J., and Citron, P.: Patient-initiated rapid atrial pacing to manage supraventricular tachycardia, Am. J. Cardiol. **38**:200-204, 1976.

Kastor, J. A. and Leinback, R. C.: Pacemakers and their arrhythmias, Prog. Cardiovasc. Dis. **13**:240, Nov., 1970.

Kos, B. A. and Culbert, P. A.: Teaching the patient with a pacemaker, Cardiovasc. Nurs. **6**:57, Nov.-Dec., 1970.

Lewis, K. B., et al.: Early clinical experience with the rechargeable cardiac pacemaker, Ann. Thorac. Surg. **18**:490-493, 1974.

Lie, K. I., et al.: Factors influencing prognosis of bundle branch block complicating acute anteroseptal infarction. The value of His bundle recordings, Circulation **50**:935-941, 1974.

Lillehei, R. C., et al.: A new solid-state, long-life, lithium-powered pulse generator, Ann. Thorac. Surg. **18**:479-489, 1974.

Luceri, R. M., et al.: Threshold behavior of electrodes in long-term ventricular pacing, Am. J. Cardiol. **30**:184-188, 1977.

Martini, E. L., et al.: A recommended protocal for pacemaker follow-up: Analysis of 1,705 implanted pacemakers, Ann. Thorac, Surg. **24**:62-67, 1977.

Morse, D., et al.: Preliminary experience with the use of a programmable pacemaker, Chest **67**:544-548, 1975.

Moss, A. J. and Rivers, R. J., Jr.: Termination and inhibition of recurrent tachycardias by implanted pervenous pacemakers, Circulation **50**:942-947, 1974.

Moss, A. J., Rivers, R. Jr., Kramer, D. H.: Permanent pervenous atrial pacing from the coronary vein. Long-term follow-up, Circulation **69**:222-225, 1974.

Parsonnet, V., and Manhardt, M.: Permanent pacing of the heart: 1952 to 1976, Am. J. Cardiol. **39**:250-256, 1977.

Parsonnet, V., et al.: Follow-up of implanted pacemakers, Am. Heart J. **87**:642-653, 1974.

Pennock, R. S., et al.: Long-term monitoring of patients with implanted cardiac pacemakers, Heart Lung **1**:227-232, 1972.

Pittman, D. E., et al.: Rapid atrial stimulation: Successful method of conversion of atrial flutter and atrial tachycardia, Am. J. Cardiol. **32**:700-706, 1973.

Preston, T. A. and Yates, J. D.: Management of stimulation and sensing problems in temporary cardiac pacing, Heart Lung **2**:533-538, 1973.

Ritter, W. S., et al.: Permanent pacing in patients with transient trifascicular block during acute myocardial infarction, Am. J. Cardio. **38**:205-208, 1976.

Samet, P., editor: Cardiac pacing. New York, 1973, Grune & Stratton, Inc.

Schnitzler, R. N., Carata, A. R., and Damato, A. N.: "Floating" catheter for temporary transvenous ventricular pacing, Am. J. Cardiol. **31**:351-354, 1973.

Stoney, W. S., et al.: The natural history of long-term cardiac pacing, Ann. Thorac. Surg. **23**:550-554, 1977.

Thalen, H. J. T., editor: Fourth international symposium on cardiac pacing, Groningen, the Netherlands. Assen, 1973, Van Gorcum B V.

Waters, D. D., and Mizgala, H. F.: Long-term prognosis of patients with incomplete bilateral bundle branch block complicating acute myocardial infarction. Role of cardiac pacing, Am. J. Cardiol. **34**:1-6, 1974.

Weinstein, J., et al.: Temporary transvenous pacing via the percutaneous femoral vein approach. A prospective study of 100 cases, Am. Heart J. **85**:695-705, 1973.

Wright, K. E. and McIntosh, H. D.: Artificial pacemakers. Indications and management, Circulation **67**:1108-1118, 1973.

CHAPTER EIGHT

CARE OF THE CARDIAC PATIENT

Donna J. Rogers, R.N., M.S.N.
Martha E. Branyon, R.N., M.S.N.
Marguerite R. Kinney, R.N., D.N.Sc.

Care of the cardiac patient is a multifaceted undertaking. Many aspects of the knowledge and expertise of health care professionals are utilized in caring for the patient who has sustained a myocardial infarction. Health care professionals have an opportunity to collect a variety of data concerning the patient while assessing, planning, implementing, and evaluating care. Subjective data are collected from the patient and his family in the form of the chief complaint, past health history, and family and social history (Chapter 3). Objective data are collected from the physical examination, laboratory studies, observations of the patient, and information gathered from invasive and noninvasive techniques (see Chapter 3).

Before discussing care of the patient following a myocardial infarction, a brief description of the equipment used in the cardiac care unit (CCU) is appropriate. Care of the patient and the equipment will also be discussed.

Equipment
MONITORING SYSTEM

The first equipment in the CCU with which the patient is likely to come in contact is the monitoring system. For a patient who has suffered a myocardial infarction or who has had a pacemaker implanted, careful monitoring of cardiac performance is the objective of preventive care. The cardiac monitor simplifies such care by continuously displaying the cardiac rhythm, blood pressure, and other parameters not readily followed by other means. Since most arrhythmias occur during the first 48 to 72 hours after infarction and 80% to 90% of patients with myocardial infarctions experience arrhythmias, the need for constant surveillance is apparent.

Recurring arrhythmias compromise cardiac function by (1) reducing cardiac output and coronary blood flow, (2) increasing the myocardial need for oxygen, (3) predisposing the patient to the development of more serious arrhythmias, and (4) complicating therapy. Therefore prompt prevention and control of arrhythmias and the states predisposing to them (acidosis, electrolyte imbalance, early cardiac failure, pain, and anxiety) decrease the incidence of more serious arrhythmias and should improve the chances for survival after myocardial infarction. Awareness of these facts underscores the importance of detecting arrhythmias through the use of the cardiac monitor.

Components. The cardiac monitor is an instrument that displays electrical activity during the cardiac cycle as a wave pattern across a screen. Since the components of particular monitoring systems vary widely, the basic components of most cardiac monitors will be described (Fig. 8-1).

Oscilloscope. The screen on which the patient's electrocardiographic pattern appears is an oscilloscope.

Digital display. An electronic mechanism averages the number of ventricular complexes per minute, and this rate is shown on the rate scale indicator. Each contraction is also indicated by an audible beep and flashing light. If the pulse rate can be relayed to a console at the nursing station, the bedside monitor beep should be silenced so that the patient does not hear it.

Rate meter. Integrated with the alarm system is the rate meter, which signals if the pulse goes above or below predetermined limits. The limits vary according to the routine of a particular unit as based on the sensitivity of the electrodes and monitoring system. For example, the alarm may be triggered to sound at either 25 beats above or below an individual patient's average heart rate, or it may be set automatically to sound at the high-low values of 150 and 50 beats per minute.

Alarm control system. When the heart rate falls below or rises above the preset levels, audio and visual alarms alert the staff. Each time an alarm is triggered, the staff must observe, identify, and make a prompt decision regarding the cardiac rhythm.

When the CCU personnel depend on an alarm system for warning, the rate limit indicators and alarm system must be checked regularly—not only for accuracy but also to be sure that the system is operative. There are times when the limit settings are temporarily turned off in the patient's room. At these times, personnel must depend on their visual observation of the oscilloscope and the related clinical picture. For instance, the limit settings are turned off to prevent false alarms from electrical interference resulting from the use of a high-power machine (direct write-out ECG machine, portable x-ray, and so forth). False alarms may also be triggered by manipulation of the chest electrodes, from repositioning the electrodes to other sites on the chest, or from bathing the patient. The patient's welfare is endangered if the alarm limit settings remain off. It is essential to periodically check these settings.

When such an alarm system is not available, personnel must develop some other means of being alerted to changes in rhythm on the monitor oscilloscope. Only through an adequate method of observation can significant changes be identified and further rhythm disturbances prevented.

Sweep speed. The rate at which the electron beam sweeps across the screen can be controlled, and the sweep can be set at trace speeds of 25 mm per second (beam sweeps across standard screen in 6 seconds) or 50 mm per second (the 3-second sweep position). The 6-second position is generally used

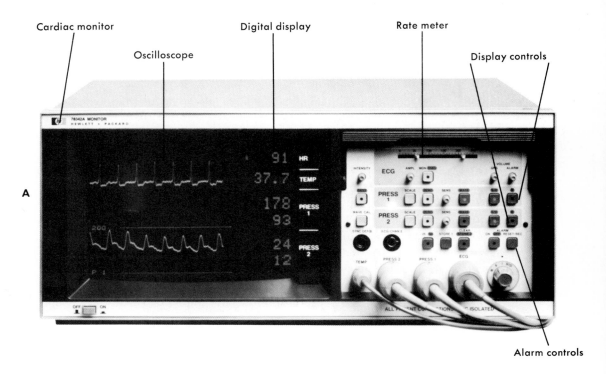

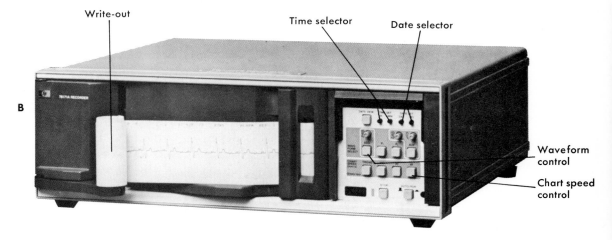

Fig. 8-1. Two sections of a cardiac monitor. **A** shows components—oscilloscope, digital display, rate meter, display control, and alarm control. **B** shows writeout, time selector, data selector, waveform control, and chart speed control. (Reprinted with permission from Hewlett-Packard Company, Palo Alto, California.)

for routine monitoring. The 3-second position often provides better interpretation of the rhythm or the pressure waveform by spreading the complexes.

Filter. The filter reduces extraneous muscular artifacts. However, when a 12-lead ECG is recorded from the monitor, the filter must be switched off, since it may distort the S-T segment.

Central console. The individual bedside monitors in a CCU are connected to a central console at the nursing station. This permits continuous visualization of the ECG patterns from all the monitors.

Additional components. Complementary parts can be added to the basic monitoring system as necessary. For example, a direct write-out ECG machine can be located in the central station; this triggered to record the cardiac rhythm automatically during alarm situations or on demand. Such recordings may be used to demonstrate the patient's response to therapy.

Some monitor systems have memory tapes that store a predetermined duration of the patient's ECG, which can then be recalled at will. This allows printing out the cardiac rhythm recorded over the previous 60 seconds, for example. Moreover, at the time of alarm some monitors write out memory storage and then current rhythm from the time of trigger. Memory mechanisms, however, erase after a period of time; therefore at the moment of an alarm, personnel must decide whether to record the stored memory information or the current rhythm. Use of 24-hour tape monitoring simplifies this problem.

The monitoring system may also include multichannel recorders to monitor central venous, pulmonary artery, pulmonary capillary wedge, and arterial pressures, and other physiologic parameters. In some research centers this information is coded for a computer where it may be stored and retrieved when needed. A pacemaking unit may be made an integral part of some monitors and may be set to trigger when the heart rate slows below a preset limit.

Electrodes. Topical electrode patches are commonly used for patient monitoring. The following steps are involved in preparing the skin and in applying the electrodes:

1. At the sites chosen for electrode placement, clean the skin thoroughly with alcohol to remove all residues. If necessary, shave the hair at these sites.
2. The skin of some patients may require abrasion at the electrode sites to obtain an adequate ECG signal. In this situation, abrade each site by rubbing the area with a gauze pad and abrasive electrode paste.
3. Apply electrode paste to the electrode and press the electrode against the skin at the prepared site. Excessive paste may ooze from under the electrode onto the skin and distort the signal.
4. Secure each electrode in place with a strip of nonallergenic tape.

PLACEMENT OF ELECTRODES. The lead that best displays upright QRS complexes and P waves (and a pacing stimulus if pacing is used) is ideal for monitoring.

A positive, a negative, and a ground electrode are required for recording one bipolar lead. The location of these electrodes determines the lead recorded by the monitor. For example, a modification of lead V_1 ($MC1_1$) is recorded by placing the negative electrode just under the outer quarter of the left shoulder and the ground electrode beneath the right clavicle, with the positive electrode being placed at the fourth right intercostal space, right sternal border (the usual V_1 position).

To avoid interfering with the physical examination the chest electrodes should be placed away from the area near the apex of the heart. For long-term monitoring, chest leads are preferable to limb leads. Placement of the electrodes on the chest reduces motion and muscle artifact and allows the patient more freedom of movement than does limb-lead monitoring.

The modified V_1 chest lead has the added advantage over other chest leads (often haphazardly positioned on the chest) of giving a maximum amount of information about rhythm disturbances and conduction. The $MC1_1$ provides an easily recognized recording of the sequence of ventricular activation and therefore furnishes maximum information to discriminate (1) between systoles originating in the right and left ventricles, (2) between right and left bundle branch block, and (3) between left ventricular systoles and right bundle aberrant beats.

Topical electrodes should be repositioned about every 8 hours, or at least daily, to prevent the occurrence of local skin sores caused by prolonged contact of the hypertonic electrode paste with one point on the skin surface.

When changing topical electrodes, the used electrodes should be replaced with clean ones. (Many institutions use disposable electrodes.) The electrodes may be washed with soap and water. A pencil eraser may help remove dried paste from the electrode. Steel wool should not be used for cleaning electrodes, since it will leave grooves in the electrode surface, which may generate recording artifacts.

The electrode wires from the patient are attached to a connecter unit pinned to the patient's gown. From this unit a cable leads to the monitor, where the electrode wires are connected to their respective terminals: positive wire to positive terminal, negative wire to negative terminal, and ground to ground. In certain machines the electrode terminals are specifically labeled. In other machines it is necessary to be familiar with the terminal connections. Incorrect matching of electrode and terminal will change the lead that is to be monitored.

Interference with monitoring. Faulty techniques probably cause over 90% of the problems encountered in the course of cardiac monitoring. The common artifacts produced by electrical interferences can be prevented.

External voltage and/or patient movement generally are responsible for interference that occurs in an efficiently running monitoring system. External voltage interference (alternating 60-cycle current) appears on the screen as a smooth thickening of the base line resulting from the 60 tiny peaks per second (Fig. 8-2, *A*). Inadequate grounding of the monitor and other equipment or

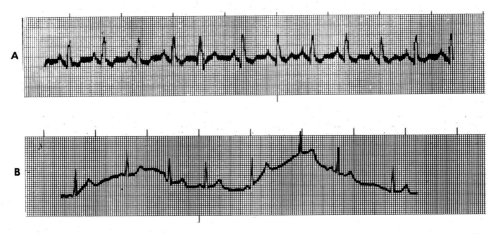

Fig. 8-2. A, ECG tracing that shows external voltage interference (alternating 60-cycle current) appearing as a smooth thickening of the base line as a result of the 60 tiny peaks per second. **B,** ECG tracing in which patient interference (coughing, turning, etc.) is shown by a wandering base line.

improper electrode placement and connection may produce this type of interference.

Since the cardiac monitor registers muscle potential, any sudden voluntary or involuntary (muscle tremor) movement by the patient can cause interference. For example, coughing or turning over in bed may precipitate a wandering base line and erratic or irregular fluctuations on the oscilloscope (Fig. 8-2, *B*). Placing the electrodes in areas of limited muscular activity will reduce this problem.

In the tense, nervous, or cold patient the monitor may display a harsh, jagged, uneven oscillation about the base line. One must be careful not to interpret these base line undulations as signifying fibrillatory waves.

Patient's feelings about the monitor. During the stay in CCU the patient is bound to experience significant psychologic stress. The intricate electronic equipment may contribute to these feelings.

The conscious patient restricted to bed rest has little to do but reflect on the experience and examine the surroundings. Since the monitor is the only continuously active object in the room, it is only natural that it draws the patient's attention. For 24 hours a day this machine displays the cardiac rhythm across the screen, flashing a light with each impulse. The patient watches the screen, soon learning to recognize delays and changes in heart rate. He also watches the faces of the professional staff as they read the monitor and, if they make the mistake of analyzing his cardiac status in his presence, he listens carefully to their discussion.

What does he think about his monitor? Is he suspicious of it? Does he wonder if it might suddenly stop running? Is he afraid of being shocked? Is he afraid to move? To bathe? Does he think the monitor paces his heart? These questions indicate some of the apprehensions patients have voiced.

Patients should be encouraged to discuss their feelings about their monitors. Continued simple explanations and reassurance should help relieve their anxieties. Families should be included, too, because they often share the patient's fears and enhance his apprehensions. The presence of the cardiac monitor is reassuring to most patients because it ensures constant surveillance.

Removal of the patient from the monitor should be explained to him as occurring only when he can be safely off the monitor for short intervals and that the removal indicates an improvement in his condition.

ARTERIAL CATHETERS

The uses and purposes of the arterial catheter are discussed in Chapter 3.

When monitoring arterial pressure directly, one must carefully observe the following precautions to obtain meaningful values:

1. Standardize, balance, and calibrate the monitoring equipment at least once every 8 hours and after position changes or movements that might alter the calibration. Instructions for this procedure accompany the individual manufacturer's equipment.
2. Flush the arterial line every hour. If Intraflo cathethers are used, flushing every 5 to 15 minutes is not necessary. A solution of 5% dextrose in water with heparin added is used for flushing. The catheter should be flushed manually every 1 to 2 hours and to clear the line after blood is drawn or if blood is in the line for any reason. The pulse waveform will become *damped or flattened* somewhat when impairment of flow occurs.
3. Prevent catheter displacement by fastening the arterial catheter securely to the skin. The catheter may be sutured to the skin after insertion.
4. Prevent blood from entering the transducer. Blood in the transducer will damp the pressure reading and may damage the transducer.
5. Observe the extremity every 1 to 2 hours for bleeding and circulatory insufficiency. The arterial catheter should be observed frequently for leakage and proper stopcock position.
6. Apply a sterile dressing to the site and change at least once every 24 hours. When the dressing is changed, note the condition of the site and the surrounding area.
7. Observe the site for infection when dressings are changed. Should the catheter remain in the artery longer than 48 to 72 hours, observation of the site at least every 8 hours is imperative. Any sign of infection should receive immediate attention.
8. Immobilize the extremity to prevent accidental dislodgment of the catheter. If an armboard or wooden device is used, proper padding will prevent stasis changes of skin and increase comfort.

9. Exercise care when drawing blood from the catheter. The stopcock must be returned to the original position to ensure proper operation and prevent leakage.

10. After removal of the catheter, apply direct pressure to the artery for 10 to 15 minutes or longer until bleeding ceases. The site should be covered with a sterile dressing for 24 hours.

11. After the catheter is removed, observe the site for signs of bleeding, infection, and circulatory insufficiency until healing is complete. If any of these are noted, immediate attention should be given to correction of the condition.

SWAN-GANZ CATHETERS

The use of Swan-Ganz catheters for measurement of pulmonary artery and pulmonary capillary wedge pressures is discussed in Chapter 4.

The use of the central venous pressure (CVP) to determine right atrial pressure (RAP) is no longer considered sufficiently accurate because the relationship between RAP and left ventricular end-diastolic pressure (LVEDP) is inconsistent. Therefore pulmonary artery end-diastolic pressure (PAEDP) and pulmonary capillary wedge pressure (PCWP), rather than CVP, should be accepted as major guides in the treatment of heart failure and shock. PCWP is also the most accurate guide in fluid management of the cardiac patient.

Pressure measurement

Pulmonary artery pressure. The pulmonary artery waveform evidences a sharp rise during ejection of blood from the right ventricle after the pulmonary valve opens. This pressure rise is followed by a slow decrease in pressure during the ejection of blood from the right ventricle until the pulmonic valve closes, indicated by the dicrotic notch. The pressure continues to decrease until systole occurs again.

Normal pulmonary artery (PA) systolic pressure is 20 to 30 mm Hg, and normal PA diastolic pressure ranges from 5 to 16 mm Hg. The normal mean PA pressure ranges from 10 to 20 mm Hg. The PA systolic pressure normally equals the right ventricular pressure (Fig. 8-3). The PA diastolic pressure should be almost equal to the mean PCWP in the absence of pulmonary vascular disease.

Elevation in PA pressure may occur during (1) increased pulmonary blood flow, as in a left-to-right shunt resulting from atrial or ventricular septal defect, (2) increased pulmonary arteriolar resistance resulting from primary pulmonary hypertension or mitral stenosis, and (3) left ventricular failure resulting from any cause.

Pulmonary capillary wedge pressure. Since there is normally a direct relationship between PAEDP, PCWP, and LVEDP, an elevated PAEDP or PCWP reflects the elevated LVEDP that occurs when the left ventricle can no longer adequately pump the blood presented to it.

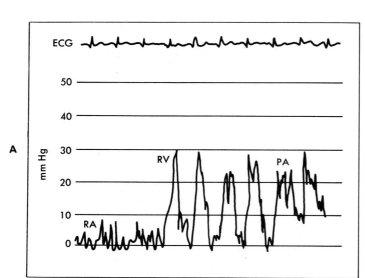

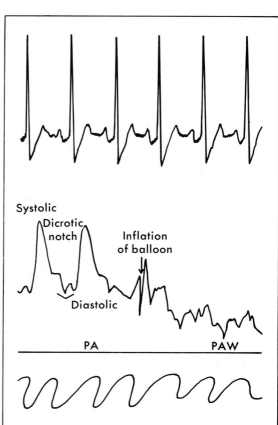

Fig. 8-3. A, After inflation of balloon at tip of Swan-Ganz catheter, intracardiac pressure identifies right atrium (**RA**), right ventricle (**RV**), and pulmonary artery (**PA**) as catheter is advanced. Right ventricle is characterized by higher systolic but similiar diastolic pressure when compared to right atrial pressure. Pulmonary artery pressure shows same systolic value as that in right ventricle, but diastolic pressure is higher than that in either right ventricle or atrium. Catheter whip or artifact is produced by exaggerated motion of catheter with inflated balloon and usually disappears with deflation of balloon. **B,** PA pressure waveform via balloon-tip catheter. Note balloon inflation and subsequent change to PAW waveform. **A,** adapted from Rackley, C. E., and Russell, R. O.: *Invasive techniques for hemodynamic monitoring,* Dallas, 1973, by permission of the American Heart Association. **B,** Adapted from Schroeder, J. S., and Daily, E. K.: Techniques in bedside hemodynamic monitoring, St. Louis, 1976, The C. V. Mosby Co.

The PCWP is normally 4 to 12 mm Hg. PCWP greater than 12 mm Hg may occur as a result of (1) left ventricular failure, (2) mitral stenosis, or (3) mitral insufficiency, in addition to other possible causes.

Measurement of PA pressure and PCWP. The method used to record PA pressure (PAP) and PCWP from the standard strain gauge pressure transducer differs among institutions. Special points to consider in maintaining the catheter and measuring pressures include the following:

I. **Recording readings**
   A. Record pressures at regular intervals as ordered and as necessary. Evaluate changes and report to the physician if not present when the reading is performed.
   B. Calibrate equipment before each reading.
   C. Irrigate line before each reading by pulling red rubber Intraflo plunger for 5 seconds, or manually if Intraflo is not used.
   D. Patient should be in same position for each reading, and position should be recorded.

II. **Maintaining catheter**
   A. Maintain patency of catheter.
      1. Pressure bag at 300 mm Hg irrigates automatically with 3 ml of saline and heparin solution per minute, using Intraflo catheter.
      2. Irrigate manually every hour by pulling Intraflo stopper for 5 seconds.
      3. Count irrigating solution used at end of each shift as part of IV intake.
      4. Change dressing every 12 hours, clean site with Betadine, and apply antibacterial ointment.
      5. Observe for signs of infection and/or phlebitis at insertion site.
   B. Observe complexes for changes in fluctuation.
      1. Flattened complexes—possible wedging of catheter in pulmonary arteriole, which could result in pulmonary infarction. Turn patient and ask him to cough and take some deep breaths; this may dislodge a catheter "stuck" in wedge. Alert physician.
      2. "Wet" complex—irregular fluctuation with no clear complex denotes need for irrigation with 10 ml syringe. If this complex continues, the catheter is probably of no value and should be removed.
      3. No complex—recalibration of transducer needed.

Care of the patient and Swan-Ganz equipment

1. Following insertion of the Swan-Ganz catheter, a sterile dressing should be applied to the site and changed at least every 24 hours. The condition of the site, including presence of active bleeding and signs of infection, should be noted.
2. The extremity should be immobilized to prevent accidental dislodgment of the catheter. Taping the catheter to the extremity will stabilize the catheter. Padding of an armboard or wooden device will promote comfort and immobilize the extremity.

3. The extremity should be observed for circulatory insufficiency and bleeding at least every hour.
4. The catheter should be observed frequently for leakage and proper stopcock position. Care should be taken to return the stopcock to the "off" position when drawing blood from the catheter.
5. The balloon should always remain deflated with a syringe attached except when the PCWP is being read.
6. After the catheter is removed the site should be observed closely for bleeding and infection until healing is complete. A sterile dressing should be applied to the site.

PHYSIOLOGIC MONITORING

A new multipurpose flow-directed pulmonary arterial catheter has been developed and evaluated on a small group of patients with acute cardiopulmonary dysfunction. This catheter permits monitoring of the bipolar atrial ECG, pulmonary arterial/wedge pressure, CVP, cardiac output, and atrial pacing. The standard Swan-Ganz thermistor catheter is modified to include two ring electrodes on the shaft at the marks for 25 and 26 mm from the tip. This change is the only visible difference between this catheter and the standard Swan-Ganz. With the catheter in the right atrium at the junction of the superior vena cava, stable ECGs of high quality were recorded in all study subjects for up to 6 days. These high-fidelity ECGs allowed rapid and accurate diagnosis of many complex arrhythmias in these unstable patients. Because of the limited noise in the ECG signal, continuous quantitative interval measurements by a computerized system are possible. In addition, the stable intracavitary electrode position provides a reliable atrial pacing site, and in the study mentioned, pacing thresholds remained stable up to 4 days. Atrial pacing in this fashion has been used to treat atrial and ventricular arrhythmias. This multipurpose catheter permits both hemodynamic and electrophysiologic monitoring plus atrial pacing that is convenient and safe for long time periods in patients with unstable cardiopulmonary problems.

Care of the patient and equipment is the same as in patients with Swan-Ganz catheters in place.

Care of the patient with a myocardial infarction

Goals of acute care of the patient who has a myocardial infarction include rapid management of existing problems, prevention and/or early detection of arrhythmias, and beginning rehabilitation.

ACUTE PHASE

The initial approach to the patient is on admission to the CCU. At this most critical time, health team members are collecting data regarding the patient, while considering priorities in data collection and subsequent actions based on these data (see boxed material on p. 292). The data collection process was discussed in Chapter 3. At this point the patient may or may not be physically able to describe any events except the presence of pain and/or shortness of breath.

Priorities in admission to the CCU

1. Immediate monitoring of cardiac rate and rhythm. Rate meter alarms should always be set. As electrodes are applied to the chest, a very brief explanation of the purpose of the electrodes should be given to the patient. Later, as he recovers, more information regarding the monitoring equipment may be discussed.

2. Establishment of a patent IV line with an indwelling catheter, preferably not a long catheter. This line is important for administration of fluid and pain medications and will prevent the necessity of establishing an IV line in an emergency, when the task is much more difficult because of circulatory insufficiency or collapse. The patent line also allows for an immediate route for treatment of arrhythmias with IV medications. A butterfly type needle should never be utilized in myocardial infarction patients, since those needles are easily dislodged from the vein.

3. Relief of pain and anxiety. The patient should be given analgesic medication immediately if he continues to complain of pain on arrival to the unit. Although morphine is the drug of choice under these circumstances, it should not be given if the patient has A-V block or sinus bradycardia because of vagotonic effects. Morphine may also decrease respiratory drive. The blood pressure, heart rate, and respiratory rate should be monitored after morphine is given to observe any untoward effects. The physician will usually write orders for analgesics and nitrates as needed for relief of pain. Pain and anxiety may potentiate the effects of each other and increase myocardial oxygen demands in an already compromised heart. Thus they should be alleviated as rapidly as possible. Explanations to the patient of all activities and equipment will assist in relieving anxiety. Often families, although well intentioned, are anxiety provoking. Visiting time should be terminated if such anxiety is noted. In other instances, however, the absence of families may produce excessive anxiety. Unit policies should be flexible enough to allow for individualization of care in each situation as judged appropriate. Other policies and procedures should be explained to the patient as necessary measures in assisting the injured heart to heal. Such an explanation assists the patient in accepting what is done as usual and necessary. Often a fact sheet with similar information for the family is helpful. (See boxed material on p. 293–294.)

4. Supplementation of oxygen. Oxygen is used to relieve dyspnea and thereby relieve anxiety. After explanation of its use and the patient's need for it, humidified oxygen should be started at 1 to 2 liters per minute with a binasal cannula. Frequent application of a lubricant or emollient to the nares will help to maintain skin integrity. Measurement of arterial blood gas levels 30 minutes after initiating oxygen

Example form for an admission note to the CCU

Stamp here with
patient's plate

Admission note

Admission status: Clinic _____ ER _____ Date _____ Time _____
Married _____ Single _____ Widowed _____ Divorced _____
Race and nationality_____ Religion _____ Age _____

Patient history

Chest pain _____ Onset _____ Duration _____ Location _____
    Radiation _____ Subjective description _____
Associated acute events:
    Loss of consciousness _____ Duration _____ Cardiac arrest _____
    Palpitations _____ GI _____ Perspiration _____ Anxiety _____
    Dyspnea _____
Medications taken or administered and time _____
Medical history and risk factors (check those appropriate):
    Myocardial infarction _____ Angina _____ Obesity _____ Weight loss _____
    Cerebrovascular accident _____ Alcohol _____ Respiratory _____
    Hypertension _____ Glaucoma _____ Diabetes _____ Smoking _____
    Prostatic hypertrophy _____ Blood transfusion _____ Gout _____
    Surgery _____ Reaction to anesthesia _____ Other _____

Personal information

    Height _____ Weight _____ Dentures _____ Glasses _____ Contacts _____
    Sleeping habits _____ Usual diet _____
    Routine medications _____
    Food, medication, environmental allergies _____
    Prostheses _____ Family history _____

Physical examination

    General appearance _____ Mental status _____
    Vital signs: Temperature _____ Pulse _____ Respirations _____
    Blood pressure: right _____ left _____
    Lungs: Aeration _____ Wheezes _____ Rales _____
    Cardiovascular: Heart sounds _____ Quality _____ Rhythm _____
        Lifts _____ Heaves _____ Thrills _____ Murmur _____ Rub _____
        Gallop _____
    Pulses (all extremities) _____ Neck veins _____ Abdomen _____
    Skin: Color _____ Temperature _____ Cyanosis _____ Edema _____
    Clubbing _____ Other _____
        Signature _____

Insert ECG strip here

Examples of fact sheet given to families of patients in coronary care unit*

CORONARY CARE UNIT INFORMATION

While you, a family member or friend, are in the CCU you may hear terms such as "coronary," "electrocardiogram" (ECG), or "congestive heart failure" and be uncertain as to what they mean about the patient's condition. This may be a time when you have a lot of questions and anxieties.

The CCU staff understands this and has prepared this information sheet to help you understand what goes on in a CCU. If you want to know more about heart disease, there is literature available in our unit on request. Also, we will be glad to try to answer any questions you may have.

The CCU Staff

Patient care

A CCU is for the "intensive" care of cardiac patients. This CCU has 11 beds and is attended 24 hours a day by registered nurses, who are specially trained to read ECGs, and recognize any early signs of complications. From the time a patient arrives in the unit until he is transferred to a room, there is a nurse near his bedside to render the care needed.

Because of the serious nature of heart disease, a patient is placed in the CCU during the critical phase of his heart's condition and remains there until this critical phase is over, usually 3 to 5 days. His progress is followed continuously with special monitoring equipment at each bedside and at the nurses' station to record the patient's ECGs. These indicate a person's heart rhythms.

While in the CCU, patients only need their necessary personal belongings. Shaving equipment (razor with nurse's approval), cosmetics, toilet articles, eyeglasses, and small change may be kept in the bedside drawer. Male patients may wear pajama bottoms. Female patients do not need their gowns as a hospital gown is worn and preferred. Patients may have a small radio and reading materials if approved by the doctor. *Television, flowers, and suitcases are not allowed.*

When the physician approves transfer out of the CCU, the patient is usually taken to a

---

*Reproduced with permission of Cooper Green Hospital, Birmingham, Al.

Continued.

therapy will give a baseline of arterial oxygenation. Such measurements may be repeated as necessary as a guide to oxygen administration and maintenance of acid-base balance.

5. Decrease in myocardial work load. The myocardium requires time, oxygen, and nutrients to recover from the injury of infarction. Decreasing the amount of work, and therefore the oxygen demand of the heart, will assist the recovery of the myocardium. The methods used to decrease demand should be adequately explained to the patient and his family. Generally accepted methods of decreasing work load of the heart include the following:

   a. Bed rest is recommended initially. After the early phase of the illness, progressive *mobilization* is considered advantageous in pre-

Examples of fact sheet given to families of patients in coronary care unit

---

CORONARY CARE UNIT INFORMATION—cont'd

room on another floor. Transferring patients is usually done during the day, but if an emergency situation arises and a bed is needed in the unit during the night, a patient may have to be moved at this time.

Because of the nature of the patient's illness, visiting times *must be limited and strictly enforced.* No more than two visitors, preferably the immediate family, will be allowed to visit the patient at any time. Visitors receive passes to the unit from the information desk.

Visiting periods for *10 minutes only* are:

10:00 AM to 10:10 AM
12:00 PM to 12:10 AM
2:00 PM to 2:10 PM
4:00 PM to 4:10 PM
6:00 PM to 6:10 PM
8:00 PM to 8:10 PM

If emergency situations exist, visitation may be refused.

Phone

There is a pay phone available. *Direct calls to the unit are not permitted.* Families may leave their phone numbers at the desk in the CCU.

Chaplain

This service is available on request at any time by contacting a CCU nurse or the chaplain's office.

Waiting rooms

The waiting room is open only until 8:30 PM. Those who wish to stay during the night must use the emergency room waiting room.

---

venting complications. Whatever limitations are imposed on activity should be discussed and reinforced with the patient, since his cooperation is important.

b. In connection with bed rest, questions of self-feeding and methods of bladder and bowel elimination arise. Many CCUs allow the patient to feed himself and to use the bedside commode with staff assistance. The physiologic stress that may result from these activities is thought to be less than the stress that results from almost total dependence on another person. The stress secondary to dependence is evident most frequently in male patients who find themselves dependent on females in a drastic reversal of roles. Assistance in maintaining some degree of independence can contribute significantly to the patient's psychologic state of self-worth and recovery. This, in turn, facilitates physical recovery.

Initially, a brief explanation by the nurse about the need for assistance in performing activities is sufficient. As the patient improves, additional information regarding the reasons for assistance in activity may be explained in greater depth to the patient and family.

Other information

Other information necessary to complete the data base may be obtained after admission to the unit and includes the following subjective and objective data.

1. Patient history (Chapter 3)
2. Physical examination (Chapter 3)
   a. *Inspection* of skin for color, diaphoresis, and other abnormalities.
   b. *Palpation* of chest area for unusual movements, thrills, excursion, cardiac enlargement, apical impulse and other signs.
   c. *Percussion* of chest for areas of dullness and of the liver for edge and size. Cardiac borders are seldom defined by percussion.
   d. *Auscultation* for normal heart sounds, gallops, and murmurs, especially the murmur of papillary muscle dysfunction, which may occur in the acute phase as a result of ischemia and/or infarction of the papillary muscle. The sound is the murmur of mitral regurgitation resulting when the injured leaflet fails to contract properly, allowing blood to be regurgitated into the left atrium during systole. The murmur is often transient, but it may be permanent if the papillary muscle does not heal completely. A ventricular septal defect murmur may also be present, resulting from perforation of the septum. This murmur usually occurs during the first 10 days after infarct and is a very loud grade 4 or 5 systolic murmur. There is usually an accompanying thrill, and the murmur is heard best along the lower left sternal border. The appearance of this murmur is an ominous event prognostically.
3. Supportive data
   a. *Twelve-lead ECG* (Chapter 5), should be performed initially in the emergency room or in the CCU. A copy should be maintained on the patient's chart for comparison with later tracings, which are performed daily for 3 days and with *every* exacerbation of chest pain and/or developing arrhythmia. Personnel in the CCU should be adept at obtaining and interpreting the 12-lead ECG in a patient with myocardial infarction. See Fig 8-4 for illustration of ECG machine and boxed material on p. 297 for procedure used in obtaining 12-lead ECG.
   b. *Serum cardiac enzyme levels* (Chapter 3), should be measured initially and then daily for 3 days to document any abnormal increase in serum levels. Should the patient have a sudden exacerbation of pain with associated ECG changes, cardiac enzyme level measurements may be indicated to assist in determining whether the previous infarction has extended.
   c. *Arterial blood gas levels* may be measured initially, then as needed,

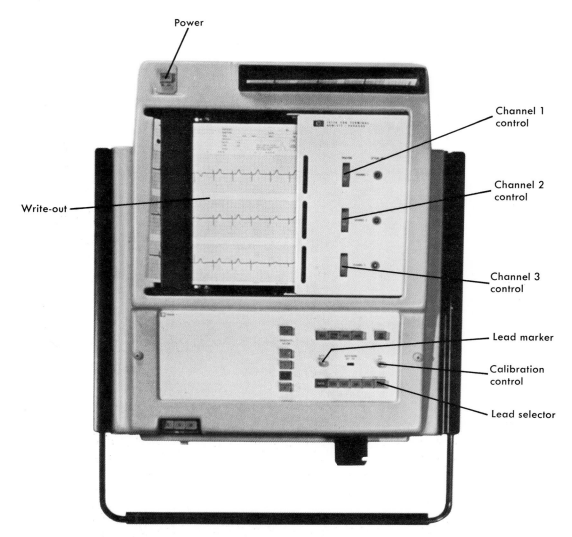

Power

Channel 1 control

Channel 2 control

Channel 3 control

Write-out

Lead marker

Calibration control

Lead selector

Fig. 8-4. Electrocardiograph machine showing components, including three channels that provide for display of three leads simultaneously. Lead selector allows choice of leads. Lead marker automatically marks which leads are being written. Calibration control allows choice of size of ECG complexes. (Reprinted with permission of Hewlett-Packard Co., Palo Alto, Calif.)

12-LEAD ELECTROCARDIOGRAM PROCEDURE FOR CCU

I. Purpose: To record an ECG for diagnostic purposes. (A graphic record of the electrical impulses causing heart action recorded by electrodes placed on the body surface.)

II. Equipment
   A. ECG machine with five-lead cable
   B. Four-limb electrode plates with rubber straps
   C. One Welsh cup electrode
   D. ECG electrode paste
   E. Cotton or gauze
   F. Alcohol sponges

III. Procedure
   A. Instruct patient regarding procedure and assure him that there is no discomfort associated with procedure.
   B. Place patient in a comfortable position on back with legs and arms adequately supported. Feet should not touch the footboard of the bed.
   C. Plug in ECG machine. Turn power switch to "on" position.
   D. Plug in five-lead patient cable to top of recorder.
   E. Select site for limb electrode placement on each extremity. Electrodes may be placed anywhere on the extremities from shoulder to hand or hip to foot. The electrode should be placed securely, so that it does not rock back and forth or move as patient breathes.
   F. Cleanse the skin area with alcohol—attempt to achieve a slight erythema by rubbing skin.
   G. Apply electrode paste and rub with electrode. Fasten electrode in place with rubber strap. Apply just the amount of tension on the strap necessary to adequately hold electrode in place. A tight electrode strap might produce muscle tremors and create artifact on tracing. Electrodes should be placed in such a way that patient cable can be attached without overbending lead wire, that is, connectors on electrodes should be pointing down on arms and up on legs.
   H. Attach each of the five-lead wires to the appropriate limb electrode. The cables are color coded and letter labeled for easy identification.
   I. Before proceeding with recording, check the instrument controls.
      1. Check the grounding of the instrument by placing the lead selector on STD position. Using one finger, touch the top of the switch marked "test." If the writing stylus vibrates, press the "test" button down. The test button is left in the position where there is *no* vibration of the writing arm when the button is touched.
      2. Adjust the "position" control so that the writing arm is centered on the ECG paper.
      3. Adjust the "intensity" to produce the necessary heat in the writing arm to give a firm, clear black line.
      4. Turn the power switch to run and check the standardization of the machine. When the button marked "STD (I MV)" is pushed, the writing arm should be deflected exactly two large squares when the "sensitivity" indicator is on "I" (see Chapter 5). Accurate standardization is important to the cardiologist, since some diagnostic and measurement criteria are meaningless without a point of reference. Note: ECGs are standardized with each lead change. ECGs are routinely run at standard "I."

Continued.

12-LEAD CARDIOGRAM PROCEDURE FOR CCU—cont'd

J. All ECGs must be identified by labeling beginning of tracing with patient's name, medical record number, date, and time.

K. A standard ECG consists of twelve separate leads. Each of these leads must be marked for the purposes of identification. This can be done by using the button labeled "marker," to create a mark in the upper margin of the paper. The following code is used for this purpose.

Lead				
I	_		V_1	_____ _
II	_ _		V_2	_____ _ _
III	_ _ _		V_3	_____ _ _ _
aV_R	_____		V_4	_____ _ _ _ _
aV_L	_____ _____		V_5	_____ _ _ _ _ _
aV_F	_____ _____ _____		V_6	_____ _ _ _ _ _ _

L. To record the first six leads:
1. Place the lead selector switch at I. Observe the writing arm; it should oscillate in the center of the strip.
2. Turn the power switch to "Run."
3. Push the "STD (I MV)" button once while the paper is running and identify the lead by pushing the "lead marker" button.
4. After recording 8 to 10 beats with a stable baseline, turn power button to "on" position.
5. Move the lead selector to lead II and proceed as above. Continue through and including lead aV_F. Be sure to mark and identify each lead. After completing aV_F, move the lead selector to the next "dot" position on the lead selector dial.

M. To record the "V" leads of the ECG:
1. Place the Welsh cup electrode on the lead marked "C" (for chest).
2. Expose the patient's chest.
3. Locate the electrode positions of leads V_1 through V_6. Cleanse the areas with alcohol sponge, rubbing to produce a slight erythema. Place a small amount of ECG paste to mark position.
4. The electrode positions are located as follows:
   V_1—fourth intercostal space at right of sternal border
   V_2—same interspace at left of sternal border
   V_3—midway between position V_2 and V_4
   V_4—fifth interspace at midclavicular line
   V_5—same level as V_4 at anterior axillary line
   V_6—same level as V_4 at midaxillary line
5. Rub the electrode paste on first chest lead (V_1) site and secure Welsh electrode cup. Turn lead selector to "V" position and power switch to run. Position stylus as necessary. Press "lead marker" to identify lead.
6. Repeat the preceding step for each of the chest lead positions on chest.

N. Disconnect the electrodes from the patient and reposition the patient for comfort. Wipe electrode paste off chest and extremities.

O. Be sure ECG is correctly labeled. See that ECG is mounted in the patient's chart.

depending on the patient's condition, to determine the adequacy of oxygenation and acid-base balance.

d. *Fluid and electrolyte balance* should be monitored. It is imperative that fluid intake and output be accurately measured. Equally important is *accurate* daily weight of the patient taken at the same time each day on the same scale. This can help to determine the minimal weight gain in the early stages of heart failure when other indicators, such as the chest x-ray film, are still normal. Personnel must be reminded to actually measure rather than estimate intake, just as all output is measured. It should also be remembered that fluids such as tube feedings, those used to flush Swan-Ganz and arterial lines, and those from any other sources must be included in the patient's total fluid intake measurement. Output should include bleeding and drainage from any site, as well as urine and stool. The patient's state of hydration may also be evaluated by the skin tone. Comparison of the initial hydration state to daily findings is helpful in evaluating fluid balance.

e. *Peripheral edema* is a late sign of congestive failure and should be added to the data base already gathered regarding the fluid balance of the patient. The extent of peripheral edema should be measured once it appears and comparative evaluations should be performed frequently to determine changes in edema noted in the periphery.

f. *Dietary regimen,* if altered from the patient's usual diet, should be explained to him and his family. Cardiac patients are usually placed on a low sodium diet for several days. In some patients, sodium restriction may be unnecessary or impractical, and these patients will be given food with the usual sodium content. A soft diet is usually prescribed with frequent small feedings. Since cardiac output levels increase following ingestion of food, the quantity of food at each serving should be kept small. Current research does not conclusively show that hot and cold liquids are detrimental and so their exclusion from diets, although routine in many CCUs, is questionable. Coffee and tea are usually permitted.

All data must be evaluated and intervention planned according to the goals that have been defined by the patient and the staff. If the goal has not been attained, revision of one or more components of the plan may be necessary to assist the patient in meeting the goals.

DAILY APPROACH TO THE PATIENT

Data collection is again the first phase in the daily approach to the cardiac patient. Data are collected utilizing the same procedures discussed in the section concerning initial contact with the patient.

1. *Subjective data* consist of information obtained from the patient and his family. These data sould supplement the subjective data obtained during the initial interview. The information may be gathered at any time and be added to the initial data base. It is appropriate for all health team members to contribute to the data base.

2. *Objective data* are obtained by the parameters discussed under intial care:
   a. Physical examination—comparison of findings with previous findings.
   b. Supportive data—cardiac enzyme levels daily for 3 days; 12-lead ECG daily for 3 days and with chest pain; other laboratory work may be indicated, such as electrolyte level measurements.
   c. Arterial blood gas levels—as needed to evaluate the status of acid-base balance.

Potential problems

Following collection of data pertinent to the patient's current status, assessment is made regarding potential problems for which personnel should be alert. These problems include development of arrhythmias, myocardial dysfunction, and psychologic disturbances.

Arrhythmias. Staff in the CCU should be skilled in arrhythmia interpretation and treatment. Most CCUs have personnel trained to give lidocaine by a preestablished protocol to patients who have ventricular arrhythmias (Appendix A).

Staff should also be certified in skills of basic cardiac life support as defined by the American Heart Association. After certification in basic cardiac life support, staff must be trained to perform other procedures, including preparation of medication, recording times of events and medication given, and assisting as necessary with activities during the resuscitation effort. In many instances, nurses who are well prepared in resuscitation techniques have been successful in returning the patient to adequate cardiopulmonary function prior to the arrival of a physician on the scene.

Some community hospitals without full-time physician coverage now encourage other health care personnel to become certified in the skills of advanced cardiac life support, which includes all the skills of basic cardiac life support in addition to the techniques of endotracheal intubation, venipuncture, arrhythmia interpretation, and drug administration.

Cardioversion. Cardioversion involves the delivery of electrical voltage to the heart by means of metal paddles placed on the intact chest or placed directly on the heart when the chest is opened, as during cardiac surgery. This procedure depolarizes the excitable myocardium, thereby interrupting reentrant circuits and discharging automatic pacemaker foci to establish electrical homogeneity. Cardioversion successfully restores sinus rhythm if the sinus node becomes the automatic focus that fires first and fastest after the electrical shock and controls the cardiac mechanism.

When a patient develops a tachyarrhythmia, slowing the ventricular rate represents the initial and frequently most important therapeutic maneuver. The patient's clinical status and the nature of the arrhythmia determine how rapidly this must be accomplished. Medical therapy involves a time-consuming and potentially dangerous biologic titration of drugs such as digitalis or quinidine; exact therapeutic or toxic levels of these drugs cannot be predicted with absolute certainty and side effects may occur. Electrical cardioversion eliminates many of these problems. Under conditions optimal for close supervision and monitoring, a precisely regulated "dose" of electricity can restore sinus rhythm immediately. The distinction between supraventricular and ventricular tachyarrhythmias, crucial to the proper medical management of arrhythmias, becomes less significant.

By synchronizing the capacitor to discharge during the downslope of the R wave or within the S wave, the ventricular vulnerable period (an interval of 20 to 40 milliseconds' duration near the apex of the T wave) may be avoided. This minimizes, but does not completely eliminate, the danger of precipitating ventricular fibrillation with the DC shock. However, if synchronization cannot be established rapidly and *immediate* cardioversion is indicated, the shock is delivered asynchronously. Immediate cardioversion using maximum voltage without synchronization (called defibrillation) is the mandatory treatment for ventricular fibrillation or ventricular flutter and for ventricular tachycardia if it produces cardiovascular collapse. Ventricular tachycardia that results in a milder hemodynamic decompensation, such as hypotension without shock, or mild congestive heart failure, may be treated initially with lidocaine, or procainamide IV. However, if the tachyarrhythmia does not terminate *promptly,* electrical cardioversion should be performed. Short self-limited bursts of ventricular tachycardia are treated medically. As a general rule, any supraventricular tachyarrhythmia that produces signs or symptoms such as hypotension, angina, or congestive heart failure and does not respond promptly to medical therapy should be terminated electrically.

A. **Elective cardioversion procedure**

An elective cardioversion may be carried out wherever resuscitative equipment such as suction, intubation equipment, medications, and experienced personnel trained in airway management are available. The steps followed are listed here.

1. Explain the procedure to the patient and obtain permission.
2. Perform a thorough physical examination, including palpation of all pulses.
3. Obtain a 12-lead ECG before and after cardioversion, as well as a rhythm strip or oscilloscopic monitoring (or both) during the procedure.
4. Withhold diuretics and short-acting digitalis preparations for 24 to 36 hours. If indicated, obtain a serum potassium or a serum digitalis level reading. Keep the patient fasting for 6 to 8 hours prior to cardioversion.
5. Maintain a reliable IV site. Allow the patient to breathe 100% oxygen for 5 to 15 minutes before, and then immediately after, DC shock.
6. Employ synchronous discharge mode on the defibrillator for elective procedures. The QRS complex recorded on the oscilloscope must be tall to ensure that it alone triggers the capacitor discharge. Determine the accuracy of synchronization by discharging several test shocks before applying the paddles to the patient.

7. Administer diazepam (Valium) or a short-acting barbiturate such as methohexital (Brevital) to produce transient amnesia or light sleep.

8. Apply electrode paste liberally but not excessively to the polished surface of the paddles, which are then placed in firm contact with the chest wall at points distant from monitoring electrodes. The paddles may be positioned anteroposteriorly, in the left infrascapular region and over the upper sternum at the third interspace, or anteriorly, to the right of the sternum at the first or second rib and in the left midclavicular line at the xiphoid level.

9. Employing the minimally effective electrical energy level reduces complications; therefore the starting level for most arrhythmias is around 50 watt-seconds or less (Fig. 8-5). The voltage necessary to terminate some arrhythmias, such as atrial flutter or ventricular tachycardia may be considerably less. If unsuccessful, this initial level may be increased to 100 watt-seconds, and then by 100 watt-second increments until 400 watt-seconds is reached. Make sure that all personnel have moved away from the patient and the bed before discharging the defibrillator.

10. Record the postshock rhythm to determine whether the procedure was successful. V_1 is preferable. An oscilloscopic interpretation is frequently unreliable.

11. Continue some form of rhythm monitoring and close observation for 2 to 3 hours after cardioversion.

B. **Emergency cardioversion procedure**

The nature of an emergency clinical situation determines which of the steps listed must be omitted. Selected procedures range from immediate

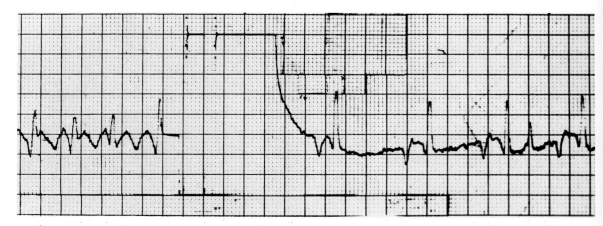

Fig. 8-5. Termination of atrial flutter. Direct current countershock was administered at 50 watt-seconds. The synchronized discharge occurred on R wave, and terminated the flutter rhythm.

cardioversion using maximum voltage without any preamble, for treating ventricular fibrillation, to omitting the delay of 6 to 8 hours after the patient's last meal to cardiovert a less threatening arrhythmia.

C. **Precautions**
   1. When digitalis excess is suspected, electrical cardioversion should be deferred and the arrhythmia treated medically initially to avoid production of serious ventricular tachyarrhythmias and failure to terminate the digitalis-related arrhythmia.
   2. Emergency drugs such as atropine, isoproterenol, and lidocaine and the emergency equipment needed for pacing, intubation, or suction must be available.
   3. Avoid coating the paddles with excessive paste or placing them too near monitoring electrodes. This may allow a spark jump and burn the skin. Local skin inflammation caused by the paddles is best treated with a topical steroid preparation.
   4. Disconnect the patient from other electrical apparatus.
   5. Certain arrhythmias may occur after cardioversion; therefore monitoring of the rhythm must continue for 2 to 3 hours. Other complications may include embolic episodes, which occur in 1% to 3% of patients cardioverted to sinus rhythm.

Resuscitation.* Circulatory arrest is potentially reversible if resuscitation begins during the first 3 to 4 minutes, before irreversible cerebral damage results. Ventricular fibrillation, rather than ventricular asystole, commonly precipitates the arrest; ventricular fibrillation occurs 25 times more commonly during the first 4 hours than it does the day after a myocardial infarction. A well-trained CCU team initiates defibrillation procedures within 30 seconds of the onset of the arrest. Prompt reversion to sinus rhythm often prevents the biochemical derangements that accompany ventricular fibrillation, eliminates the need for endotracheal intubation, and significantly increases the success rate of resuscitation attempts. After a successful resuscitation, measures must be taken to prevent recurrence of the cardiac arrest. Simple arrhythmias, such as premature ventricular systoles, may presage the occurrence of ventricular tachycardia-fibrillation. Early treatment of the former may prevent initiation of the latter.

The monitor alarm usually gives the first indication that a cardiac emergency has occurred. On occasion, personnel may observe the arrhythmia on the oscilloscope before the alarm sounds. At this time they must correlate the observed rhythm with the patient's clinical status by rapidly evaluating the patient's orientation, respirations, pupils, and carotid or femoral pulses. Loose leads can produce a rhythmic pattern simulating ventricular fibrillation. In addition, a lidocaine reaction can mimic the disoriented state seen with tachyarrhythmias asssociated with inadequate cardiac output. The importance of careful diagnosis cannot be overemphasized.

*We do not intend to describe resuscitation techniques in detail, but merely to emphasize certain points. Refer to the American Heart Association guidelines for basic cardiac life support.

A. Resuscitation procedure

1. Establish the patient's unresponsiveness and call for help.
2. Place the patient in a supine position with a board or firm mattress under the chest.*
3. Open the patient's airway by hyperextending the neck and confirm breathlessness.
4. Administer four rapid mouth-to-mouth ventilations.
5. Check the patient's carotid pulse.
6. If the patient has no palpable pulse, begin cycles of 5 external cardiac compressions and 1 ventilation if 2 people are resuscitating, or cycles of 15 compressions and 2 ventilations if only 1 person is resuscitating the patient.
7. After 4 cycles of ventilation and compression, check for return of the patient's pulse and spontaneous breathing. If there is no response, repeat the process.
8. While 1 or more people provide cardiorespiratory support, another sets up the defibrillator. If only 1 person is present, that person must decide between instituting cardiopulmonary resuscitation and attempting to defibrillate the patient. It the defibrillator is close at hand and the patient can be treated with it in 15 to 30 seconds, it is probably best for the single resuscitator to choose defibrillation rather than beginning cardiopulmonary resuscitation alone. *It is extremely critical that DC shock not be delayed while cardiopulmonary resuscitation is begun, intubation attempted, an ECG recorded, a physical examination (other than a brief palpation of pulses and so forth) performed. Rapid application of DC shock is usually the most important therapeutic maneuver in this situation.*
9. IV fluid is started if it is not already running.
10. It is helpful to have a drug list such as the one shown in Table 8-1 taped to the emergency cart. Those medications most likely to be needed are prepared at the first opportunity.
11. If there is time and a sufficient number of people and if the mechanism of the arrhythmia producing the cardiac arrest is unknown, an ECG is done before cardioversion. However, this should never detract from resuscitative measures. If necessary, an ECG is done after DC shock. Certain defibrillators have monitoring capability; their paddles act as electrodes that record the rhythm disturbance immediately prior to emergency cardioversion.
12. As soon as the defibrillator is made ready (this should not take more than 30 seconds), the patient is shocked at a peak energy level (400 watt-seconds) (Fig. 8-6). If this is not successful, defibrillation is repeated; the shock may be repeated again after lidocaine or procainamide administration.

*An initial precordial thump is not currently recommended by the American Heart Association as a necessary component of cardiopulmonary resuscitation.

Table 8-1. Essential emergency cardiac drugs*

Drug	How supplied	Dosage
Sodium bicarbonate	44.6 mEg/50 ml prefilled syringe	1 mEg/kg initially; may be repeated every 5 minutes twice, thereafter based on arterial blood gas levels
Epinephrine	1 mg/10 cc (1:10,000 dilution) in prefilled syringe	0.5 mg (5 ml of 1:10,000 solution) IV every 5 minutes during resuscitation; may be given via intracardiac route by *trained* personnel if IV route not established
Atropine	1 mg/10 ml (0.1 mg/ml) in presyringe	0.5 mg IV as a bolus; repeated at 5-minute intervals until pulse rate is greater than 60, *total* dose should *not* exceed 2 mg except in third-degree AV block, where larger doses may be necessary
Lidocaine	100 mg/5 ml (2%) in prefilled syringe	50 to 100 mg IV bolus every 3 to 5 minutes not to exceed 200 to 250 mg initially with infusions of (2 gm/500 ml dextrose in water) 1 to 4 mg/min
Calcium chloride	1 gm/10 ml (10%)	2.5 to 5.0 ml of 10% solution (200 to 500 mg) estimated from patient's weight, may be repeated every 10 minutes; Repeated large doses may elevate blood levels of calcium with detrimental effect

*See Appendix A for in-depth description of drugs and American Heart Association recommendations for essential cardiac drugs used in emergencies.

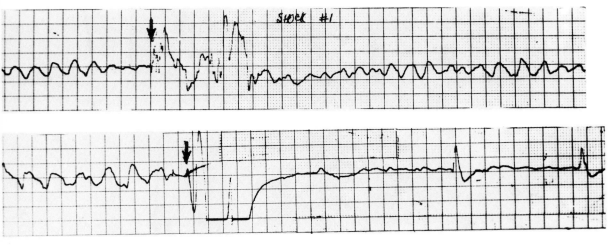

Fig. 8-6. Ventricular fibrillation was treated with application of countershock at 400 watt-seconds in top strip, noted by arrow. Since countershock was unsuccessful, as noted in continuous strip, countershock was again applied at 400 watt-seconds (arrow in second strip). Rhythm then converted to idioventricular mechanism.

13. Defibrillation, if done quickly, is a worthwhile first effort in treating asystole. Occasionally, patients with asystole may respond to the shock with the initiation of spontaneous cardiac beating. However, pacing equipment and drugs stimulating pacemaker discharge are usually necessary to treat asystole.

14. Ventricular fibrillation and ventricular tachycardia producing cardiovascular collapse are defibrillated immediately. Failure to restore an effective rhythm after delivery of a properly administered shock at high intensity suggests that complicating problems such as hypoxia, acidosis, or drug toxicity may be present. If possible, these conditions should be corrected before the next shock is delivered. Cardiopulmonary resuscitation must be continued between defibrillations or other procedures, since even a short interruption results in inadequate perfusion and increased anoxia. These complications in themselves may prevent successful resuscitation.

15. At the first opportunity an episode sheet (Fig. 8-7) is completed and clinical events and a drug tally are recorded.

B. Environment

Regulation of the environment facilitates the rapidity and efficiency of the resuscitation procedure. The corridor to the patient's room must be free of obstacles. The patient's room should have adequate lighting with electric outlets visible from the door. Furniture should not block traffic from the room door to the patient's bed. Flowers should be set on a shelf away from the bed, so that they will not be knocked off the table during an emergency.

C. Postresuscitative care

In the aftermath of a successful resuscitation, it seems natural for ward personnel to relax. Yet, meticulous attention to the patient's hemodynamic status, blood gas levels, and electrolyte balance continues to be important in maintaining clinical stability. This is a time, too, when the patient's family should be counseled about the patient's response to resuscitation, and the family should be encouraged to visit the patient when appropriate.

Myocardial dysfunction. Myocardial dysfunction may be evaluated using several methods (Chapter 3). Measurements made through noninvasive techniques include blood pressure, heart rate, temperature, ECG, echocardiogram, and myocardial scans. Invasive measurements include CVP readings, PA pressure measurements, PCWP, and cardiac outputs (Chapter 4).

Psychologic alterations. Psychologic alterations may be noted at any point during the illness of the patient and should be evaluated on a continuing basis. Already mentioned is the loss of independence, primarily affecting male patients who find they must now depend on females in many activities. Also important is the grieving process that many patients experience. The patient is grieving over the loss of a body part and the consequent changes in his life. He must be given the same understanding and comfort as the person who experiences an obvious external loss. Understanding attitudes on the part of per-

Time	Atropine	Calcium	Epinephrine	Pronestyl	Bicarbonate	Xylocaine			Pulse	Blood pressure	DC setting	Rhythm	Time of episode	Doe, John 9 A.M. / 7/27/67 P.M.
													Mechanism	*Ventricular fib*
9⁰²											400	*fib*		
9⁰³					500							*ↄ*	*I.V. drip*	
9¹⁰									90	110/70		NSR	*Pt. awake, alert*	
9¹⁵						50 mg						PVCs		
9¹⁷									90	110/70		NSR		
Summary														

Fig. 8-7. Coronary care unit episode sheet.

sonnel involved in the patient's care will assist in moving the patient toward acceptance of the illness and its sequelae. The patient who has suffered a myocardial infarction often feels well after the pain ceases and his temperature returns to normal. If he is in the denial stage of the grieving process at this time, it is difficult for him to believe that he has had death of myocardial tissue because he feels well. Health care professionals can best assist the patient by having a helpful and understanding attitude that encourages awareness of the realities of illness. Information about stages of the healing process and associated limitations may be shared with the patient as his readiness to receive it permits.

On some occasions, professional counseling may be necessary for assisting the patient who is working through psychologic alterations. A clinical specialist in mental health nursing is an excellent person to employ in this situation, in addition to psychiatrists or psychologists. Some patients may have difficulty accepting the psychiatrist because of previous stereotyping of "insanity" as the reason for consultation with a psychiatrist. Acceptance of the idea by the patient is often more successful if the psychiatrist is presented as a counselor or a person who will "talk with you and help with the feelings you are experiencing." Unfortunately, counseling is often neglected or postponed until the patient is deeply enmeshed in these psychologic problems, making the recovery process more lengthy and difficult.

Components of daily care

Once potential problems have been assessed, daily care of the patient can be based on the data obtained. Important components in daily care of the patient include relief of his anxiety and pain, monitoring of blood gas levels and fluids, decreasing the myocardial work load, and continuation of dietary recommendations.

Relief of anxiety and pain. This aspect of care has been previously discussed and is applicable in daily care. If the patient experiences pain, it is important to note the frequency, duration, quality, quantity, location, associated factors such as diaphoresis and dyspnea, and alleviating factors. This information should be recorded on the patient's chart, accompanied by an ECG rhythm strip. In addition, a 12-lead ECG should be obtained and evaluated for changes from the initial ECG, and the patient's physician should be notified. If the physician has left orders for nitrates and analgesics, these should be given as ordered, making sure that the patient's vital signs and respiratory characteristics are being monitored. If pain is not relieved, the physician should be notified so that the duration of pain and, thus, increased oxygen demand and work load of the heart can be decreased as soon as possible.

Methods of reducing anxiety have been discussed and are continuously applicable throughout hospitalization.

Evaluation of blood gas levels. The need for supplemental oxygen, once established, should be evaluated at least daily during the acute phase of the illness. Arterial blood gas samples should be drawn only by persons who are skilled in the technique.

Flow sheets that record many values are useful in maintaining a graphic representation of the patient's progress (see Fig. 8-8). Some units prefer a separate flow sheet for arterial blood gas levels, especially for people who require frequent arterial blood gas analysis.

Reduction of myocardial work load. Decreasing myocardial work continues to be an important component of daily patient care. Activities should gradually be increased according to the physician's plan in light of the patient's stage of recovery. Patients are now being mobilized earlier than they used to be, since prolonged bed rest may not prevent but may actually increase development of complications following myocardial infarction. The patient must, however, be assisted in all activities, especially during the acute phase of the illness.

Continuation of dietary recommendations. Initial dietary recommendations are usually maintained throughout the acute phase of illness and often throughout hospitalization and convalescence.

Evaluation of fluid and electrolyte balance. Fluid and electrolyte balance is very important during the acute phase of the myocardial infarction, as previously discussed. Accurate measurement of intake and output levels, daily weight readings, evaluation of hydration, the presence of pulmonary findings such as rales and any edema are all very important components in the evaluation of fluid and electrolyte balance.

• • •

Each of these considerations should be evaluated, with care planned on the basis of the evaluation. Goals should be set *with* the patient for his care. Reevaluation and further planning are performed in relation to changes in the patient's status.

		Date:						
		Time	7-3	3-11	11-7	7-3	3-11	11-7
Chest	Chest pain R$_x$ and response Gallops/murmurs Edema Jugular venous distention Breath sounds Rales Cough Dyspnea Cyanosis Other							
Abdomen	Nausea/vomiting Appetite/diet Bowels/guiac Abdominal distention Hepatomegaly Other							
Rhythm	Basic rhythm Arrhythmias Conduction defect							
	Emotional status							
	Other							
Vital signs	Bath/activity level Temperature/weight Apical/radial pulse Respirations Blood pressure							
	Time							
Laboratory data	Enzymes Blood gases Other							

I and O	Intake Oral
	            IV
	            Total
	            Total 24 hrs.
	
	Output Urine
	            Emesis/Gomco
	            Total
	            Total 24 hrs.							

	Signature							

Stamp here with patient's Addressograph plate

Fig. 8-8. Example of CCU summary flow sheet.

COMPLICATIONS

The complications most frequently encountered in patients who have had a myocardial infarction are thromboembolic events, congestive heart failure, and arrhythmias. The following sections outline methods of preventing these complications.

Thromboembolic events

Anticoagulants. The need for anticoagulation therapy in patients with a myocardial infarction continues to be controversial. Many physicians use anticoagulants for patients in the acute phase following an infarct to minimize abnormal clotting events and resultant complications. Initially, heparin may be administered continuously by an IV infusion pump at a rate of 400 units per hour. Clotting times or partial thromboplastin times should be monitored while the patient receives anticoagulant therapy. Any tendencies toward bleeding should be noted and treated immediately. Once the patient is out of the intensive care unit, oral anticoagulants may be prescribed to replace heparin if anticoagulation therapy is to be continued.

Exercise program. An exercise program can help prevent the complications engendered by inactivity and aid the patient psychologically. Exercise therapy helps prevent respiratory complications, venous stasis, joint stiffness from immobility, and the weakness resulting from loss of muscle tone. Furthermore, it promotes relaxation by decreasing tension.

An exercise program should be planned jointly with the patient for use throughout hospitalization and after discharge. Appropriate program goals and priorities for implementation should be planned with the patient. In planning this program the physical therapist and occupational therapist are useful consultants. The exercise program should be structured in progressive stages and individualized according to the patient's tolerance. Initially the patient may be assisted in performing passive exercises. A footboard is useful for the patient to exersize his leg muscles. Tolerance to exercise at each stage is observed, evaluated, and recorded. When the patient first gets out of bed, supine and standing blood pressures should be noted.

Elastic bandages or elastic stockings. Elastic supports may also be used to prevent venous stasis. They must be applied with equal pressure from the foot to above the knee, checked frequently, and removed two or three times a day. Lotion or powder may then be applied to the skin. The patient should be instructed not to cross legs or ankles. Somtimes the elastic stockings roll down over the knee and create a tourniquet effect on the leg. If this occurs, it should be corrected promptly. Should any evidence of embolization be observed, the patient's physician should be notified. The legs should be observed for redness, swelling, heat, red streaks, and a positive Homan's sign.

Congestive heart failure

Techniques are aimed at the prevention and early detection of congestive heart failure, such as recording accurate intake and output measurements and daily weight. Intake of routine IV fluids should be kept to a mimimum 20 ml per hour in the postmyocardial infarction patient unless dehydration is present. All fluids, except in an emergency, should be administered via microdrip, and drugs such as lidocaine should be placed in a reliable automatic drip control device and checked frequently to ascertain whether the proper amount of fluid is being delivered (see Chapter 4).

Assessment of the patient should be made frequently to check for signs of possible congestive heart failure. The examination should include the following points:

1. Examination of the heart, listening closely for the presence of an S_3, indicative of heart failure, as well as for the other usual components in the cardiac examination (discussed in Chapter 3). Special notice should also be given to the development of any tachyarrhythmias. These should be treated immediately after notification of the physician.
2. Examination of the lungs, listening for rales and, if present previously, comparison of location, type, and amount. The presence of rhonchi that do not clear with coughing is also important to note.
3. Examination for peripheral edema or ascites. Although both of these are late signs, they can be correlated with other earlier evidence of congestive failure.
4. Evaluation of dyspnea, an early sign of left ventricular failure in the absence of other obvious causes. Congestive failure should be suspected in the patient who has had myocardial infarction and then develops dyspnea without other known etiology.
5. Evaluation of jugular veins may reveal congestion and filling from below (see Chapter 3). The neck veins may also become distended when sustained pressure is applied on the liver (hepatojugular reflux). Systemic venous pressure is often abnormally elevated and may be recognized most easily by observing the extent of distention of the jugular veins, especially in relation to rest and exertion.

Arrhythmias

The improved management of arrhythmias constitutes a significant advance in the treatment of myocardial infarction. The prevention of serious and life-threatening arrhythmias depends on early recognition and aggressive management of their precursors. The most frequent arrhythmias noted in the acute phase of myocardial infarction are premature ventricular systoles, ventricular tachycardia, and ventricular fibrillation (see Chapter 6).

PSYCHOSOCIAL RESPONSES

Another aspect of preventive care and rehabilitation is the recognition and treatment of the patient's emotional responses to the myocardial infarction. After such an experience, psychologic stress is normal and to be expected. For the patient experiencing a myocardial infarction, the feeling is terrifying. The pain is often described as nothing ever experienced before. It in itself conveys some of the oppressive deathlike qualities inherent in the illness. Once the experience is realized, the individual must develop certain responses or psychologic means of coping with the fears and anxieties created by this event.

The defenses that were used in coping with everyday frustrations before the heart attack are relied on to handle the emotional impact of the illness. Patient responses that are commonly observed after a myocardial infarction include denial, anger, anxiety, regression, fear of dying and invalidism, and depression. These responses are manifested in certain behavioral patterns.

PATTERNS OF PATIENT RESPONSE

Denial. Denial is a defense mechanism that is often used. The patient may present two significant forms of denial. The first, *denial of the fact,* is a "this really didn't happen to me" feeling or a refusal to admit that the event actually did happen. It also exists when the patient attempts to find another excuse for the event: "It must be gas pains." In addition, when the patient ignores activity restrictions or talks about immediate return to work, the patient is using denial of the fact.

The second form of denial, *denial of the feelings associated with the heart attack,* is a refusal to admit fear or other normal emotions that might be associated with such a traumatic experience. The patient exhibits a reluctance to discuss feelings. *Hospital euphoria* is one mode of behavior associated with this form of denial. The happy-go-lucky patient who relates well with all staff and jokes lightly regarding his condition is probably one who is not realistically integrating the experience and will most likely have difficulty in future adjustment.

Anger. Anger is another manifestation of the experience. "Why should this happen to me?" *Anger* may be directed at the family, staff, or treatment program. A person who has a great deal of unresolved anger may continually complain about the nursing care or the therapeutic measures being implemented.

Anxiety. Myocardial infarction is an *anxiety*-producing event. Patients try to deal with this immediate event as well as with preillness problems. Overtly the patient may admit apprehension or nervousness. Less overt manifestations of anxiety are bad dreams, constant talking, a demanding intellectual curiosity, hypochondriasis, and projection of feelings to others.

Intellectual curiosity may be demonstrated by an intense interest in obtaining information about coronary heart disease or by constant questioning about the many physical and laboratory routines. These questions obviously indicate the patient's concern regarding the treatment program and the reasons for it.

Hypochondriasis is the transfer of the feelings of anxiety and fear into somatic complaints such as chest pain. It is important to be able to differentiate anginal pain from psychogenic pain. Usually psychogenic pain is more localized—for example, around the nipple on the left side of the chest. The patient can locate the pain by pointing to the area with his finger. The pain may be described as sharp, fleeting or stabbing, and persisting—all descriptions not characteristic of anginal pain.

Projection of feelings is demonstrated when the patient protects his ego concept through projecting his feelings and subconsciously attributing his own fears to other people. Typical sentiments expressed are "You think I've had a heart attack," "My son thinks I'm going to die," and "My wife thinks I won't be able to go back to work."

Regression. Regression may be manifested by a total dependence on others, beyond the point at which absolute activity limitation is no longer necessary. The patient is not interested in assuming any responsibilities of self-care but curls up in bed, pulls up the covers, and portrays the picture of helplessness.

Fear of dying and invalidism. Myocardial infarction threatens the patient's total integrity as well as his sense of personal adequacy and worth to others. If the threat to self-image is overwhelming, the patient may try to protect the little he thinks remains by resigning himself to a life of dependency. Moreover, the male patient who feels a loss of masculinity and fears invalidism may react by exposing his chest, flirting, and bragging.

If the patient care plan from the acute phase is not revised, the patient may retain certain fears. These include (1) fear of activity, (2) fear of recurrent heart attacks and sudden death, and (3) fear of a "fragile heart." Furthermore, these fears may be reinforced by a family member whose own feelings about the illness have not been resolved. Unresolved fear could result in the patient's becoming a cardiac invalid.

Depression. Depression is a natural initial reaction to the occurrence of a myocardial infarction. At first the patient experiences a mourning period over the loss of health. Anorexia, insomnia, apathy, withdrawal, and crying are signs of this grief period. Periodically the patient experiences feelings of depression. This may be more evident after the return home. However, it is not natural for the patient to remain depressed.

VARIABLES AFFECTING PATIENT RESPONSE

The development and the magnitude of these reactions to stress are influenced by the following variables.

Staff-patient relationship. Many studies emphasize the staff-patient relationship as one of the most important factors in the rehabilitation process. Staff who communicate frequently and frankly with the patient and the family are likely to engender feelings of reassurance and trust. The patient who does not have such rapport with the staff may be quite anxious.

Family-patient relationship. The patient's family also have feelings to resolve. Their ability to be supportive in the patient's rehabilitation process depends on their previous relationship with the patient and the extent to which they are integrated into the patient's rehabilitation program.

Age. Older people may adjust to the emotional impact of the illness more easily than younger people. They place less emphasis on physical abilities and may have fewer family and social responsibilities, for example, the retired person as compared with a father supporting a family of young children.

Socioeconomic status. Financial worries provoke stress reactions. Hospitalization is very expensive, often augmenting debts the patient may have accrued before becoming ill. In addition, society makes certain demands of the patient after illness such as the employer's attitude regarding cardiac disease and the type of work the patient will be expected to perform.

Educational background and previous experience. Previous contacts and information the patient has had about myocardial infarction influence his psychologic reactions. If he has known people who have died or been critically ill with a myocardial infarction, he may have the same expectations of himself. If the patient has experienced a previous myocardial infarction, his reaction will depend on the success or failure of his rehabilitation. On the other hand, if the patient has experienced his first myocardial infarction and has a family history of death resulting from heart disease, he is quite likely to be apprehensive. Misinterpretation of medical terminology or equipment can affect the patient's response to his illness. The cardiac monitor and other specialized equipment may be frightening to a patient who misconstrues or distorts the information given him.

Severity of illness. Complications, such as cardiac arrest or pulmonary edema, can precipitate a serious emotional setback. Patients commonly sleep poorly after a resuscitation experience. Months afterward they may still have nightmares.

Persistence of cardiac symptoms. Shortness of breath, angina, and other symptoms may cause the patient to voluntarily restrict activities and to fear attempting new activities.

Patient's medical history. Both the physical condition of the patient at the onset of this illness and previous illnesses influence his responses.

● ● ●

The stress that the patient experiences immediately after the myocardial infarction can adversely affect long-term adjustment. Acute emotional upsets may precipitate serious complications in patients with coronary artery disease through the effects of sympathetic nervous system stimulation and catecholamine release. Catecholamines increase the work load of the heart by increasing the heart rate, the force of myocardial contraction, and metabolic demands. In patients with coronary artery disease, the rigid coronary vessels may not be able to dilate in response to increased myocardial metabolic requirements. The amount of oxygen delivered to the myocardium may be inadequate. Arrhythmias, angina, myocardial infarction, heart failure, and pulmonary edema can be provoked in this manner. Thus the patient's emotional responses may significantly influence the outcome of the illness.

ROLE OF HEALTH TEAM IN PATIENT'S ADJUSTMENTS

It is important that the health team recognize a patient's need for defenses or coping responses. However, the staff must be able to differentiate constructive from destructive psychologic mechanisms. The emotional responses described may be useful as long as they do not interfere with the treatment program or ultimate rehabilitative goals for the patient.

Within the rehabilitative plan the staff must learn to *anticipate* stress responses, *recognize* the varied behavior manifestations, and *reduce* or prevent the impact of the stress on the patient's well-being. This can be accomplished through three approaches: (1) promoting rest, (2) alleviating anxiety, and (3) reinforcing feelings of effectiveness and competence.

Promote rest. Patients suffering a myocardial infarction need both physical and emotional rest to regroup their defenses. Provide care in a calm manner, and keep the general atmosphere quiet. Floor carpeting enhances this atmosphere; the bedside monitor beep should be silenced and the alarm sound relayed to the central station. Family members should be informed frequently about the patient's progress. In a few CCUs the family is telephoned each morning.

Incorporate rest periods as part of the daily routine. A scheduled "quiet hour" each day guarantees the patient rest without interruption. At this time the lights are dimmed and the shades are drawn. Schedule tests and procedures so as not to conflict with the "quiet hour."

Adjust visiting hours to the individual needs of the patient and family. Limit the number of visitors in the room to a few persons at a time. The patient's attitude toward visitors is an important consideration. The patient may view visiting restrictions as a protective measure. In fact, he may not wish certain members of his family to see him "incapacitated." Respect these feelings and be flexible. To some patients, the presence of a spouse may be disturbing; to others, it may be quite comforting.

The patient may need sedation to help him rest. Enough sedation should be given to alleviate anxiety. However, excessive sedation may interfere with integrating the realities of the event—a necessary step toward successful rehabilitation—and initiate medical complications. Careful observation of the patient's response to sedation and regulation of dosage accordingly contribute to optimum rest and adjustment.

Alleviate anxiety. Anxiety can be diminished by actively listening to what the patient says and by encouraging the patient to verbalize, depending on his readiness and willingness to talk. To fully adjust to the heart attack the patient must experience the realities of the event. Usually this is best accomplished by "living" the experience with someone—that is, by expressing the feelings and anxieties incurred and taking constructive steps to deal with them. Once the patient begins to integrate the experience, he attempts to find a cause for the event. *Overwork, overeating,* and *overtiredness* are convenient situations on which to place the blame. The patient attempts to find a familiar excuse for the event that has disrupted his life. This allows him the comfort of making changes in his way of life to prevent the event from occurring again.

Provide thorough yet simple explanations. Fear of the unknown is disabling and the anxious patient draws his own conclusions. The patient can be educated about his illness without avoiding "charged" topics or words, such as "heart attack" and "death." Since the patient may not discuss these things freely with his family for fear of upsetting them, therapeutic ward relationships are crucial.

The patient enduring a prolonged critical stage of illness receives intense around-the-clock treatment. Sensory overload and deprivation are pitfalls of any intensive care environment. Activity in the room is constant; room lights may not be dimmed for days. These circumstances may confuse the patient as to time and day. Provide measures to orient the patient to the environment. Periodically remind the patient of the day and time; also place a calendar and clock on the wall in the room. Television may effectively orient as well as occupy the patient, although some CCUs discourage the use of TV because of electrical safety problems and concern about patient reaction to some TV programs.

The CCU offers the patient continuous exposure to varied health personnel. Consistent patient assignments minimize the number of superficial relationships the patient must form and provide the reassurance of familiar faces. Not only does this facilitate orientation, but it also fosters the development of effective therapeutic relationships. The patient should be allowed to keep one or two small personal belongings as reminders of reality. It is debatable whether objects such as the defibrillator and emergency drugs in the patients room actually engender anxiety or are reassuring. Discussion of the patient's therapy or clinical progress should *not* be held in his presence unless he is included in the conference. Information misconstrued by an innocently eavesdropping patient may provoke undue and unnecessary anxiety.

Certain recent studies have described patients with angina and myocardial infarction as driving and struggling to succeed, yet not enjoying success. They may be unable to express their feelings and therefore need encouragement. These patients may indicate a sense of time urgency and impatience. By informing them of the ward activities, adhering to time schedules and routines, and anticipating many of their needs, the staff can often reduce patient's anxieties.

Additional methods to alleviate anxiety include permitting the patient as much independence as his condition safely allows, such as feeding himself, early ambulation, and "armchair management." These activities provide an outlet for the excess energy caused by apprehension. Forced immobility and dependency reduce the ability of the individual to interact with his environment. This may decrease the quality and quantity of sensory stimulation and reduce the accuracy of perception. When a patient is restricted to bed rest, he is more inclined to distort time and this may compound his anxiety. Physical restriction can aggravate feelings of helplessness, vulnerability, and depression. The patient cannot manipulate his environment to control his anxieties; he must wait to be approached. Therefore the health team should encourage early ambulation as tolerated as well as involvement in suitable activities.

The family's anxiety can impede or facilitate the patient's recovery. Working with family members by answering their questions and by educating them about the patient's illness can lessen their insecurity. The benefits from family education and rehabilitation often go unrecognized. What a family member learns from this experience will be applied to similar situations in the future.

Reinforce feelings of effectiveness and competence. Control and manipulation of the environment give rise to feelings of effectiveness and competence. Encourage the patient to direct the environment by letting him plan and participate in his own care. With the simple matter of a bath, the patient can recommend when he would like it. If food selection is possible on the daily meals, he can make these decisions. Emphasize the patient's capabilities. Throughout the therapeutic program in the hospital and at home the patient should be encouraged to participate, within prescribed limits, in physical activities, diet, sexual activity, and his occupation.

Attitudes of nurses, physicians, and the patient's family may have deleterious or beneficial influences on the patient's mental outlook. An overprotective approach by health personnel may produce regression, a rigid approach may produce frustration, and indifference may create anxiety. An approach that is realistic, honest, positive, and forward looking will show favorable results.

Electrical safety for patient and equipment operator

The varied electronic equipment harbored by a CCU increases the potential of electrical shock hazard for both the patient and the equipment operator. Consequently, CCU personnel should have a basic understanding of the principles of current flow, current source, and grounding.

If all ground connections of equipment are not at the same potential (zero volts or a few millivolts above zero), leakage current may flow between the source and its ground. Current will flow through the patient if he serves as a link in this circuit. Skin offers resistance to current flow and therefore protects the heart from electrical shock. If the voltage is high enough or skin resistance has been lowered or eliminated, ventricular fibrillation may result. On some equipment, built-in isolation circuits isolate the patient from the ground and the power line, thus preventing any conductive pathways. However, an intracardiac catheter or fluid column bypasses the skin and the protection from current flow that it affords, making the patient highly vulnerable to electrical shock. Alternating current (AC) power line current levels of only millionths of amperes, undetectable when applied to the skin, can induce ventricular fibrillation if contact with the myocardium is made.

Any AC power line–operated device from which some of the current flows through the metal frame, case, or other exposed parts may serve as a current source. It may be an electric bed with a broken or missing ground connection or any device with two-wire power cords (two-pronged plugs) such as TV sets, bed lamps, or electric fans. The patient may lie in the path between the "current source" and ground directly by touching the electrical device or ground indirectly by making physical contact with another person who touches the defectively grounded instrument. Either situation causes the patient to become a conductive pathway and allows current to flow through him to ground.

Equipment operators should be cautious when using electronic equipment near water, steam pipes, radiators, or plumbing fixtures. Such pipes and fittings are excellent electrical grounds. Consequently, any electrical device near them, including the power cords, plugs, and wall receptacles, that exposes the user to live current can be extremely hazardous if the operator simultaneously contacts both the device and a grounded pipe, faucet, and so forth. The operator then becomes the "link" between the current source and the ground that the current seeks. The resultant shock may not be fatal, but serious injury can result from violent muscular reaction in "letting go" (Table 8-2).

Ward personnel may detect "tingling" sensations when touching or brushing against a piece of electronic equipment. The voltage necessary to produce this sensation is only one thousandth of an ampere. Under ordinary circumstances this is harmless; however, this voltage is nearly fifty times the amount necessary to produce ventricular fibrillation if current flows directly to the patient's heart.

Clearly, many considerations are necessary to provide electrical safety. Awareness of potential hazards, prompt correction of faulty equipment, and regular safety inspection checks are all needed. Personnel should be thoroughly briefed in the following safety precautions.

RULES FOR ELECTRICAL SAFETY IN THE CCU

1. All equipment should be grounded. This means that a pathway of least resistance is available for the currents within the machine to flow to ground.
   a. All equipment must have three-pronged plugs (which connect the hospital ground to the equipment chassis).

Table 8-2. Effects of electric current

60-cycle current (1-second duration) delivered through skin		60-cycle current (1-second duration) leading to heart	
Milliamperes	Effects	Microamperes	Effects
1	Threshold of perception; tingling	20 to 50	Ventricular fibrillation
16	"Let go" current; muscle contraction		
50	Pain; possible fainting; mechanical injury		
100 to 3000	Ventricular fibrillation		
6000 or greater	Sustained myocardial depolarization followed by normal rhythm; temporary respiratory paralysis; burns		

    b. Adaptors fitting a three-pronged plug into a two-slot electrical outlet should not be used.

    c. Extension cords should not be used to connect electronic equipment. If extensions are necessary, use only three-pronged grounding-type cords.

2. Wet surfaces conduct current. Therefore such hazards as wet sheets and wet floors should be eliminated.

3. Safety inspection checks should be routine. A qualified electrical technician should check all equipment for faulty or missing ground connections and hazardous voltages. (Remember that equipment can still operate with defective ground connections.)

4. When two instruments are in use near a patient, connect them to the same power receptacle.

5. Never plug or unplug equipment, turn on a light, and so forth, while your hand or other part of your body is in contact with water, steam pipes, radiators, or plumbing fixtures.

6. Prevent equipment cords from kinking, draping on pipes and plumbing, or lying on wet surfaces.

7. Report "tingling" sensations emitted from a bed frame, instrument case, and so forth. Unplug the equipment that is not necessary to life support of the patient; correct this condition immediately in equipment necessary for life support.

8. When using an intracavitary lead, connect the electrode catheter to the V lead of the ECG machine, since this circuit has a high electrical resistance in relation to ground. Anyone or anything electrically grounded must not touch the V lead electrode terminals.

9. Additional precautions should be taken for patients with temporary cardiac pacemakers.

    a. The electrodes at the end of the pacemaker should be well insulated. On older models, a rubber glove is used to cover the exposed terminals at the junction with the external power source. Most newer models are adequately insulated, however.

    b. When possible, use external battery pacemakers that are isolated from the power line sources.

    c. Personnel should wear rubber gloves when connecting or disconnecting the battery pacemaker and when adjusting electrodes at the end of the catheter.

    d. Personnel should not wear leather-bottomed shoes on conductive or carpeted floors.

10. Patients should wear bedroom shoes at all times on conductive floors.

11. Patients should use battery-operated electric razors.

Transfer from CCU

    Patients tend to become dependent on the CCU atmosphere during the acute phase of their illness. Comfort is derived from sophisticated equipment and the individualized care provided by personnel in constant attendance. The concern expressed by physicians, nurses, and other health personnel adds to the developing patient dependence on the CCU. Not unexpectedly, the patient may have both emotional and physiologic reactions to transfer if adequate preparation and follow-up arrangements are not included in his care.

Health personnel, especially the primary nurse, have a responsibility to ease the reaction of the patient in the transition from CCU to the intermediate care unit. Personnel should not force or attempt to impose desired behaviors on the patient, but should strive for a working relationship that will allow the patient to rely on the nurse and other health personnel for assistance and information as he progresses in the adaptation process. Acting on behalf of the patient, guiding and teaching him in a supportive manner, and helping him to adjust to the physical changes in his new environment are all ways by which health personnel can ease the patient's transition.

Acting on behalf of the patient. Health personnel should actively assist the patient once the transfer is anticipated. Calling the patient's family to notify them of the move is helpful to both, since the patient will know that he will not be "lost" to his family, and the family will not be unduly alarmed at finding an empty bed at the next visiting time.

During daily care in the CCU the nurse has an opportunity to discuss areas of concern with the patient. Financial concerns are often the first worries mentioned by the patient. Discussing these concerns with the patient and securing assistance for him, such as a visit from the social worker, can be helpful in alleviating emotional upset. The social worker and other appropriate personnel can assist in the transition phase by rechanneling the patient's energies toward adaptation and planning for recovery.

Guiding, supporting, and teaching the patient. Beginning in the early phase of CCU care, the nurse should prepare the patient for transfer by telling the patient that the CCU is an area in which he is to receive temporary care. Once he has improved sufficiently, care can be maintained in a unit that provides intermediate care. This explanation prepares the patient for the move well in advance and helps him to realize that improvement in his condition is the primary determinant for the move.

Since the actual transfer may be planned or sudden, the patient should be informed about the elements of transfer prior to anticipated time of transfer. The patient should be aware that staff in the intermediate care unit will be given a verbal report concerning his illness, his progress, and potential problems for which they should be alert, in addition to charted information gathered throughout the CCU phase. The CCU nurse should accompany the patient to the intermediate care unit and introduce him to the primary nurse responsible for his care so that he is familiar with the person to call should he need assistance. Any information that the patient requests regarding the new unit can then be answered by the intermediate care unit nurse.

Positive and realistic reinforcement of the patient's progress is a necessary component in his adaptation. Information regarding his status and improvement should be discussed as his condition evolves. Reassurance by health personnel along with factual information about his progress, will assist the patient in looking forward to the transfer and his return to a "normal life."

Assisting the patient's adaptation to environmental changes. The possible dependence of the patient on the monitor has been mentioned previously. The use of the monitor and its limitations should be described to the patient initially and periodically thereafter. Patients have been known to think that their heartbeat depended on the monitor. If such inaccuracies in the patient's perceptions can be dispelled early, potential anxieties related to discontinuation of the monitor may be prevented. If possible, the patient should be "weaned" from all equipment, including the monitor, prior to transfer.

Continuity in the plan of care for the patient should be discussed with the intermediate care unit staff. The patient should be made aware that such communication has taken place and that such continuity is planned. The clinical nursing specialist can be an asset in the coordination of planning and implementation to provide maximum continuity for the patient.

INTERMEDIATE PHASE

Several terms have evolved to describe an area designed to allow closely supervised convalescence for patients who have left the CCU. This area provides more intense observation and care than a routine medical ward, but less than that provided in a CCU. Synonyms for this area include step-down unit, liberalized cardiac unit, and intermediate care unit. Regardless of the name selected, this unit has multiple purposes:

1. Continued patient monitoring to allow for immediate recognition of cardiac arrhythmias and conduction disturbances
2. Immediate cardiopulmonary resuscitation
3. Safe, supervised, early mobilization
4. Reduction in costs of acute care practices in hospitalization
5. Environment conducive to psychologic and physical recovery
6. Education and reeducation concerning abilities and disabilities related to heart disease
7. Continuation of the planned rehabilitation program

Studies have shown that some patients who suffer acute myocardial infarction continue to be at risk even after surviving the first hazardous days after onset. In fact, mortality during the later hospital phase of the illness, when the patient is usually no longer being cared for in the CCU, may be as high as that in the CCU for some groups of patients. This fact is the basis for the concept of intermediate coronary care, whereby patients can be located in an area that is usually close to the CCU. This unit has monitoring and resuscitative equipment and is staffed with personnel adequately prepared to provide routine as well as cardiopulmonary emergency care.

The following groups of patients have been shown to be at increased risk of catastrophic cardiac events during hospitalization and after discharge from the CCU:

1. Patients with anterior infarctions involving large portions of the left ventricle and interventricular septum
2. Patients who exhibit circulatory failure in the form of cardiogenic shock, pulmonary edema, and congestive heart failure while in the CCU
3. Patients with preexisting cardiovascular disease, prior infarction, and fascicular block
4. Patients who exhibit arrhythmias that are primarily ventricular in origin or are indicative of heart failure, for example, atrial fibrillation or flutter and/or persistent sinus tachycardia

Although current data support the fact that people who fall within the categories listed above have a two to six times greater chance of late in-hospital sudden death, this cannot be predicted with complete accuracy. However, these patients have had a slightly longer stay in the CCU (1 to 2 days longer) and tend to be 3 to 4 years older than their counterparts who survive hospitalization. These facts alone support the need for accurate assessment and interpretation of data to prevent and/or treat the complications that contribute to the high late in-hospital mortality.

RECEIVING PATIENT FROM CCU

The following suggestions will ease the patient's transition from the CCU to the intermediate care area:

1. Having the intermediate care area prepared with all the equipment needed by the patient and locating it close to bathroom facilities, nurses' station, and emergency equipment
2. Monitoring cardiac activity by telemetry to provide continuity and rapid detection of potential arrhythmic problems
3. Providing a proposed guideline for educational activities in which the patient will participate during the remainder of hospitalization
4. Providing patient and family with information on routines appropriate to efficient operation of the unit, such as visiting policies, educational opportunities, activity routines, and purpose of specialized equipment

ASSESSMENT OF PATIENT

The evaluation process initiated on admission to the CCU should be continued in the intermediate care unit. This evaluation can be easily divided into three phases: (1) initial or admission assessment, (2) assessment of health needs, and (3) preparation for discharge.

Initial assessment. Initially the person with primary responsibility for providing care to the patient should complete a health assessment. This entails collecting data, making a plan of care based on the assessment of the data, carrying out the plan, and, finally, evaluating the effectiveness of the care.

First, when the patient arrives at the intermediate care area, a brief history can be obtained by direct questioning. This limited interview provides a basis for a therapeutic relationship and yields information needed for making judgments about appropriate care. Additional information can be obtained from the clinical record and from CCU personnel.

Second, a brief physical examination concentrating on the cardiopulmonary system and using inspection, palpation, percussion, and auscultation will provide baseline information by which to evaluate and reevaluate progress.

Assessment of health needs. The second phase of evaluation involves assessment of the individual's health needs. Attention should be given to activity tolerance, educational strengths and deficits, and the physical and psychologic status of the individual.

One goal of intermediate care is supervised early mobilization. Consistent with this expectation is a gradual increase in physical activity during the remainder of hospitalization, enabling the patient to reach the activity levels required for self-care when he returns home. The activities allowed include progressively increased self-care, increasing time spent sitting up in a chair, and body motion and strength-building exercises. The patient should increase his ambulation daily until he can walk about the hosptial unit without tiring.

These physical activities are alternated with rest periods. Exercise should always be avoided after meals, when a large percentage of cardiac output is being used to digest food. Criteria for decreasing the level of activity include the following:

1. Chest pain or dyspnea
2. Heart rate greater than 120 beats per minute
3. Occurrence of a significant arrhythmia
4. Decrease in systolic blood pressure of 20 mm Hg
5. Increased S-T segment displacement on the ECG or monitor

Assessment of the patient's educational strengths and deficits should be determined soon after admission to the intermediate care unit so that planned teaching can be completed prior to discharge. In many instances, personnel with special knowledge and skill in psychologic evaluation can be of tremendous assistance in determining how to best motivate patients and facilitate learning. For some patients denial, depression, and despair are patterns of behavior that prevent optimal benefit from educational efforts. People with psychologic expertise can be of particular assistance with these exceptional patients and their families. This period of time immediately following the CCU experience has been recognized as the time when patients are most receptive to accepting changes in life-style. Lifelong habits can be changed at this point more easily than they can be later, when the emotional impact of the acute event has subsided. The personnel *must* take full advantage of this receptive period.

Preparation for discharge. Preparing the patient and his family for the time when he leaves the hospital should be a primary focus of care during the intermediate phase. All of the following items should be considered in a discharge planning program.

Intervention. Intervention must be based on individualized prescriptions

Table 8-3. Classes of organic heart disease: guide for evaluating impairment of the whole person*

Class I prime (none)	Class I (minimal)	Class II (moderate)	Class III (severe)	Class IV (very severe)
Energy expenditure over 7 calories per minute	Energy expenditure continuous up to 5 calories per minute intermittent to 6.6 calories per minute	Energy expenditure continuous up to 2.5 calories per minute intermittent to 4 calories per minute	Energy expenditure continuous up to 2 calories per minute intermittent to 2.7 calories per minute	Energy expenditure up to 1.5 calories per minute
No symptoms with any type of activity	No symptoms with ordinary activity	Slight symptoms with ordinary activity; none at rest	Less than ordinary activity causes symptoms; none at rest	Symptoms even at rest
Walking, climbing stairs freely, and all activities of daily living do not produce symptoms	Walking, climbing stairs, and usual activities of daily living do not produce symptoms	Walking on level, climbing one flight of stairs (average pace), and usual activities of living do not produce symptoms	Walking more than one block on level or climbing one flight of stairs (average pace) or usual activities of daily living produce symptoms	Performance of any activities of daily living beyond personal toilet or its equivalent produces increased discomfort Symptoms increase with emotional reaction, any physical activity increases discomfort
Continuous (3 minutes or longer), very severe (rapid action or mass musculature) physical exertion, hurrying, hill climbing, severe or competitive recreation do not produce symptoms	Intermittent (2 minutes or less), severe physical exertion, hurrying, hillclimbing, active recreation, and marked emotional stress do not produce symptoms	Emotional stress, hurrying, hill climbing, active recreation, or similar physical activities produce slight symptoms	Emotional stress, hurrying, hill climbing, active recreation, or similar activities produce marked symptoms	
Signs of congestive heart failure are not present	Signs of congestive heart failure are not present	Signs of congestive heart failure are not present	Signs of congestive heart failure may be present, and if so are usually relieved by therapy	Signs of congestive heart failure, if present, are usually resistant to therapy

*Adopted with revisions from the American Heart Association (New York Heart Association). From Hellmuth, G. A.: Work and heart disease, J.A.M.A. **198:**13, Dec. 26, 1966, and American Medical Association (Committee on Medical Rating of Physical Impairment). From Guides to the evaluation of permanent impairment: The cardiovascular system, Committee on Medical Rating of Physical Impairment, J.A.M.A. **172:**1049-1060, March 5, 1960.

for care. This includes activity, diet, and educational pursuits. It is important that the family be included in all planning. The following components are included as minimum requirements in planning a coronary rehabilitation program.

ILLNESS. Help the patient gain insight into his illness or condition. Provide information about the disease process, risk factors, and symptoms.

MEDICATIONS. Explain prescriptions and details of the drug program to the patient and responsible family member; knowledge of the drugs' actions and side effects is helpful to patients. Prescriptions should be labeled. Help the patient adjust the medication schedule to the usual life-style at home in order to ensure maximum adherence to the regimen.

NUTRITION. Explain dietary modifications of calories, fats, and/or sodium. Demonstration of food preparation consistent with the dietary regimen and the patient's eating preferences and habits is desirable.

PHYSICAL ACTIVITY. Prescribe recommendations related to the type and magnitude of exercise, based on the patient's prior level of activity and job requirements. It is the responsibility of the health team to prescribe and initially supervise the type of exercise, to determine its duration and schedule, and to forewarn about signs of overexercising.

For the first 10 to 12 weeks after myocardial infarction, the patient's energy expenditure level may be 4 to 5 calories per minute. Thereafter the maximum level depends on the patient's functional tolerance based on the classification system of the American Heart Association (Tables 8-3 and 8-4). A class I (functional classification according to New York Heart Association) patient requires no physical limitation, whereas a class IV patient is greatly restricted.

A patient having slight symptoms during ordinary activity, emotional stress, or active recreation and no symptoms at rest is designated as being in class II. According to the guide for evaluating impairment in Table 8-3, the prescribed energy expenditure level for class II patients should not exceed 2.5 calories per minute of continuous activity or 4.0 calories per minute of intermittent activity. Continuous activities of 2.5 calories per minute or less include watch repairing, painting, and machine sewing. These may be interspersed with brief periods of window cleaning, car driving, or horseback riding, that is, activities of 4.0 calories per minute or under.

In prescribing exercises, swimming, jogging, and bicycling are commonly used conditioning activities. Less appreciated is the value of walking, yet walking is practical to do and is within the tolerance level of most cardiac patients. Walking can be done throughout the year, since enclosed shopping centers can be used during periods of inclement weather.

As previously mentioned, many physicians now employ treadmill testing and other techniques of stress testing. This is done periodically to determine functional tolerance limits as a guide to prescribing graded levels of activities throughout the duration of the coronary rehabilitation program.

SMOKING. Health care personnel should set an example by not smoking.

Table 8-4. Average energy expenditure levels of various activities

Activity	Cost, calories per minute	Activity	Cost, calories per minute
		Housework activities	
Hand sewing	1.4	Scrubbing floors	3.6
Sweeping floor	1.7	Cleaning windows	3.7
Machine sewing	1.8	Making beds	3.9
Polishing furniture	2.4	Ironing, standing	4.2
Peeling potatoes	2.9	Mopping	4.2
Scrubbing, standing	2.9	Wringing by hand	4.4
Washing small clothes	3.0	Hanging wash	4.5
Kneading dough	3.3	Beating carpets	4.9
		Recreational activities	
Painting, sitting	2.0	Swimming, 20 yards per minute	5.0
Playing piano	2.5	Dancing	5.5
Driving car	2.8	Gardening	5.6
Canoeing, 2.5 miles per hour	3.0	Tennis	7.0
Horseback riding, slow	3.0	Trotting horse	8.0
Volleyball	3.5	Spading	8.6
Bowling	4.4	Skiing	9.9
Cycling, 5.5 miles per hour	4.5	Squash	10.2
Golfing	5.0	Cycling 13 miles per hour	11.0
		Industrial activities	
Watch repairing	1.6	Carpentry	6.8
Radio assembly	2.7	Binding sheaves	7.3
Sewing at machine	2.9	Mowing lawn by hand	7.7
Shoe repairing	3.0	Felling tree	8.0
Bricklaying	4.0	Shoveling	8.5
Plastering	4.1	Ascending stairs, 17 pounds load, 27 feet per minute	9.0
Tractor ploughing	4.2		
Wheeling barrow 115 pounds., 2.5 miles per hour	5.0	Planing	9.1
		Tending furnace	10.2
Horse ploughing	5.9	Ascending stairs, 22 pounds load, 54 feet per minute	16.2

Clinics are offered by many communities to assist people in stopping smoking.

SEXUAL ACTIVITY. Most people having an uncomplicated myocardial infarction can resume sexual activity while increasing other usual activities. For most individuals, resumption occurs 4 to 8 weeks after myocardial infarction. Sexual activity can be viewed, in part, as a form of exercise. The physiologic costs in the home setting are small for normal, middle-aged, long-married individuals. Studies have shown that the oxygen cost is less than that required to perform a single Masters two-step test or climb two flights of stairs.

Instruct the patient to report anginal pain before or during intercourse, palpitations lasting more than 10 to 15 minutes after intercourse, and excessive fatigability the day of or day after intercourse. The choice of a position for intercourse is dictated by what the patient personally prefers and finds less taxing. Situations that merit caution are (1) environmental extremes of temperature, (2) intercourse immediately postprandially, (3) intercourse after consuming alcohol (alcohol dilates blood vessels and reflexly increases heart rate), and (4) intercourse when the patient is already fatigued and tense.

COMMUNITY RESOURCES. The local heart association, vocational rehabilitation center, Veterans Administration, and other such organizations may be of help to the patient.

Resource people. Other people, such as the social worker, public health nurse, dietitian, physical therapist, chaplain, occupational therapist, and psychologist may be asked to help in the planning. Many communities have now developed "coronary clubs," in which interested postmyocardial infarction patients, their families, and health care workers meet at a regular time for guidance in care and education. This offers an opportunity to teach basic cardiac life support to the former patient and his family. Guest speakers may discuss topics such as nutrition, exercise, sexuality, basic cardiac life support, and antismoking techniques.

Information and reassurance. Finally, assure the patient that help is readily available if it is needed again. Inform the patient about when to seek help and where to obtain it. This can be done by "reliving" with the patient the symptoms and the action taken prior to the last heart attack. Next, warning symptoms other than those previously experienced can be discussed. Finally, alternative ways of reaching help can be explored.

Problems. Intervention should be aimed at the prevention and treatment of health problems, and personnel should be especially aware of the following potential complications.

ARRHYTHMIAS. Most postmyocardial infarction patients have some type of occasional premature systole. However, the rhythms of cardiac ischemia and heart failure, such as premature ventricular systole, ventricular tachycardia, atrial flutter, and atrial fibrillation, warrant immediate and accurate diagnosis and instigation of appropriate therapy (see discussion of arrhythmias, Chapter 6).

HEART FAILURE. Heart failure is a frequent complication of a myocardial infarction (see Chapter 4).

PULMONARY DYSFUNCTION. Pulmonary dysfunction is noted frequently as pulmonary embolism, chronic obstructive pulmonary disease (COPD), and/or pneumonia requiring early detection and intervention.

POSTMYOCARDIAL INFARCTION SYNDROME. As emphasized by Dressler, postmyocardial infarction syndrome occurs in a small percentage of patients. The cause is unknown, but it has been attributed to a hypersensitivity reaction in which the antigen is necrotic cardiac muscle. The disorder usually occurs a few weeks or months after myocardial infarction, but it has been observed within 1 week after infarction. The syndrome is characterized by pericardial-type pain, pericardial friction rub, and fever. It may last days to weeks and must be differentiated from a recurrent myocardial infarction, pulmonary infarction, and congestive heart failure. The condition is treated with corticosteroids, aspirin, and indomethacin.

MYOCARDIAL ISCHEMIA AND/OR MYOCARDIAL INFARCTION. Some patients will sustain further myocardial damage as a result of extension of a previous infarction or development of a new area of infarction. Personnel must be alert to this possibility and arrange for immediate transfer to the CCU for treatment of the acute episode. Although data reported in the literature provide some conflicting statistics, it is generally accepted that the following factors provide evidence for predicting the increased possibility of reinfarction:

1. *Age.* The risk of reinfarction is generally greater for those people over the age of 65 years.
2. *ECG readings.* Assessment of site and extent of infarction can help in anticipating further problems. Anterior infarctions carry a greater risk, especially when associated with bundle branch block. The larger the area of infarction, the greater the chance of reinfarction.
3. *Systolic blood pressure on admission.* People with systolic blood pressures 85 mm. Hg. or below with clinical signs of shock and heart rates above 100 beats per minute are at increased risk of reinfarction.
4. *Heart size determined by x-ray film.* Cardiomegaly recognized as an increased cardiothoracic ratio usually reflects chronic heart disease.
5. *Degree of pulmonary congestion determined by x-ray film.* Acute left heart failure noted as confluent lung densities in the central lung fields and increased pulmonary vascularity connotes an increased risk of reinfarction.
6. *Previous history of cardiac ischemia.* The risk of reinfarction increases when a person has a history of angina pectoris and/or one or more myocardial infarctions.

Evaluation. Evaluation must be a part of care to ensure intervention that facilitates reaching the goals established by the patient, his family, and health care personnel. Accurate assessment, planning, intervention, and evaluation during hospitalization will allow the discharge process to proceed with minimal problems.

DISCHARGE PLANNING. The actual discharge planning will require little time if the goals established for the patient during hospitalization have been met. To ensure that all points have been covered, a checklist that includes the following considerations should be initiated prior to discharge.

1. *Activity.* The prescription will depend on the patient's physiologic and emotional limitations.
2. *Diet.* Dietary modifications, particularly of calories, fats, and sodium intake should be recommended and recorded.
3. *Medications.* Information about actual medication prescribed, including drug name, dosage, desired effects, and possible adverse effects should be thoroughly explained to the patient.
4. *New or recurrent symptoms.* Chest pain is particularly important. Intensive education instructing the patient to seek immediate medical care is mandatory to decrease deaths from recurrent myocardial infarction. Personnel should provide the family with a telephone number for

assistance at any hour. Many communities have available the universal emergency number *911.*

5. *Follow-up care.* An appointment should be given to the patient for a visit to his physician. A second appointment should be made to get the patient and family active in a "coronary club."

6. *Return to employment.* Studies now show that a majority of people under the age of 65 years will return to their former work after recovering from a myocardial infarction. For those unable to achieve their former level of physical activity, special centers for evaluating the work capacity of the individual are available in most medical complexes. In either event the goal of health personnel should be to restore the person to as full and useful a life as possible. A positive attitude on the part of the personnel and patient will do much toward improving the patient's quality of life.

Rehabilitation phase
GOALS OF THE POSTHOSPITAL RECOVERY PHASE

Each year more than one-half million people survive acute myocardial infarctions and leave the hospital to face substantial changes in their life-styles. Many with an initial infarction have not sustained major mechanical damage and may be totally asymptomatic. The goal of the patient and health professionals assisting him should be to achieve full recovery, if possible, and to introduce into the patient's life-style those changes that may alter the progression of the disease process.

Although primary prevention, begun in childhood and continued throughout life, is the ideal means of achieving cardiovascular health secondary prevention programs for people with clinical manifestations of coronary artery disease must be implemented if the so-called "black plague of the 20th century" is to be controlled. A secondary prevention program is tantamount to entering into a partnership with the patient and his family and viewing them as full participating members of the health care team.

POTENTIAL PROBLEMS OR RISKS

Patients who survive an initial acute myocardial infarction and are discharged from the hospital have an increased risk for morbidity and mortality primarily because of further manifestations of ischemic heart disease. Additionally, psychologic responses to the disease have been shown to be significantly related to posthospital morbidity and mortality.

Physical risks. The incidence of sudden death is highest in the first 6 months after myocardial infarction and decreases progressively following that initial period. The first 2 months following discharge from the hospital have, in fact, been referred to as the "vulnerable period." Deaths during this period of time have been attributed to residual ischemia, electrical instability, or mechanical dysfunction, coupled with increased physical and psychosocial demands.

Fatal and nonfatal reinfarctions occur in a significant number of persons during the first 2 years after initial infarction. The risk of suffering a new nonfatal reinfarction has been shown to increase with the occurrence of each infarction. Additionally, the mortality related to reinfarction is pronounced.

Other physical problems that may require management following myocardial infarction are angina pectoris, arrhythmias, and congestive heart failure.

Psychosocial problems. The occurrence of a myocardial infarction brings with it a psychosocial upheaval for the patient and his family. Progress has been made in the past decade in assisting the patient to adjust during the period of hospitalization. However, discharge from the hospital is a major psychologic event. It is a mixed blessing because of the many uncertainties that accompany leaving the safety of the hospital environment.

It has been said that after myocardial infarction there are many more problems in the mind than in the heart. Psychologic factors may well be the culprits that impede resumption of a full and normal life. Emotional problems may hamper the patient in returning to his place in family, work, and society.

Anxiety, fear of sudden death, fear of another heart attack, lack of confidence, and loss of motivation are frequently reported psychologic problems following myocardial infarction. Psychologic responses to heart disease can result in cardiac invalidism with serious socioeconomic sequelae.

The psychologic response of the patient to his myocardial infarction during the hospitalization phase may be useful in planning care that will promote successful rehabilitation. Some patients may disregard the seriousness of their disease and be unwilling to modify their life-style. Others may view their disease objectively and realistically and make changes in their social, family, and work life that are consistent with their physical condition. Still other patients may exaggerate their condition and become altogether nonadaptive, responding with early retirement from work, loss of sexual functioning, and even complete withdrawal from routines of daily living.

INTERVENTION

Rehabilitative perspectives have increasingly broadened to consider not only the quantity of life but the quality as well. Rehabilitation ideally achieves a return to the preillness stage in the physical, psychologic, and social spheres, and/or achieves maximum function in the psychologic and social spheres consistent with the patient's physical limitations.

An individualized program of rehabilitation can be prescribed based on data that depict functional capacity, knowledge, and attitudes about coronary artery disease, marital and family adjustments, socioeconomic status, vocation, hobbies, and personality traits. Treadmill exercise testing may be employed to determine functional capacity and prescribe physical activity. An individually tailored program of physical activity can be designed to improve cardiac function. Early evaluation of functional capacity and a return to normal physical activity may also be useful in alleviating anxiety and depression. Many communities offer programs in which the activity prescription can be implemented under supervision.

Knowledge about coronary artery disease can be determined through interviews or self-reporting measures. It is important that the patient gather information related to function of the normal heart as a basis for understanding how myocardial infarction affects cardiac function. Although knowledge alone will not guarantee that the patient will follow the prescribed regimen, understanding may favorably influence compliance with the rehabilitation regimen.

It is equally important to determine how the spouse and other family members react to the disease and how they treat the patient. They are also victims of the cardiac event and should not be disregarded. It is just as important to prepare the family for the patient as to prepare the patient for return to the family. Discouragement from family members has often been found to be a significant factor in patients' failure to return to work. Additionally, serious fluctuations in a family's interpersonal life interfere with successful rehabilitation. Therefore it is important to include in a cardiac rehabilitation program an analysis of the family's interpersonal situation, with identification of and intervention in maladaptive behaviors and an effort to develop more adaptive family relationships.

Sexual counseling for the patient and his spouse or partner is an important aspect of rehabilitation but one that has been neglected in the past. It should not be assumed that because the patient or spouse does not ask questions he or she has no concerns related to sexual activity. Consideration should be given to the patient's level of sexual activity before the infarction rather than to age or marital status.

Myocardial infarction changes the manner of living of the patient and his family. Therefore educational programs should be offered to them that provide information about life-style factors that increase the risk of disease progression and the benefits that may result from changes in lifestyle. Even though there is no conclusive evidence that such secondary prevention programs alter the risk of suffering another cardiac event, failure to address risk factors is likely to encourage resumption of the life-style that may have initially contributed to the development of cardiac disease. When appropriate, information should be offered related to dietary alterations, cessation of smoking, control of associated disease when present, all medications prescribed, emotional tension, and appropriate responses to symptoms that may occur.

Proper attention should be given to the so-called "cardiac environment," which compromises physical, psychologic, human, social, and cultural elements. Many of the problems in rehabilitation arise because of insufficient attention to the cardiac environment in the form of inadequate communication, lack of vocational guidance or family counseling, or inattention to the patient's reaction to his illness. Health professionals must focus on the entire cardiac environment, not just selected parts, if the patient is to find his place in his working, playing, and social worlds.

Summary

Increasing concern about the quality of life following myocardial infarction has resulted in increased scrutiny by health professionals of the cardiac environment, with assessment and intervention beginning in the CCU and continuing until the patient returns to his maximal functioning. Although many questions remain concerning the effects of secondary prevention programs on morbidity and mortality, reducing the level of invalidism following myocardial infarction seems a goal worthy of attention from health professionals.

REFERENCES

Abraham, S. A., et al.: Value of early ambulation in patients with and without complications after acute myocardial infarction, N. Engl. J. Med. **292**:719, 1975.

Alderman, E. L., et al.: Hemodynamic effects of morphine and pentazocine differ in cardiac patients, N. Engl. J. Med. **287**:623, 1972.

American Heart Association: Coronary care: rehabilitation after myocardial infarction, New York, 1973, The Association.

American Heart Association: Exercise testing and training of individuals with heart disease or at high risk for its development: a handbook for physicians, New York, 1975, The Association.

American Heart Association and National Academy of Sciences–National Research Council: Standards for cardiopulmonary resuscitation (CPR) and emergency cardiac care (ECC), J.A.M.A. **227**:833, 1974.

Baden, C. A.: Teaching the coronary patient and his family, Nurs. Clin. North Am. **7**:563, 1972.

Barry, E. M., Knight, S. M., and Acker, J. E.: Hospital program for cardiac rehabilitation, Am. J. Nurs. **72**:2174-2177, 1972.

Baxter, S.: Psychological problems of intensive care. Part two, Nurs. Times **71**:63, 1975.

Bruhn, J. G., et al.: Psychological predictors of sudden death in myocardial infarction, J. Psychosom. Res. **18**:187-191, 1974.

Christensen, D., et al.: Sudden death in the late hospital phase of acute myocardial infarction, Arch. Intern. Med. **137**:1675, 1977.

Cosby, R. S., et al.: Late complications of myocardial infarction, J.A.M.A. **236**:1717, 1976.

Crate, M.: Nursing functions in adaptation to chronic illness, Am. J. Nurs. **65**:72, 1965.

Croog, S. H. et al.: The heart patient and the recovery process, Soc. Sci. Med. **2**:111, 1968.

DeBusk, R. F.: How to individualize rehabilitation after myocardial infarction, Geriatrics **32**:77, 1977.

Eliot, R. S., and Forker, A. D.: Emotional stress and cardiac disease, J.A.M.A. **236**:2325, 1976.

Epstein, S. E., et al.: The early phase of acute myocardial infarction: pharmacologic aspects of therapy, Ann. Intern. Med. **78**:918-936, 1973.

Forrester, J. S., Chaterjee, K., and Swan, H. J. C.: Hemodynamic monitoring in patients with acute myocardial infarction, J.A.M.A. **226**:60-62, 1973.

Foster, S., and Andreoli, K.: Behavior following acute myocardial infarction, Am. J. Nurs. **70**:2344, 1970.

Foster, S. B.: Pump failure, Am. J. Nurs. **74**:1830, 1974.

Fournet, K. M.: Patients discharged on diuretics: prime candidates for individualized teaching by the nurse, Heart Lung **3**:108, 1974.

Fox, S. M., Naughton, J. P., and Gorman, P. A.: Physical activity and cardiovascular health. III. The exercise prescription: frequency and type of activity, Mod. Concepts Cardiovasc. Dis. **41**:25, 1972.

Friedman, G. D., et al.: A psychological questionnaire predictive of myocardial infarction: results from the Kaiser-Permanente epidemiologic study of myocardial infarction, Psychosom. Med. **36**:327, 1974.

Gentry, W. D., Foster, S., and Haney, T.: Denial as a determinant of anxiety and perceived health status in the coronary care unit, Psychosom. Med. **34**:39, 1972.

Gentry, W. D., and Haney, T.: Emotional response and clinical severity as early determinants of six-month mortality after myocardial infarction, Heart Lung **4**:730, 1975.

Gentry, W. D., and Williams, R. B., editors: Psychological aspects of myocardial infarction and coronary care, St. Louis, 1975, The C. V. Mosby Co.

Germain, C. P.: Exercise makes the heart grow stronger, Am. J. Nurs. **72**:2169, 1972.

Gorfinkel, J. J., Haider, R., and Lindsay, J.: Diagnosis and treatment of hemodynamic abnormalities after acute myocardial infarction, Med. Ann. D.C. **43**:395, 1974.

Grace, W. J., and Chadbourn, J. A.: The first hour in acute myocardial infarction, Heart Lung **3**:736, 1974.

Granger, J. W.: Full recovery from myocardial infarction: psychosocial factors, Heart Lung 3:600, 1974.

Green, H. L.: Hazards of electronic equipment in critical care areas: a research approach, Cardiovasc. Nurs. 9:1, 1973.

Griffith, G. C.: Sexuality and the cardiac patient, Heart Lung 2:70, 1973.

Hurst, J. W.: Ambulation after myocardial infarction, N. Engl. J. Med. 292:746, 1975.

Hurst, J. W., et al.: The heart—arteries and veins, ed. 4, New York, 1978, McGraw-Hill Book Co.

Jenkins, C. D., Rosenman, R. H., and Zykanski, S. J.: Prediction of clinical coronary heart disease by a test for the coronary-prone behavior pattern, N. Engl. J. Med. 290:1271, 1974.

Kentals, E., and Sarna, S.: Sudden death and factors related to long-term prognosis following acute myocardial infarction, Scand. J. Rehabil. Med. 8:27, 1976.

Kjoller, E.: Long-term prognosis after acute myocardial infarction, with special reference to the long-term survival, the risks of re-infarction and cardiac arrest, Dan. Med. Bull. 23:238, 1976.

Kleiger, R., Shaw, R., and Avioli, L. V.: Postmyocardial infarction complications requiring surgery, Arch. Intern. Med. 137:1580, 1977.

Klein, R. F.: Behavioral and psychological processes in ischemic heart disease, Arch. Intern. Med. 137:1672, 1977.

Klein, R. F., et al.: Transfer from a coronary-care unit—some adverse responses, Arch. Intern. Med. 122:104, 1968.

Kones, R. J.: Oxygen therapy for acute myocardial infarction: basis for a practical approach, South. Med. J. 67:1322, 1974.

Lawson, M.: Progressive coronary care, Heart Lung 1:240, 1972.

Lethbridge, B., Somboon, O., and Shea, H. L.: The transfer process, Can. Nurse 72:39, 1976.

Mallaghan, M., and Pemberton, J.: Some behavioral changes in 493 patients after acute myocardial infarction, Br. J. Prev. Soc. Med. 31:86, 1977.

Mantle, J. A., et al.: A multipurpose catheter for electrophysiologic and hemodynamic monitoring plus atrial pacing, Chest 72:285, 1977.

Martin, S. P., et al.: Inputs into coronary care during 30 years: a cost effectiveness study, Ann. Intern. Med. 81:289, 1974.

Mason, D. T.: Digitalis pharmacology and therapeutics: recent advances, Ann. Intern. Med. 80:520, 1974.

Medical Division, Glasglow Royal Infirmary: Early mobilization after uncomplicated myocardial infarction; prospective study of 538 patients, Lancet 1:346, 1973.

Merrill, S. A.: A nursing contribution to cardiac rehabilitation programs, Milit. Med. Feb.:129, 1977.

Meltzer, L. E., and Dunning, A. J.: Textbook of coronary care, Bowie, Md., 1972, The Charles Press Publishers, Inc.

Meltzer, L. E., Pineo, R., and Kitchell, J. R.: Intensive Cardiac Care, a manual for nurses, ed. 10, Philadelphia, 1969, The Charles Press Publishers, Inc.

Moss, A. J., DeCamilla, J., and Davis, H.: Cardiac death in the first 6 months after myocardial infarction: potential for mortality reduction in the early posthospital period, Am. J. Cardiol. 39:816, 1977.

Nielsen, M. A.: Intra-arterial monitoring of blood pressure, Am. J. Nurs. 74:48, 1974.

Niven, R. G.: Psychologic adjustment to coronary artery disease, Postgrad. Med. 60:152, 1976.

Obier, K., MacPherson, M., and Haywood, J.: Predictive value of psychosocial profiles following acute myocardial infarction, J. Nat. Med. Assoc. 69:59, 1977.

Orem, D. E.: Nursing: concepts of practice, New York, 1971, McGraw-Hill Book Co.

Patterson, R. H., Burns, W. A., and Jannotta, F. S.: Complications of external cardiac resuscitation: a retrospective review and survey of the literature, Med. Ann. D.C. 43:389, 1974.

Payne, S., McBarron, R. A., and O'Connor, E. J.: Implementation of a problem-oriented system in a CCU, Nurs. Clin. North Am. 9:255, 1975.

Rackley, C. E., and Russell, R. O.: Invasive techniques for hemodynamic monitoring, Dallas, 1973, American Heart Association.

Resnekow, L.: The intermediate coronary care unit: a stage in continued coronary care, Br. Heart J. 39:357, 1977.

Ross, R. S.: National heart, blood vessel. lungs and blood program, vol. 3, Report of panel chairmen, Apr. 6, 1973, Department of Health, Education, and Welfare, Public Health Service.

Schoenberger, J.: Prevention of heart disease in the asymptomatic post infarction patient, Primary Care 4:217, 1977.

Shroeder, J. S., and Daily, E. K.: Techniques in bedside hemodynamic monitoring, St. Louis, 1976, The C. V. Mosby Co.

Shannon, V. J.: The transfer process: an area of concern for the CCU nurse, Heart Lung 2:364, 1973.

Shapiro, R. M.: Anticoagulant therapy, Am. J. Nurs. 74:439, 1974.

Stern, M. J., Pascale, L., and Ackerman, A.: Life adjustment postmyocardial infarction, Arch. Intern. Med. 137:1680, 1977.

Stern, M. J., Pascale, L., and McLoone, J. B.: Psychosocial adaptation following an acute myocardial infarction, J. Chron. Dis. 29:513, 1976.

Stocksmeier, U., editor: Psychological approach to the rehabilitation of coronary patients, New York, 1976, Springer-Verlag New York, Inc.

Swan, H. J. C.: The role of hemodynamic monitoring in the management of the critically ill, Crit. Care Med. **3:**83, 1975.

Thompson, P., and Sloman, G.: Sudden death in hospital after discharge from coronary care unit, Br. Med. J. **4:**136, 1971.

Thorn, G. W., et al., editors: Harrison's principles of internal medicine, ed. 8, New York, 1977, McGraw-Hill Book Co.

Thornley, P. E., and Turner, R. W. D.: Rapid mobilization after acute myocardial infarction: first step in rehabilitation and secondary prevention, Br. Heart J. **39:**471, 1977.

Vedin, A., et al.: Deaths and non-fatal reinfarctions during two years' follow-up after myocardial infarction, Acta Med. Scand. **198:**353, 1975.

Vedin, A., et al.: Prediction of cardiovascular deaths and non-fatal reinfarctions after myocardial infarction, Acta Med. Scand. **201:**309, 1977.

Weil, M. H., and Carlson, R. W.: Priorities governing the care of the critically ill, Hosp. Prac. **11:**67, 1976.

Weinberg, S. L.: Intermediate coronary care: the failure of a concept? Am. J. Cardiol. **37:**181, 1976. (Abstract.)

Wenger, N. K.: Patient and family education after myocardial infarction, Postgrad. Med. **57:**129, 1975.

Wilhelmsson, A. V., et al.: Symptoms, disablement and treatment during two years after myocardial infarction, Scand. J. Rehabil. Med. **8:**85, 1976.

Wilson, C., and Adgey, A. A. J.: Survival of patients with late ventricular fibrillation after acute myocardial infarction, Lancet **2:**124, 1974.

Wishnie, H. A., Hackett, T. P. and Cassem, N. H.: Psychological hazards of convalescence following myocardial infarction, J.A.M.A. **215:**1292, 1971.

Zipes, D. P. The clinical application of cardioversion, Cardiovasc. Clin. **2:**239, 1970.

Zyzanski, S. J., et al.: Psychological correlates of coronary angiographic findings, Arch. Intern. Med. **136:**1234, 1976.

CARDIOVASCULAR DRUGS

This section will present in some detail some of the significant drugs mentioned in the text as well as additional drugs used to treat cardiac disorders.

The drugs are as follows:

Digitalis
Quinidine
Procainamide hydrochloride (Pronestyl hydrochloride)
Lidocaine (Xylocaine)
Phenytoin (Dilantin)
Calcium
Potassium
Edrophonium chloride (Tensilon)
Atropine
Nitroglycerin (glyceryl trinitrate)
Diazepam (Valium)
Sodium bicarbonate (NaHCO$_3$)
Glucagon
Dopamine (Intropin)
Dobutamine
Heparin
Warfarin sodium (Coumadin)
Sympathomimetic drugs
    Alpha adrenergic receptor stimulating drugs (alphamimetic)
        Methoxamine (Vasoxyl)
        Phenylephrine (Neo-Synephrine)
    Beta adrenergic receptor stimulating drugs (betamimetics)
        Isoproterenol (Isuprel)
        Mephentermine (Wyamine)
    Alpha and beta adrenergic receptor stimulating drugs
        (alpha-betamimetics)
        Norepinephrine (levarterenol, Levophed)
        Epinephrine (Adrenalin)
        Metaraminol (Aramine)
    Alpha adrenergic receptor blocking drugs (alphalytics)
        Phenoxybenzamine (Dibenzyline)
        Phentolamine (Regitine)

335

Beta receptor blocking drugs (betalytics)
Propranolol hydrochloride (Inderal)
New or investigational antiarrhythmic agents
Bretylium tosylate (Bretylol)
Amiodarone (Cordarone; Atlansil)
Aprindine (Fiboran; Fibocil)
Disopyramide (Norpace; Rhythmodan)
Ethmozin
Mexiletine (Mexitil)
Tocainide
Verapamil (Isoptin; Iproveratril; Cordilox)
Vasodilator agents
Sodium nitroprusside (Nipride)
Isosorbide dinitrate (Isordil)
Hydralazine (Apresoline)
Prazosin (Minipress)
Nitroglycerin

DIGITALIS

Cardiac glycosides are derived from several plants, including *Digitalis purpurea* (digitoxin and digitalis leaf), *Digitalis lanata* (lanatoside C and digoxin), and *Strophanthus gratus* (ouabain).

Actions. The fundamental action of digitalis is its ability to increase the contractile state of the ventricle (called positive inotropic action). The rate at which tension or force develops is also increased. This direct action occurs in both the failing and the normal heart. Cardiac output rises in the failing heart but not in the normal heart; in the latter situation the mild direct arteriolar constrictive effects of digitalis increase peripheral resistance, and compensatory mechanisms prevent a rise in cardiac output. Arteries and veins dilate when digitalis is administered to a patient with heart failure, since the better pumping action induced by digitalis allows a relaxation of the sympathetic tone, which counters the mild direct vasoconstrictor effect of the drug. Digitalis increases oxygen consumption, but in heart failure the improved contractility reduces the total myocardial oxygen needs, cardiac efficiency rises, and heart size diminishes. Heart rate slows during sinus rhythm—a result, in part, of a direct effect of the drug, and also a result of an increase in vagal tone and a decrease in sympathetic tone as the degree of heart failure diminishes. Improvement in heart failure may occur before or without a reduction in heart rate; however, in a normal patient the heart rate may not slow. Digitalis slows the ventricular rate during atrial fibrillation through vagal and extravagal effects that prolong the effective refractory period of the A-V node to block more atrial impulses.

The electrophysiologic effects of digitalis are complex and differ according to the type of myocardial fiber studied. Some pertinent properties will be noted briefly. (See Fig. A-1.) The refractory period of the atria shortens but

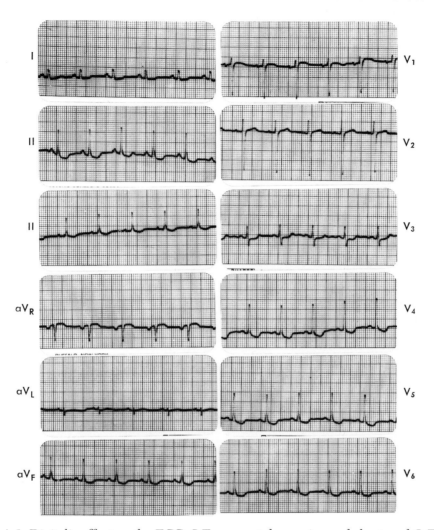

Fig. A-1. Digitalis effect on the ECG. S-T segment depression and shortened Q-T interval commonly occur with digitalization. This event should not be equated with digitalis intoxication. S-T segment depression is present in leads I, II, III, aV$_F$, and V$_3$ to V$_6$. Note characteristic "sagging" of S-T depression.

that of the A-V node increases. After atropine administration, digitalis lengthens the atrial refractory period and has a reduced effect on the A-V node. Digitalis shortens the refractory period of the ventricle, which is apparent in man as a shortened Q-T interval. Automaticity, especially in the Purkinje fibers, is increased and may account for many digitalis-induced tachyarrhythmias. Excitability and conduction velocity of atria and ventricles increase with small doses, but decrease with larger doses of digitalis.

Table A-1. Digitalis preparations

Drug	Initial dose*	Subsequent doses	Time of action			Total digitalizing dose	Daily maintenance dose
			Onset	Peak	Dissipated		
For emergency use—all given intravenously							
Lanatoside C (Cedilanid)	0.8 to 1.0 mg	0.4 mg every 2 to 4 hours for total dose < 2.0 mg in 24 hours	5 to 10 minutes	½ to 2 hours	3 to 5 days		
Digoxin (Lanoxin)	0.50 to 1.0 mg	0.25 mg every 2 to 4 hours for total dose < 1.5 mg in 24 hours	10 to 15 minutes	½ to 4 hours	3 to 5 days		
Ouabain (G-strophanthin)	0.25 to 0.5 mg	0.1 mg every 30 to 60 minutes for total dose < 1.0 mg in 24 hours	5 minutes	½ to 1 hour	24 hours		
For oral use (digitalization over 24 to 48 hours) (average figures)							
Digitalis leaf, U.S.P.	0.5 to 0.8 gm	0.1 to 0.2 gm every 6 to 8 hours				1.2 to 1.4 gm	0.05 to 0.2 gm
Digitoxin	0.5 to 0.8 mg	0.1 to 0.2 mg every 6 to 8 hours				1.2 to 1.4 mg	0.05 to 0.2 mg
Digoxin	0.5 to 1.0 mg	0.25 to 0.5 mg every 6 to 8 hours				2 to 3 mg	0.125 to 0.5 mg

*These values are to be used as guidelines only.

Uses

1. To increase the contractility and efficiency of the heart in congestive heart failure or other states characterized by a reduction in cardiac contractility.
2. To treat supraventricular rhythms, including atrial fibrillation, atrial flutter, and paroxysmal atrial and A-V junctional tachycardia (provided the arrhythmias are not caused by digitalis overdose).
3. At times, some ventricular tachyarrhythmias may respond to digitalis administration, particularly in the setting of congestive heart failure (see discussion of arrhythmia treatment, Chapter 6).

Precautions

1. Digitalis route of administration, loading, and maintenance dosage must be determined for the individual patient and the clinical situation (Tables A-1 to A-3). "Full digitalizing doses" are often not indicated, at least acutely, since a smaller amount of the drug will still produce a a positive inotropic effect. Many times, when mild heart failure is pres-

Table A-2. Digitalis intoxication

Cardiac	Neurologic	Gastrointestinal	Other
Changes in rhythm (effects on cardiac automaticity and conduction) Ventricular premature contractions, coupled rhythm (bigeminy) Ventricular tachycardia; precursor of ventricular fibrillation; may be mechanism of sudden death in digitalis intoxication Nonparoxysmal A-V junctional tachycardia with or without A-V block Atrial tachycardia with or without block; most frequently seen in patients with associated potassium deficiency caused by concurrent use of thiazide diuretics Virtually *any* arrhythmia may be produced by digitalis excess Effect on conduction system Prolonged P-R interval Slow heart rates including sinus bradycardia and first-, second- (type I Wenckebach), and third-degree A-V block Cardiac failure	Mental depression and personality changes Abnormal visual sensations Color (especially brown, yellow, and green) Scotoma Blurred or dimmed vision Photophobia Cerebral excitation manifested as headache, vertigo, increased irritability, convulsions Peripheral neuritis Generalized muscular weakness	Anorexia Nausea Vomiting Diarrhea	Gynecomastia Allergic manifestations such as skin rash

Table A-3. Serum concentrations of drugs

Drug	Usual range of therapeutic serum concentration*
Digoxin	0.9 to 2.0 nanogram (ng)/ml
Digitoxin	14 to 24 ng/ml
Phenytoin	10 to 20 microgram (μg)/ml
Lidocaine	1.5 to 4.0 μg/ml
Procainamide	4 to 8 μg/ml
Quinidine	3 to 6 μg/ml
Propranolol	20 to 50 ng/ml

*These values are to be used as guidelines only.

ent, a loading dose may not be necessary or may be given over a few days.

2. Renal function must be examined. Renal failure predisposes to digitalis toxicity, particularly with a short-acting preparation such as digoxin.
3. Hypokalemia sensitizes the heart to the toxic effects of digitalis. Electrolyte levels should be determined frequently, especially if potassium-wasting diuretics are administered.
4. Digitalis should be given with caution to patients with A-V conduction disturbances.
5. One should be familiar with the toxic manifestations of digitalis (Table A-2).
6. Serum levels of digitalis and other antiarrythmic agents may provide useful guidelines for drug administration (Table A-3).

QUINIDINE

Quinidine, like quinine, is found in cinchona bark. Quinidine, however, is the cinchona alkaloid of choice in the treatment of various cardiac arrhythmias.

Actions. The cardiac actions of quinidine are as follows:

1. Prolongs the effective refractory period of the atrial and ventricular muscle.
2. Decreases myocardial excitability, thereby decreasing the ability of the ventricle to respond to a stimulus.
3. Prolongs conduction time in cardiac muscle, Purkinje fibers, and A-V conduction tissue.
4. Decreases automaticity of all pacemaker cells, which depresses or abolishes ectopic impulse generation. However, the vagal blocking action of quinidine may actually increase the rate of sinus discharge in man or the intact animal.
5. Elevates the threshold to electrically induced ventricular fibrillation.
6. Depresses myocardial contractility.

Uses. Quinidine has been successfully used to prevent or correct virtually all arrhythmias, including atrial fibrillation, atrial flutter, paroxysmal supra-ventricular and ventricular tachycardia, and premature systoles.

Preparations and administration. Quinidine sulfate is available in 100, 200, and 300 mg tablets and is administered orally in maintenance doses of 0.2 to 0.4 gm, four to six times daily. It is also available in long-acting preparations. Quinidine is rapidly absorbed orally and in about 15 minutes can be detected in the serum. In some patients, absorption may be poor, making it a good policy to check serum levels if the arrhythmia appears unresponsive to quinidine. Usually, maximum serum levels are reached from 2 to 4 hours after administration of a single oral dose.

Quinidine gluconate can be administered parenterally as well as orally; however, parenteral routes present a considerably greater risk of toxicity than oral administration and are generally avoided if possible.

Toxic effects. Quinidine is a potentially dangerous drug, and deaths have occurred from its use.

1. Hypersensitivity to the drug is not uncommon and may be manifested by severe hypotension, respiratory depression, convulsions, and even death in some individuals. An allergic reaction to quinidine may at times produce thrombocytopenic purpura.
2. In large doses, quinidine can cause cinchonism, characterized by nausea, vomiting, diarrhea, tinnitus, vertigo, and visual disturbances.
3. Quinidine depresses myocardial contractility as well as impulse formation and conduction; therefore, with large doses or in patients with severe myocardial damage, the drug can make heart failure worse and can cause S-A or A-V block, and cardiac asystole. Quinidine can cause idioventricular rhythms, as well as death from ventricular fibrillation.
4. With large doses the ECG effect of quinidine demonstrates a prolonged Q-T interval and increased duration of the QRS complex because of increased duration of electrical systole, refractory period, and intraventricular conduction time.

Treatment of quinidine toxicity

1. Stopping the drug or reducing the dosage may be sufficient to combat toxic effects. Absolute withdrawal is indicated in a hypersensitive reaction.
2. For overt quinidine toxicity, molar sodium lactate or sodium bicarbonate may be effective. Isoproterenol (Isuprel) may be needed to treat conduction disturbances, and norepinephrine (Levophed) or metaraminol (Aramine) to treat vascular collapse.

Precautions

1. When quinidine is used in the treatment of atrial flutter or atrial fibrillation, it slows the atrial rate and may establish 1:1 A-V conduction with a sudden increase in the ventricular rate when atrial rates around 200 beats per minute are reached. The vagal blocking action of quinidine enhances A-V conduction and may contribute to increasing the number

of conducted atrial beats. Prior administration of digitalis is mandatory to reduce this hazard by depressing A-V conduction.

2. Serum concentration of quinidine should be followed in patients, since clinical effects and toxicity are better correlated with this value than with dosage per se.
3. Since hypersensitivity to quinidine is not uncommon, a test dose of the drug may be given before instituting intensive therapy.
4. The dose should be reduced in patients with renal disease.

Contraindications. Quinidine is contraindicated in patients known to be allergic to it. It must be used cautiously or not at all in patients with conduction disturbances. "Quinidine syncope" refers to ventricular tachyarrhythmias produced by quinidine, causing loss of consciousness, and has been reported in 1% to 3% of patients receiving maintenance quinidine therapy. Should this complication occur, quinidine therapy is discontinued.

PROCAINAMIDE HYDROCHLORIDE (PRONESTYL HYDROCHLORIDE)

Procainamide is a synthetic antiarrhythmic drug with cardiovascular actions similar to those of quinidine. Like quinidine, it possesses anticholinergic properties; procainamide may be given IV.

Actions
1. The refractory period is prolonged more significantly in the atrium than in the ventricle.
2. Excitability is depressed in the atrium and ventricle.
3. Conduction time is prolonged in cardiac muscle, *Purkinje fibers,* and A-V conduction tissue.
4. Automaticity of pacemaker cells is decreased.
5. In the atrium and ventricle the threshold to electrically induced fibrillation is elevated.
6. Myocardial contractility may be less depressed by procainamide than by quinidine.

Uses
1. The main indication for procainamide is the treatment of premature ventricular systoles and ventricular tachyarrhythmias, particularly when IV medication is required and lidocaine has been employed without success.
2. Procainamide appears less successful than quinidine in the treatment of atrial arrhythmias. However, many investigators consider the drugs interchangeable. One drug may be effective when maximal doses of the other have not been. At times, low-dose combinations of multiple antiarrhythmic agents may be needed.

Preparations and administration
1. Procainamide is available in 250 or 500 mg capsules. The usual dose is 500 mg given orally four to six times a day after a loading dose of 500 mg to 1 gm. Procainamide has a shorter duration of action than quinidine. Larger, more frequent doses (every 3 hours) may be necessary in some

patients with refractory arrhythmias. When taken orally, procainamide is readily and almost completely absorbed from the gastrointestinal tract and the drug's plasma concentration becomes maximal in about 60 minutes.

2. Procainamide is available in solution for injection (100 mg per milliliter). Continuous IV administration of procainamide in 5% glucose in water (2 to 6 mg per minute) may be used to control acute arrhythmias following suppression of the arrhythmia with a loading dose. When given IV its action is almost immediate.

3. Usually, procainamide is given orally or IV, although it can be administered intramuscularly. After IM injection, peak plasma levels are reached in 15 to 60 minutes.

Side effects and toxicity

1. When the drug is given orally, untoward effects include anorexia, nausea, vomiting, and diarrhea.

2. Flushing and central nervous system disturbances (giddiness, mental depression, and psychosis with hallucinations) have been described. In addition, bone marrow depression, allergic reactions, and a lupuslike syndrome have been reported.

3. With IV administration, hypotension can occur and may result in cardiovascular collapse, convulsions, and coronary insufficiency. This effect is related to the rate of infusion.

4. Large doses of procainamide can cause A-V block and the appearance of premature ventricular systoles, which may proceed to ventricular fibrillation.

5. The anticholinergic effects of procainamide and quinidine may accelerate the normal heart rate. During atrial flutter or fibrillation the ventricular rate may suddenly increase as the atrial rate is slowed and the degree of A-V block lessened; digitalization may reduce this danger.

6. ECG changes most often include widening of the QRS complex; prolonged P-R and Q-T intervals and changes of the T wave occur less regularly.

Precautions

1. Procainamide should not be administered when complete A-V block is present, and in the presence of partial heart block it should be used cautiously, if at all, because of the danger of asystole or of advancing the degree of block.

2. When given IV, the drug should be administered slowly at a rate of 50 to 100 mg per 1- to 3-minute period with continuous observation of the ECG and frequent blood pressure measurement. The medication should be stopped if the QRS is excessively widened. Vasopressors, such as norepinephrine, should be available in the event of hypotension.

3. Frequent blood tests during long-term procainamide therapy are important, since fatal agranulocytosis has been reported. Over 80% of patients

may develop abnormal laboratory evidence suggestive of systemic lupus erythematosus (SLE). Many of these patients may develop signs or symptoms of SLE.

4. It is well to remember that virtually all antiarrhythmic agents (except bretylium) depress myocardial contractility. All, except possibly phenytoin, slow conduction velocity, and they *all* may of themselves *cause* arrhythmias.

5. Doses may need to be reduced in patients with congestive heart failure or renal disease.

LIDOCAINE (XYLOCAINE)

Lidocaine is a rapidly acting antiarrhythmic agent that has been used for some time to produce anesthesia locally. The drug, given IV, has proved to be an excellent, and safe antiarrhythmic agent. It is generally the initial drug of choice for suppressing premature ventricular systoles that occur in the CCU setting.

Actions

1. Lidocaine depresses automaticity of Purkinje fibers (to suppress ectopic discharge) and shortens the refractory period and action potential duration. The latter shortens more than the former. Except in high doses or in abnormally depressed tissue, it does not slow conduction velocity or depress excitability. In contrast to procainamide, equivalent doses of lidocaine cause little if any fall in blood pressure or decrease in myocardial contractility.

2. Its onset of action is rapid (within 45 to 90 seconds) and duration of action brief (effects are dissipated within 20 minutes) to allow close titration of its effect.

Uses. Lidocaine suppresses ventricular arrhythmias of any etiology, but primarily those associated with acute myocardial infarction, cardiac surgery, or digitalis toxicity. It is less effective in suppressing atrial arrhythmias.

Preparation and administration

1. Lidocaine may be administered in single or multiple doses, by IV infusion, or by a combination of both. A priming dose must be given to achieve adequate blood levels. Arrhythmias, which may be suppressed by an initial bolus injection, may return unless the blood level is maintained by IV drip.

2. Lidocaine, 25 to 100 mg, may be given IV in a bolus injection that may be repeated two to three times per hour if necessary; 1.0 to 4.0 mg per minute is a usual dose administered IV to an average patient. Rarely is more than 3 mg per kilogram as a bolus or more than 400 mg in a single hour necessary; 300 mg IM (3 ml of a 10% solution) has also proved to be an effective antiarrhythmic dose. Care should be taken not to give the drug into fatty areas such as the buttocks, which retard absorption.

Side effects. Side effects are related to the dosage and size of the patient.

1. Early toxic effects are initial stimulation of the central nervous system

followed by depression. Early signs appear as sleepiness, dizziness, paresthesias, dysphagia, blurred or double vision, and sweating.

2. More severe signs include hypotension, convulsions, and coma.
3. At the first sign of toxic effects the dosage should be decreased, and it should be stopped if more severe effects occur.

Contraindications. Lidocaine is given cautiously, if at all, to patients with slow heart rates or block. The dose is reduced in patients with liver disease or low cardiac output.

Precaution. The cardiac rhythm of all patients receiving IV lidocaine should be monitored.

PHENYTOIN (DILANTIN)

Cardiac actions
1. Depresses automaticity of pacemaker cells.
2. Does not depress excitability in normal tissue. The refractory period and action potential duration of atrial or ventricular muscle and the specialized conduction system shorten, the latter more than the former.
3. Does not slow conduction velocity and, in fact, may improve conduction if it is abnormally depressed.
4. Depresses contractility less than comparable doses of quinidine or procainamide.

Cardiovascular uses. Phenytoin appears to be most effective against digitalis-induced arrhythmias such as atrial tachycardia with block, premature ventricular systoles, or nonparoxysmal A-V junctional tachycardia. It is more effective against ventricular than atrial arrhythmias, whether or not they are digitalis related. It is not effective in treating atrial flutter or fibrillation.

Preparations and administration. Phenytoin is supplied as 30 and 100 mg capsules for oral use and as a powder of 100 or 250 mg, which, when dissolved in the solvent provided, makes a solution of 50 mg per milliliter.

Oral doses are generally 100 mg four times daily. A loading dose of 1 gm the first day has been recommended to achieve adequate blood levels.

IV doses are probably best given by multiple increments of 50 to 100 mg, administered slowly every 5 to 10 minutes until the arrhythmia terminates, toxic symptoms develop, or 1000 mg has been given.

Precautions and side effects. Ataxia, vertigo, nystagmus, seizures, behavioral changes, nausea and vomiting, peripheral neuropathy, confusion, skin eruptions, and gum hyperplasia are some of the many possible side effects reported from the use of phenytoin.

1. Rapid IV administration may produce significant hypotension; the drug must be administered slowly. Cardiac arrest resulting from phenytoin has been reported.
2. IV administration in a small vein elicits severe pain if the solution is not well diluted and may produce phlebitis. The solution is extremely alkaline.

3. Phenytoin should be used cautiously, if at all, in patients with sinus bradycardia or S-A or A-V block.

4. Oral anticoagulants retard the metabolism of phenytoin, thereby reducing the required dose or making a previously effective dose into a toxic dose.

CALCIUM

Calcium is important in the body for the growth of bone, regulation of nerve, muscle, and gland activities, maintenance of cardiac and vascular tone, and normal coagulation of blood. A decrease in the serum calcium level decreases the threshold requirement for stimulation and prolongs ventricular systole; an elevated calcium level has the opposite effect. For the purpose of this discussion, we will concentrate on calcium therapy, its cardiovascular actions, uses, preparations, and precautions.

Actions

1. Calcium has a direct effect on myocardial contractility, increasing the strength of myocardial contraction.

2. Calcium administration may slow spontaneous rhythm and ultimately block impulse conduction. At times it may increase automatic discharge.

3. In general, calcium opposes many of the actions of potassium on the heart. Low calcium levels may attenuate, whereas elevated calcium levels may enhance, digitalis toxicity.

4. Recent observations suggest calcium may play an important role in impulse formation or conduction in certain cell types (sinus and A-V nodes) or in cells during certain pathologic conditions, often called the "slow response."

Uses. In the setting of a cardiac arrest, an intracardiac injection, 3 to 5 ml of a 10% solution of calcium gluconate, may be used to increase myocardial tone and contraction or make ventricular fibrillation movements more "coarse" (larger amplitude). This is indicated if there is no return of heart tone or if fibrillatory movements remain "fine" (of small amplitude) after massage and adequate ventilation have been carried out for a brief period.

Preparations and precautions

1. Calcium chloride is usually given IV in a concentration of 5% to 10%. Injection rate should be slow (not to exceed 1 to 2 ml per minute). This drug is intensely irritating to tissue and will cause painful sloughing if extravasation occurs during IV therapy.

2. Calcium gluconate can be given IM and IV. Although lower in ionized calcium content than the chloride, calcium gluconate is less irritating to the subcutaneous tissue. For parenteral use, it is administered as a 10% solution IV (5 to 30 ml).

3. ECG manifestations of hypocalcemia include prolongation of the S-T segment and Q-T interval, without changing the duration of the T wave. The polarity of the T wave may shift, however. Elevated calcium level shortens the S-T segment and the Q-T interval. (Fig. 6-75.)

Side effects. A moderate fall in blood pressure resulting from vasodilation may attend calcium injection.

POTASSIUM

Potassium is the principal cation within the cells. Renal function provides the major regulation of body potassium; some disease states and drug therapy can alter the normal level. Certain metabolic diseases, kidney diseases, diarrhea and vomiting, diuretic therapy, or infusions of potassium-free fluids, that increase extracellular fluid volume may all reduce serum levels of potassium. Hypokalemia affects the skeletal and cardiac muscles and may be manifested by weakness to paralysis, changes in gastrointestinal and kidney function, and abnormalities of the myocardium with conduction defects, increased automaticity producing both supraventricular and ventricular tachyarrhythmias, and a sensitivity to digitalis. A low extracellular potassium level is synergistic with digitalis and enhances ectopic pacemaker activity.

Actions

1. Potassium administration initially enhances and then depresses conduction velocity and the excitability of the heart.
2. Potassium administration also depresses ectopic impulse generation by suppressing automaticity and adds to the depression of A-V conduction produced by digitalis. It is important to remember that the effects of potassium administration relate critically to the speed of administration, the preexisting potassium level, and the ratio of intracellular and extracellular potassium concentrations.

Uses, preparations, and administration

1. For patients receiving both digitalis and thiazide therapy, the routine prophylactic use of potassium salts orally in doses of 1 to 2 gm four times daily has been recommended. More commonly used potassium chloride is available in 300 and 500 mg as well as 1 gm tablets. Liquid potassium chloride does not produce the small-bowel ulcers attributed primarily to potassium-coated diuretics.
2. In severe potassium depletion or in the treatment of arrhythmias secondary to digitalis toxicity, potassium chloride should be given IV in a dosage of 30 to 60 mEq initially, administered in 500 to 1000 ml of 5% glucose in water at a rate of about 0.5 mEq per minute during close observation. Potassium administration will often correct arrhythmias caused by digitalis intoxication, even in the presence of normal serum levels of potassium.
3. Since sodium chloride (salt) restriction may be imposed on the patient with chronic heart failure, it is important that a source of chloride be made available to him. This can be accomplished with potassium chloride. Potassium can be found in some "salt substitutes," bananas, and citrus fruits or drinks.
4. Potassium salts are indicated in the treatment of those conditions producing hypokalemia, as described previously. Furthermore, potassium may effectively suppress ectopic activity not caused by digitalis excess.

Side effects and toxicity

1. Rapid potassium infusion produces bradycardia, depression of pacemakers, and slowing of conduction to the point of block.
2. Adverse symptoms reported with potassium therapy are nausea, vomiting, diarrhea, and abdominal discomfort.
3. Hyperkalemia may occur following administration of potassium salts, especially in patients with impaired renal function. This is recognized by unexplained lassitude, weakness, paresthesias of the extremities, decreased blood pressure, and ECG changes (Fig. 6-73). Cardiac arrhythmias, from heart block to cardiac arrest, may occur because of ventricular fibrillation or ventricular asystole.
4. ECG manifestations of hyperkalemia include a narrowed, peaked T wave and a shortened Q-T interval. The QRS complex may widen as toxicity increases; the P-R interval may lengthen and the P wave may diminish in size or disappear. The S-T segment may shift. Hypokalemia decreases T wave amplitude, depresses the S-T segment and creates prominent U waves. The duration of the Q-T interval (measured to the end of the T, not the U, wave) does not increase; the duration of the QRS complex increases slightly, whereas the duration of the Q-U interval increases prominently. (See Figs. 6-73 and 6.74.)

Precautions

1. Potassium should be administered cautiously, since a potassium-depleted myocardium is unusually sensitive to sudden increases in potassium concentration.
2. Potassium administration to normokalemic patients in an attempt to control digitalis-induced premature systoles is potentially dangerous because potassium intoxication may ensue. Furthermore, the effect is transient, and termination of the infusion may allow arrhythmias to begin again.
3. Rapid infusion of potassium chloride may cause burning or pain at the infusion site.
4. When electrolyte alterations are expected, ECG monitoring often reveals early manifestations of the anticipated change.
5. Rapid IV potassium replacement only to the point of normal serum potassium levels in patients with very low potassium levels may dangerously suppress impulse formation and conduction.

Contraindications

1. The presence of second-degree A-V block is generally a contraindication for the use of potassium salts. However, in patients manifesting digitalis-induced atrial tachycardia with A-V block, cautious potassium administration may slow the atrial rate and restore sinus rhythm without worsening the A-V block. Similarly, when digitalis has produced first-degree A-V block and premature systoles, cautious administration of potassium may suppress the premature systoles without advancing the A-V conduction disturbance.

2. Potassium is contraindicated in patients having severe renal impairment with oliguria or azotemia, untreated Addison's disease, acute dehydration, heat cramps, acidosis, and hyperkalemia from any cause.

EDROPHONIUM CHLORIDE (TENSILON)

Edrophonium chloride is a short-acting cholinergic drug with a rapid onset of action.

Actions

1. Edrophonium chloride inhibits or inactivates acetylcholinesterase at sites of cholinergic transmission. Consequently, its cardiac effects result from accumulation of acetylcholine at the myoneural junction, which potentiates the action of the vagus. This results in bradycardia and a decrease in strength of contraction, resulting in a fall in cardiac output. At the same time, the effective refractory period of atrial muscle fibers is shortened, and the refractory period and conduction time of the specialized conducting tissue in the A-V node are increased.
2. After injection, edrophonium chloride's effect is manifest within 30 to 60 seconds and lasts a few moments.

Use. Edrophonium chloride may be used to treat attacks of paroxysmal supraventricular tachycardias that are unresponsive to carotid sinus massage, gagging, or Valsalva's maneuver.

Preparation and administration. Edrophonium chloride injection is available in ampules containing 10 mg per milliliter and the entire dose is usually given as an IV bolus. A test dose of 3 to 5 mg IV may be given initially. A continuous infusion of 0.25 to 2.0 mg per minute edrophonium may provide a titratable, longer-lasting effect.

Side effects and toxicity. Toxicity resulting from overdosage of a reversible agent such as edrophonium chloride usually persists for only a matter of minutes. Momentary side effects include nausea, perspiration, salivation, bronchiolar spasm, slow pulse, and hypotension.

ATROPINE

Atropine is a drug that inhibits the actions of acetylcholine and is used in cardiology for the treatment of certain arrhythmias and conduction defects.

Cardiovascular actions. Atropine blocks vagal stimulation of the heart, which results in:

1. Increased discharge rate of the S-A node.
2. Shortened refractory period and increased speed of conduction through the A-V node.

Uses

1. Atropine therapy is indicated when increased vagal tone contributes to the production of *symptomatic* sinus bradycardia, for example, occurring in early acute myocardial infarction.
2. In certain cases of partial heart block, such as A-V Wenckebach, in which vagal activity may be an etiologic factor, atropine frequently lessens the degree of block.

3. Atropine may be given with morphine to counteract vagomimetic effects of the latter.

Preparations and administration. Initial atropine dose administered IV should be in the range of 0.5 mg. Generally the dose should then be titrated by increments of 0.3 to 0.5 mg to a total of 2.0 mg, or until the desired effect is achieved. Atropine may be administered IM to produce a less intense but longer-lasting effect; 1 mg IV may be roughly comparable in peak effects to 2 mg IM. However, it should be remembered that even 2 mg IM may elicit an initial vagomimetic effect. Similarly, smaller doses given IM or subcutaneously may provoke a transient slowing of heart rate that does not occur when the drug is administered rapidly IV.

Side effects and toxicity

1. When only one or two doses of atropine are given, there are few complications. After atropine administration, inability to void is common for several hours, particularly in older men who have prostatic enlargement.
2. Other side effects include dryness of mouth and skin, flushing, and dilation of pupils.
3. Mental confusion and acute glaucoma are uncommon unless large and repeated doses are administered. Elderly patients appear more prone to developing these side affects.
4. Reduction in bronchial secretions may lead to pulmonary complications.
5. Less commonly, premature ventricular systoles or ventricular tachycardia may accompany the increased heart rate produced by atropine in patients with myocardial infarction.

Precautions. The side effects noted occur more commonly with repeated doses of atropine. Therefore prolonged administration must be undertaken cautiously.

NITROGLYCERIN (GLYCERYL TRINITRATE)

Nitroglycerin is a rapidly acting nitrate and, therefore, the drug of choice for treating angina pectoris.

Action. The most important pharmacologic action of nitroglycerin relates to its relaxing effect on the vascular smooth muscle. This vasodilating effect reduces vascular resistance and blood pressure to decrease the work load of the heart. Larger coronary vessels dilate, but coronary resistance does not alter significantly in patients with angina pectoris, and coronary blood flow may actually *decrease* in parallel with the reduced blood pressure.

Several theories have been advanced to explain the action of nitroglycerin in the relief of angina pectoris. Two major concepts are stated here: (1) Studies have demonstrated that nitroglycerin increases both collateral coronary flow and myocardial Po_2 in the ischemic areas of the myocardium. This effect probably occurs either through selective vasodilation of collateral vessels bypassing areas of constriction or through alternation of the mechanical factors exerted on them by the heart muscle so as to reduce their resistance to flow. (2) Nitroglycerin improves the oxygenation of the myocardium by its peripheral vascular actions. Dilation of the veins with pooling of blood in the venous system may reduce heart size and decrease the diastolic filling pressure of the ventricles, thereby reducing oxygen consumption. Peripheral arteriolar dilation also reduces ventricular work and oxygen consumption.

Use. Nitroglycerin is useful in the treatment of angina pectoris but generally does not relieve the prolonged pain of acute myocardial infarction. Nitroglycerin-induced hypotension should be avoided in patients with an acute myocardial infarction. Preventive use of nitroglycerin can often be even more valuable than treatment of the actual anginal attack. Since angina often follows a recurring pattern, the prophylactic use of nitroglycerin tablets taken *before* precipitating events such as climbing stairs or sexual intercourse or taken *after* "heavy meals" may completely forestall feared attacks.

Nitroglycerin has also been used recently as a vasodilator agent to provide afterload reduction in patients with severe congestive heart failure. In this setting, it may be given sublingually or IV.

Preparation, dose, and administration. Nitroglycerin is available in tablets of 0.2, 0.4, and 0.6 mg. The usual sublingual dose is 0.4 mg; the smallest effective dose appears preferable. When taken sublingually, the drug appears in the blood in about 2 minutes; peak blood level is reached in 4 minutes; the effect begins to disappear in 10 minutes and is virtually dissipated within 30 minutes. Most anginal episodes are relieved within 2 to 3 minutes. Fall in blood pressure occurs in 1 to 5 minutes after administration and maximum fall occurs in 5 to 10 minutes. There is a return to initial blood pressure readings within 15 to 40 minutes.

If ischemic pain is not relieved in 3 to 5 minutes, the dose may be repeated. If pain persists after 3 or more tablets have been taken, the physician should be notified. Unusually severe or "different" chest pain should provoke a prompt call to the doctor or trip to the emergency room. However, some patients take as many as 30 or more tablets a day without harm. Headache is frequently the limiting factor.

Side effects. The vasodilating action of nitroglycerin causes side effects. Headache, hypotension, flushing of the skin, nausea and vomiting, and vertigo may appear. Patients vulnerable to vascular headaches may not tolerate therapeutic doses of nitroglycerin. Such individuals may improve tolerance by taking aspirin to raise their headache threshold.

Tolerance. Tolerance to long-acting nitroglycerin compounds may begin to appear within a few days and is well established within a few weeks. Tolerance to nitrate-induced headache is generally more prominent than tolerance to its other effects. However, tolerance may be broken by stopping administration temporarily, thereby making the patient more susceptible to the effects of the drug. Fortunately, in patients taking nitroglycerin sublingually to terminate or prevent angina pectoris, the development of tolerance is rarely a problem and patients should be encouraged to use the nitroglycerin liberally.

They should be told that the drug is not habit-forming and be advised to use it at the very onset of chest *discomfort,* not just chest *pain,* including tightness, pressure, fullness, "indigestion," and so forth.

Precautions (patient teaching). To ensure the effectiveness of this drug, certain precautions are observed. Patients must realize the importance of holding the tablet beneath their tongue until absorbed. The failure of some patients to respond has been related to swallowing the pill. Fresh tablets produce a tingling sensation beneath the tongue. Since the drug has a hypotensive effect, especially when the patient is in an erect position, he should be instructed to take the medication in a supine or sitting position, *particularly if taking more than one tablet.* During hospitalization patients with angina must be instructed to carry pills with him whenever he leaves the ward for tests or therapy.

Nitroglycerin deteriorates rapidly when exposed to air, light, or heat; consequently, it should be kept in a tightly sealed brown glass bottle and protected from heat, particularly the warmth of an inside pocket. Fresh tablets should be procured every 4 to 6 months. The patient should store his supply in a cool, dark place, carrying only a few tablets with him. These tablets should be easily available and taken *promptly* at the earliest sense of chest discomfort, for nitroglycerin is more effective at this early stage than at the height of pain.

Recent tests showed less than 5% loss of potency for tablets stored at room temperature in tightly sealed clear or amber glass vials for 201 days. Storage in strip-packaging polystyrene vials or pill boxes each demonstrated increased loss of potency. Improved manufacturing of some brands assumes stability and uniform potency.

DIAZEPAM (VALIUM)

Action. Diazepam depresses the central nervous system, producing drowsiness, sleep, and amnesia.

Cardiovascular uses. Diazepam provides effective relaxation and amnesia for elective cardioversion. As with the short-acting barbiturates, the onset of action is within 3 minutes of administration. However, diazepam prolongs the prompt recovery from anesthesia noted with short-acting barbiturates.

Dosage. Incremental IV doses of 2.5 to 5.0 mg at 30-second intervals are used for an average dose of 10 to 15 mg. This dosage is reduced if heart failure, hypotension, or liver disease is present.

Precautions

1. As with barbiturates, increased cough reflex and laryngospasm may occur.
2. Compared with barbiturates, diazepam administration lacks a distinct end point: speech becomes slurred but the patient is easily aroused and still responds to verbal commands. He frequently cries out and clutches his chest at the moment of shock, since pain is perceived. Amnesia prevents recollection of this event.
3. Diazepam is contraindicated in patients with glaucoma.

SODIUM BICARBONATE (NaHCO₃)

Action and use. Sodium bicarbonate is an inorganic buffer used to correct metabolic acidosis, which may be produced by ventricular fibrillation or cardiac arrest, as well as by other causes.

Preparation and administration. Sodium bicarbonate is available in 44 mEq per vial or 500 ml IV bottle; during a cardiac arrest, 3 to 5 vials are given initially if the patient is not immediately resuscitated and 1 vial is given every 5 minutes until effective cardiorespiratory action is restored. Blood gas and pH are monitored and subsequent doses of sodium bicarbonate are adjusted accordingly.

Precautions

1. Treatment of acidosis with alkaline infusions does not alter the underlying defect causing the acidosis, such as perfusion failure.
2. Overdosage may produce a metabolic alkalosis.
3. Large amounts of sodium administration may worsen the congestive heart failure frequently seen in these patients.

GLUCAGON

Glucagon is a pancreatic hormone that, in small amounts, helps regulate hepatic glycogen metabolism. Large amounts exert inotropic and chronotropic effects on the myocardium.

Action. Glucagon increases heart rate, decreases A-V conduction time, and augments cardiac contractility. The latter effect results even after full digitalization, catecholamine depletion, or beta adrenergic receptor blockade. Myocardial oxygen consumption and coronary blood flow also increase. Glucagon reportedly produces less arrhythmia than isoproterenol, but its positive inotropic effect is less than that produced by isoproterenol, especially in the failing heart. Doses that produce effective cardiac stimulation usually initiate nausea and vomiting.

Uses. Glucagon is used as an adjunct to conventional therapy for treating patients with intractable congestive heart failure, cardiogenic shock, or myocardial depression and to reverse bradycardia and myocardial depression caused by beta adrenergic receptor blocking agents.

Administration

1. Dissolve glucagon in 5% dextrose and water. Administer at a dose of 2.5 to 15 mg per hour IV.
2. Investigational for cardiac uses; little testing done now, primarily because of side effect 9 following.

Side effects and toxicity

1. Arrhythmias.
2. Nausea and vomiting.
3. Hypokalemia.
4. Hyperglycemia; secondary hypoglycemia may result.

5. Contraindicated in patients with pheochromocytoma.
6. Contraindicated in patients with uncontrolled arrhythmias.
7. Starting dose reduced by one tenth in patients receiving monamine oxidase inhibitor.
8. Glucagon may have adverse effects in the patient with hypovolemia. The latter should be corrected prior to glucagon administration.
9. Gel-like particles with characteristics resembling glucagon have been found in the lungs of dogs receiving the drug for long periods.
10. Enhances the anticoagulant effects of warfarin.

DOPAMINE (INTROPIN)

Dopamine is the immediate precursor in the enzymatic synthesis of norepinephrine in the body.

Actions

1. Increases myocardial contractility by a beta adrenergic receptor stimulating action and by norepinephrine release.
2. Produces mild vasoconstriction, predominantly in skeletal muscle by an alpha adrenergic receptor stimulating effect.
3. Increases cardiac output and stroke volume.
4. Directly dilates mesenteric and renal vessels to increase blood flow. Increased diuresis and natriuresis results in patients with congestive heart failure.

Uses. Dopamine can correct hemodynamic imbalance present in the shock syndrome and chronic cardiac decompensation, as in congestive heart failure and is particularly useful in light of the following characteristics.

1. Superior to isoproterenol when peripheral vascular resistance is low, since dopamine in larger doses increases peripheral vascular resistance.
2. May be useful when digitalis administration is contraindicated.
3. May avoid the tachycardia associated with isoproterenol administration.
4. May produce less myocardial oxygen consumption than isoproterenol.

Administration. Dissolve 1 ampule (5 ml, 200 mg) into 250 ml (800 μg per milliliter) or into 500 ml (400 μg per milliliter) of normal saline solution or 5% dextrose in water. Begin with 2 to 5 μg per kilogram per minute. Seriously ill patients may require up to 20 to 50 μ per kilogram per minute.

Contraindications and precautions

1. Contraindicated in patients with pheochromocytoma.
2. Contraindicated in patients with uncontrolled arrhythmias.
3. Reduced dosage in patients receiving monamine oxidase inhibitors.
4. Inactivated if added to an alkaline solution.
5. Correct hypovolemia prior to drug administration.

Side Effects

1. Ectopic arrhythmias
2. Nausea and vomiting.
3. Anginal pain

4. Dyspnea
5. Headache
6. Hypotension

DOBUTAMINE (DOBUTREX)

Dobutamine is a synthesized sympathomimetic amine derived by modifying isoproterenol's chemical structure to reduce its chronotropic, arrhythmogenic, and vascular side effects.

Actions

1. Increases myocardial contractility by a direct stimulatory action on $beta_1$ adrenergic cardiac receptors.
2. Stimulates alpha and $beta_2$ vascular receptors only slightly.
3. Exerts less than one fourth of the chonotropic effect of isoproterenol at equivalent inotropic doses.

Uses. Dobutamine can be used to treat states characterized by cardiac decompensation, as in congestive heart failure or cardiogenic shock. Dobutamine appears superior to isoproterenol, since it does not result in vasodilation; it appears superior to norepinephrine, since it does not excessively elevate peripheral vascular resistance and arterial blood pressure. Dobutamine may be used to increase myocardial contractility without having an arrhythmogenic effect or producing a significant increase in heart rate; it does not act on dopamine receptors to cause renal and mesenteric vasodilation.

Preparations and administration. Dobutamine is infused IV at rates of 1 to 40 μg per kilogram per minute. It has recently been approved for clinical use.

HEPARIN

Controversy still exists regarding the benefits of anticoagulation in patients with acute myocardial infarction. Although anticoagulant therapy does not significantly affect clotting in the arterial system in a patient with an acute myocardial infarction, it is thought to prevent venous clotting complications and reduce subsequent thromboembolic episodes. Anticoagulants may decrease the incidence of venous thrombosis, pulmonary emboli, mural thrombosis, and systemic emboli. At the present time, anticoagulation is not generally a routine procedure in every patient with acute myocardial infarction, but it may be recommended for patients with (1) a large infarction, (2) a history of previous infarctions, (3) a history of previous thromboembolic complications, (4) congestive heart failure, and (5) complications requiring a prolonged period of bed rest. Since it is unlikely that intravascular clotting produces complications in patients with questionable or small myocardial infarction who are at bed rest for only short periods of time, anticoagulation is not recommended for those patients. Because a significant risk from major bleeding exists in patients receiving anticoagulant therapy, this therapy is contraindicated in patients with suspected or proved gastrointestinal tract lesions that are likely to bleed, liver disease, azotemia, severe hypertension, or any other disease predisposing to hemorrhage.

Low-dose heparin (5000 units subcutaneously three times daily) has been shown to reduce the incidence of venous thromboses in patients postoperatively and in patients with myocardial infarction. In a related study, patients anticoagulated with heparin (40,000 IU per day by continuous IV infusion for 48 hours) and then switched to sodium warfarin exhibited a decrease in the frequency of calf-vein thrombosis. When a policy of early mobilization was followed, critically important emboli did not occur in either anticoagulated or nonanticoagulated patients. In that study, it was suggested that anticoagulation may be reserved for patients with evidence of thrombosis of veins above the knee or patients who are confined to bed for more than a week.

Some studies indicate that anticoagulant therapy may reduce the mortality rate during the first 1 or 2 years after an acute myocardial infarction, when given on a long-term basis.

Actions

1. Complex, but heparin basically acts by retarding the formation of thrombin and fibrin. Onset of action is immediate.
2. Decreases platelet clumping.
3. Increases lipoprotein lipase clearing factor, which clears the plasma of postprandial lipemia.

Uses. Heparin is used to produce anticoagulation.

Preparations and administration. The heparin dose is determined by the clotting time, which is maintained between 25 to 30 minutes or two to three times the normal control clotting time, usually determined 4 hours after the last heparin dose. The anticoagulent effects of heparin may be reversed by administering protamine.

1. Heparin must be administered parenterally, subcutaneously, IM, or IV.
   a. *IV administration.* In a continuous infusion, heparin may be given daily in a solution of 20,000 to 40,000 units per 250 to 1000 ml 5% dextrose in water. A loading dose of 5000 units may be necessary to achieve an immediate effect. Heparin may be administered intermittently via a heparin lock secured in the vein in a dose of 5000 to 7500 units every 4 hours, 10,000 units every 6 hours, or 15,000 units every 8 hours, depending on the weight and response the patient.
   b. *IM injection.* An initial IV dose of 5000 to 10,000 units is recommended, followed by a dose of concentrated heparin solution, 20,000 to 40,000 units IM. The effects usually last from 8 to 10 hours but may last longer. This route of administration may produce bleeding into muscle and should generally be avoided.
   c. *Deep subcutaneous (SC) injection.* Initial dose of 5000 to 10,000 units IV is recommended, followed by a dose of 15,000 units SC every 12 hours. Smaller doses may be given more often: 5000 to

10,000 units every 6 to 8 hours. Care must be taken to avoid bleeding or bruising. A short narrow-gauge needle should be used. It should be cleared of the drug before administration and the drug should be given in a slow, steady manner. The skin is not pinched or rubbed after administration.

2. Sodium heparin is available in solutions containing 1000, 5000, 10,000, 20,000 or 40,000 USP units per milliliter. Respiratory forms of heparin contain a concentrated solution of heparin (20,000 to 40,000 USP units per milliliter).

Toxic effects

1. Hemorrhage.
2. Thrombocytopenia.
3. Rarely, hypersensitivity and anaphylactoid reaction.
4. Severe asthma, giant urticaria, rhinitis, lacrimation, and fever.
5. Heparin is contraindicated in patients with bleeding tendencies, suspected hemorrhage, threatened abortion, and so forth.

WARFARIN SODIUM (COUMADIN)

Action. Opposes the action of vitamin K in the liver to inhibit synthesis of prothrombin and other clotting factors. This takes 24 to 36 hours to occur.

Uses. Warfarin sodium is used to produce anticoagulation. Since it takes 24 to 48 hours to produce the desired effect, heparin is frequently started at the same time warfarin is given and the former is then stopped 24 to 48 hours later when the warfarin is producing an anticoagulant effect. However, existing data do not support the need for beginning heparin as the initial anticoagulant approach before the warfarin drugs begin to have effect.

Preparations and administration. Warfarin usually produced hypoprothrombinemia in 24 to 36 hours, with a duration of action that may persist 4 to 5 days. The administration and dosage of warfarin, as with heparin, must be individualized for each patient according to the particular patient's sensitivity to the drug as indicated by the prothrombin time. An initial oral dose of 40 to 50 mg for the average adult or 20 to 30 mg for elderly and debilitated patients is reasonable, followed by a maintenance dose of 2 to 10 mg daily. For patients with liver disease, a loading dose may not be necessary. The dose of warfarin is regulated according to the prothrombin time, which is maintained at about 25 to 30 seconds or 10% to 30% of normal. Vitamin K reverses excessive anticoagulation caused by warfarin sodium. Warfarin sodium is available as 2, 5, 7.5, 10, and 25 mg and also as a powder for the preparation of a parenteral solution.

Toxic effects. Warfarin, like heparin, may cause hemorrhage resulting from excessive anticoagulation. The following instances may be associated with increased risk of hemorrhage: pregnancy, prolonged dietary deficiency, hepatic and renal insufficiency, various gastrointestinal diseases, severe trauma of the head, surgery, hypertension, and other states. The patient receiving anticoagulants should be observed for signs of bleeding such as hematuria, excessive bruising, melena, purpura, hematoma, epistaxis, bleeding gums, or hematemesis. An electric razor may be preferable for shaving.

Precautions

1. Numerous factors alone or in combination may influence the response of the patient to anticoagulants. It is essential to obtain frequent prothrombin time determinations whenever medications are added or discontinued or doses are changed. The following factors are hypoprothrombinemic; that is they may be responsible for *increased* prothrombin time response: carcinoma, collagen disease, congestive heart failure, diarrhea, hepatic disorders, vitamin K deficiency, alcohol allopurinol, anabolic steroids, antibiotics, chloral hydrate, chlorpropamide, dextrothyroxin, diazoxide, indomethacin, diuretics, phenylbutazone, quinidine, quinine, salicylates, thyroid drugs, glucagon, tolbutamide, colfibrate, broad-spectrum antibiotics, methyldopa (Aldomet) and guanethidine (Ismelin). These drugs *enhance* the action of warfarin sodium. Warfarin sodium can also affect the metabolism of other drugs such as tolbutamide (Orinase) and phenytoin (Dilantin).

   The following factors may be responsible for *decreased* prothrombin time response: diabetes, edema, adrenocortical steroids, alcohol, antacids, antihistamines, barbiturate, chloral hydrate, cholestyramine, high vitamin K diet, diuretics, glutehimide, griseofulvin, meprobamate, oral contraceptives, paraldehyde, rifampin, and others. These drugs *attenuate* the action of warfarin sodium.

2. Oral anticoagulants pass through the placental barrier and the danger of fetal hemorrhage exists. Even if the maternal prothrombin level is in the accepted therapeutic range, fetal hemorrhage in utero may occur. Warfarin drugs may pass into the milk of lactating mothers and cause a prothrombinopenic state in the nursing infant.

Contraindications

1. Hemorrhagic blood states; recent or contemplated surgery of the central nervous system, eye, or traumatic surgery resulting in large open surfaces; active ulceration or overt bleeding of the gastrointestinal, genitourinary, or respiratory tracts; cerebral vascular hemorrhage; aneurysms; pericardial effusions; and subacute bacterial endocarditis are contraindications for the use of warfarin.

2. The prothrombin time of the patient receiving anticoagulant therapy must be monitored at all times, and the patient must be observed carefully for the development of bleeding tendencies, such as hematuria, bleeding gums, and purpura. In general, when use of the drug is stopped, dosage should be tapered over a period of a few weeks rather than abruptly terminating anticoagulation.

Sympathomimetic drugs

Drugs that mimic the action of sympathetic nervous system stimulation are called sympathomimetic. The hormones norepinephrine and epinephrine, which are secreted by the adrenal medulla, are sympathomimetic amines (also called catecholamines). According to Ahlquist's (1948) classification, sympathomimetic drugs affecting the cardiovascular system are subdivided by their action on peripheral nerve receptor sites. The vascular system has *alpha* and *beta* adrenergic receptors. Alpha receptors are contained in the smooth muscle structures of the blood vessels. Those drugs that stimulate the alpha nerve receptors are said to have alpha action. Systemic arterial vasoconstriction is produced by stimulation of alpha receptors. Beta receptors are contained in the myocardium and in the blood vessels of skeletal muscle. Beta receptors in the heart are called beta$_1$, whereas those in the smooth muscle of blood vessels are called beta$_2$ receptors. Drugs that stimulate beta nerve receptors are said to have beta action. Stimulation of the beta$_2$ receptors of blood vessels produces vasodilation, whereas stimulation of beta$_1$ receptors produces increased rate and force of cardiac contraction. Both alpha and beta receptors are found in other areas of the body as well.

Sympathomimetic amine action that affects the heart *rate* is called chronotropic. Sympathomimetic amine action that affects the *strength* of cardiac contraction is called inotropic. Drugs may have positive (increase) and negative (decrease) inotropic or chronotropic actions.

Most sympathomimetic drugs have combined alpha and beta actions, although one action usually dominates.

ALPHA ADRENERGIC RECEPTOR STIMULATING DRUGS (ALPHAMIMETIC)

Alpha adrenergic receptor stimulating drugs have a pure alpha stimulating action that produces peripheral vasoconstriction. This results in increased arterial resistance and arterial pressure and reduced venous return. Cardiac output remains unchanged or may be reduced. The pressor action (elevated blood pressure) may reduce the heart rate by reflex vagal stimulation and sympathetic inhibition. Most vascular beds constrict, reducing blood flow to the brain, kidneys, skin, and viscera. Coronary blood flow is usually not reduced. Generally, there is no place for pure alpha adrenergic receptor stimulating agents in the treatment of cardiogenic shock.

Methoxamine (Vasoxyl)

Action. Methoxamine increases blood pressure rapidly as a result of vasoconstriction and resultant increase in peripheral vascular resistance.

Cardiovascular uses. Methoxamine may be used to:
1. Reverse excessive hypotension caused by ganglion-blocking agents.
2. Treat patients in shock who develop a low peripheral resistance with a normal or elevated cardiac output.
3. Terminate paroxysmal atrial tachycardia by reflexly stimulating vagal discharge.

Administration. The usual dose is 10 to 20 mg IM or 5 to 10 mg IV. Doses should be titrated according to the observed response.

Side effects

1. Excessive dosage may produce headache, pilometer stimulation, and projectile vomiting.
2. Prolonged administration may reduce plasma volume (hematocrit rises), and patients should be observed for signs of hypovolemia.

Phenylephrine (Neo-Synephrine)

Action. As in methoxamine.

Cardiovascular uses. As in methoxamine.

Administration. The usual dose is 0.5 to 1.0 mg IV or 5 to 10 mg SC or IM. Doses should be titrated.

Precautions

1. Marked reflex bradycardia produced by phenylephrine may be blocked with atropine.
2. Use caution when treating patients having hyperthyroidism, slow heart rate, heart block, or myocardial disease.

BETA ADRENERGIC RECEPTOR STIMULATING DRUGS (BETAMIMETIC)

The drugs included here have a pure beta stimulating action. They produce arteriolar vasodilation, decreasing peripheral vascular resistance. Their effect lessens venous pooling, returning more blood to the heart. Furthermore, betamimetic drugs increase the strength of myocardial contraction and increase heart rate. These combined effects increase cardiac output. However, hypotension may result if the blood volume is reduced.

Isoproterenol (Isuprel)

Action. Isoproterenol stimulates beta adrenergic receptors to relax smooth muscle in the bronchi, skeletal muscle vasculature, and alimentary tract. Stimulation of beta adrenergic receptors in the heart increases heart rate and contractility. Isoproterenol lowers peripheral vascular resistance and decreases diastolic pressure. Positive chronotropic and inotropic cardiac actions and increased venous return raise the cardiac output. Systolic pressure may increase, whereas the mean arterial pressure may lessen. Myocardial oxygen consumption rises, and myocardial efficiency decreases.

Cardiovascular uses

1. In cardiogenic shock, isoproterenol may counteract intense vasoconstriction, causing perfusion failure, and may increase cardiac output.
2. Isoproterenol enhances pacemaker automaticity and facilitates A-V conduction during heart block to increase ventricular rate.
3. In bronchospastic lung disease and emphysema, isoproterenol may be useful to produce bronchodilation.

Administration. Isoproterenol may be given 10 to 15 mg sublingually every 2 to 6 hours; however, absorption is variable and unreliable. Also, one may use 0.5 to 4.0 μg per minute by IV solution. Dose is titrated according to clinical response. Oral preparations (to be swallowed) and inhalants are available.

Side effects

1. Arrhythmias such as sinus tachycardia, premature ventricular systoles, ventricular tachycardia, or ventricular fibrillation may result. When ventricular ectopic beats result from a slow heart rate, increasing the rate with isoproterenol may eliminate the ectopic beating.
2. In the presence of hypovolemia, hypotension may occur because of the vasodilating effect.
3. Headache, flushing of skin, anginal pain, nausea, tremor, dizziness, weakness, and sweating may result.

Mephentermine (Wyamine)

Action. Although mephentermine stimulates beta adrenergic receptors primarily, it has a weak alpha adrenergic receptor stimulating effect. Pressor effects last 30 to 60 minutes following subcutaneous administration and for 4 hours after IM administration. Increased strength of cardiac contraction may increase cardiac output and blood pressure. Peripheral resistance may increase in normal patients but decrease or remain unchanged in hypotensive patients. Cerebral and coronary blood flow and venous tone increase.

Uses. Hypotensive states.

Administration. Mephentermine may be given in doses of 10 to 30 mg SC or IM; IV dose is titrated according to desired effects.

Side effects. Similar to isoproterenol.

ALPHA AND BETA ADRENERGIC RECEPTOR STIMULATING DRUGS (ALPHA-BETA MIMETIC)

The following drugs have combined alpha and beta adrenergic receptor stimulating action.

Norepinephrine (levarterenol) (Levophed)

Action. Predominantly acts on alpha adrenergic receptors peripherally, increasing systolic, diastolic, and pulse pressures and total peripheral resistance. Centrally, it has betamimetic actions similar to epinephrine. Cardiac output remains unchanged or decreased because of the increased peripheral resistance and slowed heart rate. Reflex vagal activity slows the heart. Coronary blood flow and stroke volume increase, whereas renal, cerebral, visceral, and skeletal muscle blood flow diminishes.

Uses. Norepinephrine is used to treat hypotensive states, especially when the peripheral vascular resistance is low and the cardiac output is normal or slightly elevated. It represents one of the major drugs used in treating cardiogenic shock. Positive inotropic and chronotropic effects occur, but are less than those produced by epinephrine, probably because these effects are attenuated by the peripheral alpha adrenergic receptor stimulating effects.

Administration. A dose of 2 to 4 μg per minute of a solution containing 4 to 8 mg per 1000 ml in 5% dextrose in water is best administered in "piggyback" manner into an exisiting IV line. Titration of the drug controls the pressor response.

Side effects

1. Anxiety, respiratory difficulty, and transient headache may result.
2. Overdosage may cause severe hypertension with headache, photophobia, stabbing retrosternal and pharyngeal pain, intense sweating, and vomiting.
3. Many varied arrhythmias may be produced.

Precautions

1. Blood pressure should be monitored frequently. Systemic blood pressure should not be raised higher than the pressure necessary to restore effective perfusion.
2. The site of administration should be observed frequently. Extravasation of drug at infusion site may cause pain and tissue sloughing as a result of vasoconstriction. Local phenotalamine (Regitine, 10 mg) infiltration may prevent this from occurring.

Epinephrine (Adrenalin)

Action. Epinephrine acts directly on beta adrenergic receptors of the heart to increase heart rate and the force of myocardial contraction, as well as cardiac output. Stroke volume and coronary blood flow also increase. Small doses of epinephrine stimulate beta adrenergic receptors primarily (and lower blood pressure by their vasodilator action on skeletal muscle vessels), whereas larger doses activate alpha adrenergic receptors also. This effect elevates blood pressure and peripheral resistance, reducing blood flow to the skin and kidneys.

Cardiovascular uses

1. Initiate cardiac rhythm in cardiac arrest by its stimulating effect on pacemaker cells.
2. Lessen the degree of heart block, since conduction in the A-V node, His bundle, Purkinje fibers, and ventricle improves. In general, isoproterenol is preferable for this use.
3. Raise blood pressure in larger doses. However, norepinephrine is more frequently used for this purpose.

Administration. Epinephrine is given 0.1 to 0.5 mg SC; 1 to 8 μg per minute IV infusion, titrated according to patient response; 0.25 to 0.5 mg IV; or 0.25 to 0.5 ml of a 1:1000 solution intracardiac during emergency situations. Although epinephrine stimulates pacemaker activity, frequently simply stimulating an arrested heart with a needle will initiate spontaneous beating.

Side effects

1. Ventricular arrhythmias may result.
2. Such disturbing reactions as fear, anxiety, and tension may occur and aggravate symptoms in psychoneurotic individuals.
3. May precipitate angina because of the inability of coronary blood flow to meet the increased oxygen requirement of the heart.

4. May produce throbbing, headache, tremor, and weakness.
5. Renal blood flow, glomerular filtration rate, and sodium excretion are usually reduced after administration of epinephrine.

Precautions

1. Isoproterenol and epinephrine decrease the amount of cardiac work done relative to oxygen consumption (cardiac *efficiency* decreases). These drugs increase oxygen consumption by increasing the heart rate and degree of contractility.
2. Epinephrine has a number of undesirable metabolic effects, among which are an elevation of blood sugar and free fatty acid levels and increased body metabolism.
3. Prolonged administration of norepinephrine and epinephrine may damage the arterial wall and endocardium.
4. Acidosis reduces the effectiveness of many catecholamines.

Metaraminol (Aramine)

Action. Metaraminol has actions similar to those of norepinephrine but they are less potent and more prolonged. Vasoconstriction increases systolic and diastolic pressures, accompanied by a reflex bradycardia. The force of myocardial contraction also increases. In normotensive patients, reflex bradycardia prevents an increase in cardiac output. Atropine eliminates the bradycardia and cardiac output increases.

Uses

1. Treat hypotensive states from many causes.
2. Terminate supraventricular tachycardias by reflex vagal stimulation.
3. Serve (like norepinephrine) as one of the first drugs of choice when immediate blood pressure elevation is indicated (see Chapter 4).

Administration. Metaraminol is given 2 to 10 mg IM or 15 to 100 mg diluted in 500 ml in 5% dextrose in water and titrated IV according to the patient's response. Higher concentrations may be required for some patients.

Side effects

1. Reflex bradycardia may occur.
2. Ventricular arrhythmias may result.
3. SC injections may produce tissue sloughing.

ALPHA ADRENERGIC RECEPTOR BLOCKING DRUGS (ALPHALYTIC)

Some drugs block the effect of alpha adrenergic receptor stimulation, preventing arterial and venous constriction caused by alpha adrenergic receptor stimulating agents. In that respect, their action may be likened to beta adrenergic receptor stimulation of peripheral blood vessels.

Phenoxybenzamine (Dibenzyline)

Action. The effects of alpha adrenergic receptor blockade depend on the existing sympathetic tone; in general, blood flow to the brain and coronary vessels remains unaltered, whereas renal, splanchnic, skin, and muscle blood flow may increase because of a reduction of the sympathetic tone. Phenoxybensamine reaches a maximal effect within 1 hour, with a half-life of 24 hours. Beta adrenergic receptor stimulating effects remain unaltered.

Uses

1. Inhibit or reverse pressor responses resulting from epinephrine and other sympathomimetic amines. It may be useful for maintenance therapy and during operative removal of pheochromocytoma.
2. Increase vasodilation and tissue perfusion in the presence of emboli, hypertension, shock, and pulmonary congestion or edema.
3. In treatment of patients with cardiogenic shock, alpha adrenergic receptor blocking may counteract some of the alpha adrenergic receptor stimulating effects of agents such as norepinephrine or metaraminol.

Dosage. Phenoxybenzamine is given orally, 20 to 200 mg per day, or IV, 1.0 mg per kilogram of body weight, diluted in 250 to 500 ml of 5% glucose or 0.9% sodium chloride solution and infused over 1 hour.

Precautions

1. Loss of vasomotor control may produce hypotension and reflex tachycardia. A drop in blood pressure may occur during standing (postural hypotension). In patients who are *hypovolemic,* a sharp fall in blood pressure may result. Therefore administration should be slow and constantly observed. Blood or a plasma-volume expander should be available. Central venous pressure monitoring is helpful.
2. As compensatory vasoconstriction is blocked, the hypotensive effects of narcotics and other agents may be magnified.
3. Miosis, nasal stuffiness, inhibition of ejaculation, sedation, weakness, and nausea and vomiting may result.

Phentolamine (Regitine)

Phentolamine is another alpha adrenergic receptor blocking agent with properties similar to those of phenoxybenzamine except that its action is much more transient) it is poorly absorbed from the gastrointestinal tract, and it is therefore given IV in titratable doses of 5 mg. Also, it has direct cardiac and gastrointestinal stimulating effects.

BETA ADRENERGIC RECEPTOR BLOCKING DRUGS (BETALYTIC)

Betalytic drugs block the inotropic and chronotropic actions mediated by beta receptor stimulation. They may reduce cardiac output and may increase arterial resistance.

Propranolol hydrochloride (Inderal)

Description. Propranolol is a beta adrenergic receptor blocking agent that blocks the beta adrenergic receptor stimulating actions of catecholamines.

Actions

1. Propranolol decreases heart rate and cardiac contractility; it also reduces myocardial oxygen requirements. Some newer beta adrenergic

receptor blocking agents may have antiarrhythmic properties without depressing myocardial contractility.

2. Propranolol depresses automaticity of pacemakers to slow the sinus rate and suppress ectopic beating; A-V conduction time and refractory period are prolonged. Particularly effective in digitalis toxicity, propranolol also has a "quinidine-like" antiarrhythmic action.

Uses

1. Control the ventricular response to atrial flutter, atrial fibrillation, and atrial tachycardia.
2. Suppress ectopic discharge, particularly when caused by digitalis.
3. Treat patients with angina that is unresponsive to nitrates. The mechanism of this action is not completely understood but may relate to decreasing oxygen requirements of the heart.
4. Effectively prevent or reduce attacks of recurrent paroxysmal tachyarrhythmias such as PAT.

In addition, propranolol may be used in combination with other drugs such as nitrates, for patients with angina; quinidine, for patients with ventricular arrhythmias; and digitalis, for patients with supraventricular tachyarrhythmias.

Administration. Give 0.5 to 1 mg every 1 to 3 minutes IV (up to total dose of 3 mg) or 20 to 60 mg orally three to four times daily.

Side effects. Propranolol is a myocardial depressant. It should not be used in the presence of bradycardia or A-V block. It is contraindicated in congestive heart failure, since the patient may be dependent on catecholamine effects for stimulation of force of myocardial contraction. Since propranolol blocks the bronchodilator effects of catecholamines, it should be avoided in the presence of bronchospasm or chronic lung disease. Fortunately, propranolol does not block the positive inotropic action of digitalis, and its beta adrenergic receptor blocking effects can be reversed by sufficiently large doses of isoproterenol.

Available forms. For IV use and in 20, 40, and 80 mg tablets.

Investigational drugs. A variety of other beta receptor blocking agents exist, some with a less negative inotropic effect than propranolol. However, at the present time, these other drugs are for investigational use only.

New or investigational antiarrhythmic agents
BRETYLIUM TOSYLATE (BRETYLOL)

Actions

1. Interferes with the release of norepinephrine from nerve endings and inhibits the uptake of catecholamine into nerve endings.
2. Causes a release of norepinephrine from sympathetic nerve endings and from cardiac tissue. Particularly at high concentrations, effect in the latter predominates over effect in the former to block the release of norepinephrine.
3. Has a positive inotropic effect on the heart that enhances myocardial

contractility. The release of norepinephrine from cardiac sympathetic nerves is the cause of the positive chronotropic and inotropic effects of bretylium.

4. Equally lengthens action potential duration and effective refractory period of Purkinje fibers and ventricular muscle.
5. Raises the ventricular fibrillation threshold.
6. Does not block beta adrenergic receptor stimulation. In fact, myocardial action of circulating catecholamines becomes enhanced.

Uses

1. Bretylium is generally reserved for patients with serious, recurrent ventricular arrhythmias that fail to respond to conventional antiarrhythmic drugs such as lidocaine, quinidine, procainamide, propanolol, or disopyramide.
2. At the time of this writing, bretylium is still an investigational drug, but it should be approved for use shortly.

Side effects

1. Hypotension, particularly postural.
2. Initial hypertension often followed by hypotension.
3. In some patients, transient initial increase in arrhythmias, especially digitalis-induced arrhythmias.
4. Nausea or vomiting.
5. Parotid pain after long-term oral maintenance.
6. May interact adversely with other antiarrhythmic agents such as quinidine.

Preparation and administration

1. Give 5 mg per kilogram IV over a 15-minute interval or 5 mg per kilogram IM. In patients who do not respond to 5 mg per kilogram, 7 to 10 mg per kilogram may be given. The onset of antiarrhythmic action is relatively slow, and bretylium requires 2 to 3 hours to reach peak action, although some episodes of ventricular arrhythmias can be eliminated in minutes.
2. Alternatively, one can give 600 mg IM as a loading dose, with incremental doses of 200 mg IM every 1 to 2 hours until either the arrhythmia is controlled or total of 2 gm has been given.
3. Oral therapy appears to be in the range of 600 mg every 6 hours.

AMIODARONE (CORDARONE, ATLANSIL)

Amiodarone, a benzfuran derivative with an antagonistic effect on sympathetic nerve stimulation, is used clinically in Europe and South America. It has not been approved for general investigational use in the United States.

Cardiac actions

1. Increases action potential duration in atrial and ventricular muscle and in Purkinje fibers.
2. Prolongs the effective refractory period.

3. Slows sinus node discharge rate but does not affect normal automaticity of Purkinje fibers.

Uses. Amiodarone has been used successfully to treat atrial and ventricular tachyarrhythmias. It has been extremely effective in suppressing many arrhythmias refractory to conventional drugs. It is useful in tachyarrhythmias associated with the Wolff-Parkinson-White syndrome.

Preparations and administration. Amiodarone is available in 200 mg tablets and is administered in doses from 200 to 1000 mg daily. It is also available in IV form. It has an extremely long duration of action and can be administered in one or two doses daily. Some data suggest that its anitarrhythmic action may persist for several weeks after the drug is discontinued.

Amiodarone appears to be slowly and fairly well absorbed, although somewhat variably. Its metabolites become deposited in many organs. The half-life has not been determined, although it has been estimated that the body concentration has diminished by only 16% to 34% 30 days after the drug has been stopped. Such "body stores" may in part explain the persistence of amiodarone's antiarrhythmic effect for as long as several weeks after drug administration has been discontinued. The full antiarrhythmic effect of amiodarone may take days to weeks to occur.

Toxic effects. Amiodarone is generally well-tolerated but has notable potential side effects including the following:
1. Hyperthyroidism and hypothyroidism
2. Neuromuscular side effects such as ataxia or weakness
3. Skin discoloration
4. Corneal microdeposits occur in probably 100% of adults receiving the drug, but only interfere with vision in a small percentage of patients. These microdeposits are reversible following cessation of therapy.

APRINDINE (FIBORAN, FIBOCIL)

Aprindine, an antiarrhythmic agent with prominent local anesthetic effects, is available clinically throughout most of Europe and is being evaluated as an investigational drug in the United States.

Actions
1. Shortens action potential duration and effective refractory period of Purkinje fibers. In cardiac muscle fibers, action potential duration is only slightly reduced and duration of the effective refractory period is lengthened.
2. Prolongs conduction time in all cardiac tissue.
3. Depresses automaticity of pacemaker cells.

Uses. Aprindine has been used successfully in patients with both supraventricular and ventricular tachyarrhythmias, particularly those refractory to conventional antiarrhythmic agents. Aprindine has been effective in treating digitalis toxicity and is particularly effective in treating arrhythmias in patients with the Wolff-Parkinson-White syndrome.

Preparations and administration. Aprindine is available in 10 and 25 mg capsules with daily maintenance doses ranging between 50 and 200 mg in single or divided doses administered every 8 to 12 hours. Aprindine may also be given IV. It has a half-life of approximately 20 to 30 hours.

Aprindine is well absorbed and approximately 95% of the hydroxylated metabolites undergo glucuronidation in the liver. Sixty-five percent of aprindine and its metabolites is found in the urine, with the remaining 35% in the feces. Clinically the full antiarrhythmic effect of aprindine may not occur for several days. Hemodynamic studies reveal that therapeutic doses of aprindine mildly depress myocardial function.

Toxic effects

1. Neurologic side effects are common, are related to dosage, and include most often a tremor of the hand and fingers. Dizziness, intention tremor, ataxia, nervousness, hallucinations, diplopia, memory impairment, or seizures may also occur.
2. Infrequent GI side effects.
3. Cholestatic jaundice.
4. Agranulocytosis has occurred in association with the use of aprindine and is thought to be an idiosyncratic reaction, as opposed to dose-related toxicity. This complication is reversible if the drug is continued.

DISOPYRAMIDE (NORPACE, RHYTHMODAN)

Disopyramide has recently been approved for general clinical use in the United States.

Actions

1. Prolongs action potential duration and effective refractory period of Purkinje fibers, similar to the effects of procainamide and quinidine.
2. Lengthens conduction time.
3. Decreases automaticity.
4. Exerts a vagolytic effect.

Uses. Disopyramide has been used successfully to treat patients with a variety of supraventricular and ventricular arrhythmias. Preliminary data indicate that its efficacy is comparable to that of quinidine but disopyramide is generally better tolerated.

Preparations and administration. Disopyramide is available in capsules of 100 or 150 mg and is generally taken every 6 hours. An IV preparation is not available clinically in the U.S. Oral doses appear to be 80% to 100% absorbed. Most of the dose presumably undergoes hepatic degradation with some metabolites excreted in the urine. At creatinine clearances of less than 40 ml per minute, renal clearance of disopyramide is reduced. Disopyramide mildly decreases cardiac output and increases systemic vascular resistance.

Toxic effects

1. From 10% to 40% of patients report side effects resulting from anticholinergic activity of the drug, including dry mouth or urinary hesitancy. From 3% to 9% report urinary retention, constipation, blurred vision, dry nose, eyes, or throat.

2. Marked Q-T prolongation may occur at usual maintenance doses, and disopyramide may induce ventricular tachycardia or ventricular fibrillation, as has been noted with quinidine.

3. Disopyramide appears to exert a greater negative inotropic effect than does quinidine or procainide, and worsening of heart failure or hypotension may occur, particularly in patients who have preexisting heart failure.

ETHMOZIN

Ethmozin is a phenothiazine derivative synthesized in the Soviet Union, where it is available clinically. Clinical trials have begun in the United States using the drug on an investigational basis.

Actions

1. Shortens action potential duration and effective refractory period of Purkinje fibers.
2. Lengthens effective refractory period of ventricular muscle.
3. Increases the excitability threshold.
4. Prolongs conduction time.
5. Does not alter sinus node discharge rate or A-V nodal conduction when injected into the sinus node artery and A-V node artery in dogs.

Uses. Preliminary data indicate that ethmozin is very effective in suppressing supraventricular arrhythmias and somewhat less effective against ventricular arrhythmias.

Toxic effects. The drug is extremely well tolerated, especially by elderly patients, and mild gastrointestinal side effects or skin side effects have been noted in a very small percentage of patients.

Preparations and administration. Therapeutic doses of ethmozin are still being established. Preliminary data suggest that doses in the range of 600 to 1200 mg daily in three divided doses will produce effective antiarrhythmic action and will be well tolerated.

MEXILETINE (MEXITIL)

Mexiletine is a local anesthetic with anticonvulsive properties that is similar in action to lidocaine. It has recently been approved for clinical use in Europe and Great Britain and investigational studies in patients have just begun in the United States.

Actions

1. Shortens action potential duration and the effective refractory period of Purkinje fibers.
2. Depresses automaticity.
3. Prolongs activation time.
4. Suppresses a variety of experimentally induced arrhythmias.

Uses. Mexiletine is effective for treatment of both acute and chronic ventricular arrhythmias and has been shown to exert antiarrhythmic efficacy equal to that of procainamide.

Preparations and administration. Mexiletine is available in 100 or 200 mg capsules and is administered orally in maintenance doses of 200, 300, or 400 mg every 8 hours. An IV form is not available in the United States. It is rapidly and well absorbed in normal patients, but absorption is somewhat delayed and incomplete in patients with myocardial infarction and in patients receiving narcotic analgesics that retard gastric emptying. Mexiletine is eliminated metabolically by the liver, with less than 10% excreted unchanged in the urine. Mexiletine has only mild negative inotropic effects and only slightly depresses myocardial contractility.

Toxic effects

1. Neurologic side effects include tremor, nystagmus, diplopia, dizziness, dysarthria, paresthesia, ataxia, and confusion.
2. Gastrointestinal disorders consist of nausea, vomiting, and dyspepsia.
3. Presence of antinuclear factor and thrombocytopenia have been reported but do not appear to be common problems.
4. Cardiac side effects include hypotension, bradycardia, or exacerbation of arrhythmias.

TOCAINIDE

Tocainide is a primary amine analog of lidocaine that can be taken orally.

Actions

1. Decreases action potential duration and effective refractory period of Purkinje fibers.
2. Prolongs activation time.
3. Decreases automaticity of pacemaker cells.
4. Effective against a variety of experimentally induced arrhythmias.

Uses. Tocainide has been used primarily to suppress premature ventricular systoles that occur chronically in stable patients. More recently, it has been used in patients with recurrent ventricular tachycardia or ventricular fibrillation with good results.

Preparations and administration. Tocainide is available in 200 mg capsules and is taken in doses of 400 to 800 mg every 8 hours. It appears to be rapidly and well absorbed, with peak serum levels occurring 60 to 90 minutes after administration. Renal excretion of unchanged drug averages 40%. Presumably, 60% of the drug undergoes hepatic degradation. The drug is available in oral and IV forms.

Toxic effects

1. Gastrointestinal complaints are the most frequent side effects and include anorexia, nausea, vomiting, abdominal pain and constipation.
2. Neurologic disturbances have been reported and include tremor, twitching, headache, altered hearing, sweating, hot flashes, paresthesia, blurred vision or diplopia, nervousness, anxiety, and dizziness or light-headedness and appear more related to dose than do the gastrointestinal side effects. The drug is generally well tolerated despite this relatively long list.

VERAPAMIL (ISOPTIN, IPROVERATRIL, CORDILOX)

Verapamil, a papaverine derivative, is available clinically throughout much of the world and has recently undergone investigational studies in the United States.

Actions

1. Blocks the slow channel through which calcium and possibly sodium, under some circumstances, cross the cell membrane.
2. Verapamil appears to reduce the extent of experimentally induced myocardial ischemia or infarction in animals and these conditions occurring spontaneously in people.
3. Slows spontaneous sinus node discharge rate and prolongs A-V nodal conduction time.
4. Depresses myocardial contractility.
5. In isolated tissues, at low to moderate concentrations, verapamil exerts little or no effect on action potential amplitude or other characteristics of cells with fast response characteristics (atrial and ventricular muscle, His-Purkinje system), but suppresses activity in fibers with slow response properties (sinus and A-V nodes and other abnormal tissue).

Uses. Verapamil has been used successfully IV to terminate paroxysmal supraventricular tachycardias and to slow the ventricular response in patients with atrial fibrillation or atrial flutter. Given orally, the drug is less effective, but it has been used to control the ventricular response in patients with atrial flutter and atrial fibrillation and to prophylactically prevent recurrence of paroxysmal supraventricular tachycardia. It is also a coronary vasodilator and has been used in the treatment of patients with angina pectoris resulting from coronary heart disease. Verapamil has been less effective in treating patients with ventricular arrhythmias. It exerts mild antihypertensive effects. It is rapidly and nearly completely absorbed after oral administration in humans and appears to be primarily metabolized in the liver.

Toxic effects

1. Surprisingly, in view of the calcium blocking properties of verapamil, its hemodynamic effects in man have been relatively slight and can be ascribed to a mild negative inotropic effect.
2. In data reported from over 8000 patients treated with verapamil, the drug was very well tolerated, with adverse reactions reported in only 9% of patients, with 1% discontinuation of the drug. Adverse cardiovascular effects include bradycardia, transient asystole, hypotension, development of or worsening of heart failure, and development of rhythm disturbances.
3. Central nervous system problems were primarily headache and dizziness.
4. Gastrointestinal disturbances usually included constipation and nausea.
5. The drug should be avoided or used with caution in patients with sick sinus syndrome, A-V conduction disturbances, severe congestive heart

failure, or in combination with beta adrenergic receptor blocking agents.

Vasodilator agents
SODIUM NITROPRUSSIDE

Actions. Sodium nitroprusside administered IV, as with other organic nitrates, dilates arterial and venous vascular beds by a direct relaxation of the vascular smooth muscle. This results in venous pooling, a reduction of peripheral vascular resistance (afterload), and a decrease in both ventricular filling pressure (preload) and ventricular volume. Because of this effect, blood pressure is reduced, as is myocardial oxygen consumption; ventricular function is improved. Reflex sympathetic activity following hypotension may increase the heart rate and myocardial contractility, changes that tend to offset the hypotension and reduction in myocardial oxygen consumption. Vasodilator therapy, acting on the systemic arteries, allows the ventricle to eject a larger cardiac output by reducing the resistance to ventricular emptying. As the amount of blood ejected increases, the improved cardiac output maintains blood pressure despite the lowered systemic resistance, and tissue blood flow is maintained or improved.

Uses. Vasodilator therapy has been used for the treatment of low output congestive heart failure in myocardial infarction, mitral insufficiency, and severe refractory heart failure.

Preparations and administration

1. Sodium nitroprusside is given IV at beginning rates of 10 to 15 μg per minute with the infusion rate increased until the pulmonary artery wedge pressure or mean arterial pressure declines. A constant maintenance infusion rate is then determined by serially monitoring the pulmonary wedge and systemic arterial pressures.
2. Sodium nitroprusside is light sensitive and therefore all infusion apparatus must be shielded by opaque material.

Toxic effects

1. Hypotension.
2. Accumulation of thiocyanate, producing fatigue, nausea, muscle spasm, psychotic behavior and development of hypothyroidism.

Precautions. Administration must be monitored by measuring pulmonary artery wedge pressure and systemic arterial pressure continuously or very frequently, along with frequent determinations of cardiac output. Patients with pulmonary wedge pressures below 15 mm Hg usually are not improved hemodynamically and may develop tachycardia, hypotension, and diminished cardiac output. Patients with elevated pulmonary wedge pressure should exhibit a reduction in pressure without significant reduction of arterial pressure, if previously normotensive.

ISOSORBIDE DINITRATE (ISORDIL)

Action. Isosorbide dinitrate is an organic nitrate with a peripheral vasodilator effect.

Uses

1. In angina pectoris in patients with coronary heart disease.
2. In congestive heart failure to decrease the impedence to ventricular ejection (afterload) and diminish venous return (preload).

Preparations and administration. Available in 5 to 10 mg preparations, sublingual or chewable form. Isosorbide dinitrate is administered every 4 to 6 hours.

Toxic effects

1. Hypotension
2. Headache
3. Cerebral insufficiency
4. Cutaneous flushing

HYDRALAZINE (APRESOLINE)

Actions

1. Induces peripheral vasodilation
2. Decreases peripheral vascular resistance
3. Elevates heart rate, stroke volume, and cardiac output
4. Increases renal, coronary, and hepatic circulation

Uses

1. Vasodilator therapy for treatment of congestive heart failure
2. For treatment of hypertension

Preparations and administration. Hydralazine is given in 10 mg doses orally four times daily increasing by 10 to 25 mg per dose but not exceeding a total of 200 mg/day except for brief periods.

Toxic effects

1. Headache, nasal congestion, tachycardia, nausea, vomiting, numbness, and tingling.
2. In larger doses, fever, lupus erythematosus, and other reactions have occurred.
3. Reflex effects on heart rate and cardiac output may need to be countered by propranolol.

PRAZOSIN (MINIPRESS)

Actions. Prazosin induces peripheral arterial vasodilation, possibly a result of direct effect or alpha adrenergic receptor blockade.

Uses

1. Vasodilator agent for congestive heart failure
2. Antihypertensive agent

Preparations and administration. Usual beginning dose is 1 mg three times a day, increasing to 20 mg per day given in two to four divided doses.

Toxic effects. Prazosin can cause lethargy, lightheadedness, headache, mild nausea, and syncope.

NITROGLYCERIN

See page 350.

REFERENCES

Bellet, S., et al.: Intramuscular lidocaine in the therapy of ventricular arrhythmias, Am. J. Cardiol **27**:291, 1971.

Beregovich, J. et al.: Dose-related hemodynamic and renal effects of dopamine in congestive heart failure, Am. Heart J. **87**:550, 1974.

Bergersen, B. S.: Pharmacology in nursing, ed. 13, St. Louis, 1976, The C. V. Mosby Co.

Bernstein, J. G., and Kock-Weser, J.: Effectiveness of bretylium tosylate against refractory ventricular arrhythmias, Circulation **45**:1024, 1972.

Bigger, J. T., Jr.: Antiarrhythmic drugs in ischemic heart disease, Hosp. Pract., p. 69, Nov. 1972.

Conn, H. G.: Current therapy, ed. 27, Philadelphia, 1975, W. B. Saunders Co.

Day, H. and Baconer, M.: Use of bretylium tosylate in the management of acute myocardial infarction, Am. J. Cardiol. **27**:177-188, 1971.Disintegration and storage of nitroglycerin tablets, Med. Lett. Drugs Ther. **13**:13-14, Feb. 19, 1971.

Ebert, R. V.: Use of anticoagulants in acute myocardial infarction, Circulation **45**:903, 1972.

Frieden, J., Cooper, J. A., and Grossman, J. I.: Continuous infusion of edrophonium (Tensilon) in treating supraventricular arrhythmias, Am. J. Cardiol. **27**:294, 1971.

Gallus, A. S., et al.: Small subcutaneous doses of heparin in prevention of venous thrombosis. N. Engl. J. Med. **288**:545-551, 1973.

Goldberg, L. I., Hsieh, Y. Y., and Resnekov, L.: Newer catecholamine for treatment of heart failure and shock: an update on dopamine and a first look at dobutamine, Prog. Cardiovasc. Dis. **19**:327, 1977.

Goodman, L. S., and Gilman, A.: The pharmocological basis of therapeutics, ed. 5, New York, 1974, Macmillan Publishing Co., Inc.

Hurst, J. W., and Longue, R. B.: The heart, ed. 4, New York, 1978, McGraw-Hill Book Co.

Koch-Weser, J.: Serum drug concentrations as therapeutic guides, N. Engl. J. Med. **287**:227, 1972.

Lefkowitz, R. J.: Selectivity in beta adrenergic responses: clinical implications, Circulation **49**:783, 1974. (Editorial.)

Tuttle, R. R., and Mills, J.: Development of a new catecholamine to selectively increase cardiac contractility, Circ. Res. **36**:185, 1975.

Wray, R., Maurer, B., and Shillingford, J.: Prophylactic anticoagulant therapy in the prevention of calf-vein thrombosis after myocardial infarction, N. Engl. J. Med. **288**:815-818, 1973.

Zipes, D. P., and Troup, P. T., New antiarrhythmic agents, Am. J. Cardiol. **41**:1005, 1978.

CHEST PAIN

A reasonably large number of clinical problems, in addition to acute myocardial infarction, may have the chief complaint of "chest pain." To differentiate between myocardial ischemia and these other causes of chest pain requires a systematic evaluation of the patient's symptoms. This section will briefly describe several disorders that commonly have chest pain and must be differentiated from acute myocardial infarction. In addition, the production of chest pain by the postmyocardial infarction syndrome (Chapter 4) must be considered.

Pericarditis
Vascular disorders
    Dissecting aortic aneurysm
    Pulmonary embolism with or without infarction
    Pulmonary hypertension and nondissecting atherosclerotic aneurysms
Pulmonary disorders
    Spontaneous pneumothorax
    Pneumonia with pleurisy and bronchitis
Gastrointestinal disorders
Musculoskeletal disorders
Neurologic disorders
Anxiety states
Other self-limiting problems

Pericarditis

Nearly all patients with acute pericarditis have chest pain. This pain is often quite characteristic and at other times is not. It is usually sudden in onset and sharp in quality. The pain often begins over the sternum and may radiate to the neck and down the left upper extremity. Thus it mimics very closely the pain of acute myocardial infarction. The two disorders can usually be distinguished by a careful history. In acute pericarditis the pain is usually increased by deep breathing or by rotating the chest and may be somewhat relieved if the patient sits up and leans forward. In acute myocardial infarction the pain is not usually influenced by breathing, movement, or position. The picture of chest pain in acute myocardial infarction has been discussed in Chapter 4. Some other comparative features, however, are that the patient with acute myocardial infarction only rarely describes the chest pain as sharp or knifelike; more often it is described as a heaviness, pressure, burning, constriction, or an aching across the chest.

Pericardial disease may cause a compression of the heart, either by fibrosis of the pericardium or by accumulation of pericardial fluid. When fluid accumulates in the pericardial sac, the heart is unable to fill completely and the pressures in the systemic and pulmonary veins rise. Eventually cardiac output is decreased, and syncope may occur if these events transpire rapidly. This sequence of events is called *cardiac tamponade*. If the cardiac restriction results from fibrosis rather than fluid, it is called *constrictive pericarditis*.

Patients with cardiac tamponade or with constrictive pericarditis may develop an interesting physical sign called *pulsus paradoxus*. This paradoxical pulse, an exaggeration of a normal phenomenon, is defined as an abnormal inspiratory fall in systemic blood pressure. If the blood pressure drops more than 8 or 10 mm Hg during normal breathing, the inspiratory drop of systemic blood pressure is considered to be abnormal.

Another feature of pericarditis is the pericardial friction rub, although it is

Table B-1. Differential diagnostic features of pericarditis and myocardial infarction*

	Pericarditis	Myocardial infarction
Usual age at onset	15 to 35	"Coronary age," 40 to 65 years
Preceding upper respiratory infection	Common	Infrequent
Pain syndrome		
Onset	Sudden	Sudden
Quality	Sharp, stabbing, knifelike, infrequently squeezing	Predominantly pressure, squeezing, "viselike"
Severity	Moderate to severe, rarely described as agonizing, fear of death infrequent	Severe, frequently described as agonizing, fear of death typical
Site	Wide area over base and precordium	Predominantly retrosternal
Radiation	Infrequent down right arm, or to teeth or jaw	Frequent down both arms, goes to jaw
Movement	Aggravates pain	No effect
Pleuritic pain	Common	Rare in uncomplicated cases
Fever	Appears first day, runs erratic course, low grade	Rare in first 24 hours, gradual lysis, low grade
Pericardial rub	Appears first day with fever, wide distribution over chest, may persist 7 to 10 days	Appears after 24 to 36 hours, narrow area, frequently at apex, frequently transient, lasting 2 to 6 days
Heart sounds	Normal, except with effusion	Gallop sounds, murmurs may occur
Serum enzymes	LDH normal, SGOT rarely elevated, below 100	LDH and SGOT abnormal, SGOT frequently above 100
Roentgen studies	Heart may be dilated, pericardial effusion frequently present	Heart may be dilated, effusion rare, abnormal left ventricular pulsation

*From Bishop, L. F.: Pericarditis vs. myocardial infarction, Hosp. Med. 3:9, 1967.

not always present. This rub should be searched for with the patient in various positions—for example, sitting, leaning forward with the breath expelled, and on his hands and knees in bed. A pericardial rub occurs as the heart moves. The presence of a rub does not exclude the diagnosis of acute myocardial infarction, since up to 50% of the patients with acute myocardial infarction have transitory rubs at some time early in their course.

Other physical findings include distended neck veins (increased venous pressure) and tachycardia. It is often difficult to differentiate acute pericarditis from acute myocardial infarction. This is particularly true if symptoms appear in a previously healthy individual without clinical evidence of other systemic illness and especially if the patient is in the usual coronary age group. Table B-1 may be a helpful reference in making a differential diagnosis.

The ECG of acute pericarditis is characterized by elevation of the S-T

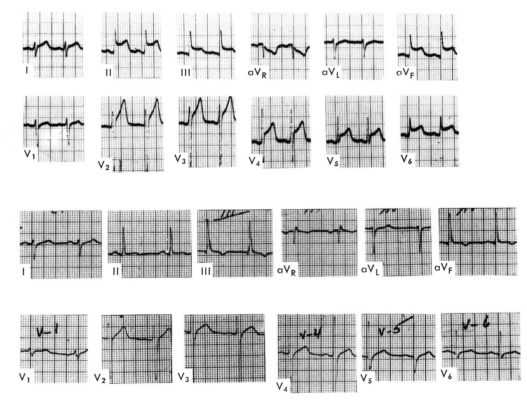

Fig. B-1. Acute pericarditis. In **A,** note S-T segment elevation in leads I, II, III, aV$_F$, and V$_1$ to V$_6$, indicating vector of S-T segment to be pointing inferiorly, slightly posteriorly, and laterally, toward the cardiac apex. In **B,** S-T segments have returned to normal and there is T wave inversion in leads II, III, and aV$_F$. Abnormal Q waves have not developed in any leads. This tracing is most compatible with acute pericarditis, which the patient demonstrated clinically. In addition to S-T and T wave changes, mean frontal QRS vector is to the right, at approximately +120 degrees.

segment (epicardial current of injury) in those leads reflecting the epicardial surface of the involved area. Ordinarily, pericarditis is a diffuse disease. Accordingly, the acute stage may show elevation of the S-T segments in two or three of the bipolar limb leads, unipoplar leads (aV_L and a V_F), and lateral precordial leads. This means reciprocal S-T segment depression in the leads facing the left ventricle usually does not occur; rather there may be depression of the S-T segments in leads V_1 and aV_R. See Fig. B-1.

After a few days or a week the S-T segment returns to normal, and the T waves become negative in leads I, II, aV_L,aV_F, and the lateral precordial leads. At this time the disorder is entering its subacute phase. It is important that this ECG be distinguished from that of acute myocardial infarction (Chapter 5). The Q waves that develop with acute myocardial infarction do not appear in patients with acute pericarditis. In the first few days of the attack the absence of reciprocal S-T depression in the limb leads is another indication of pericarditis. In acute pericarditis the T waves become negative only after the S-T segments return to the base line. In acute myocardial infarction the T waves usually become negative, whereas the S-T segments are still at least slightly elevated.

The chest x-ray film may show an enlarged heart shadow if pericardial fluid accumulates in the pericardial space. This same picture may also result if an associated myocarditis has produced cardiac dilation. Often, a pulmonary infiltrate accompanies pericarditis. Congestive heart failure with cardiac enlargement and pulmonary congestion may exhibit a similar picture.

Vascular disorders
DISSECTING AORTIC ANEURYSM

Excruciating chest pain is associated with dissecting aortic aneurysms. The pain is usually located in the anterior portion of the chest, lasts for hours, and is often of maximum intensity at the onset. It is described as developing suddenly with a tearing and knifelike quality. The pain tends to radiate into the thoracic portion of the back more often than that caused by myocardial infarction and may be felt predominantly in the back. It is not usually aggravated by deep breathing or turning. If the arteries of the abdominal viscera are involved, the pain may be located in the abdomen. Occasionally the pain appears to shift from one area in the chest to a lower portion as the dissection progresses.

The physical findings, which are compromised, are related to the aortic branch and may include a lower blood pressure in one arm than in the other, paralysis (central nervous system or spinal cord vessel involvement), the murmur of aortic insufficiency (aortic valve involvement), or pulsus paradoxus (leakage of blood into the pericardium). Since hypertension is commonly associated with dissecting aneurysm, the ECG may reveal the pattern of left ventricular hypertrophy. Usually no specific ECG changes are noted; however, the aneurysm may occlude a coronary artery, and typical infarct changes may be observed. X-ray examination usually shows widening of the aorta and occasionally a left pleural effusion.

PULMONARY EMBOLISM WITH OR WITHOUT INFARCTION

Most pulmonary emboli do not produce chest pain and that is probably why many emboli are not diagnosed. In contrast, however, the syndrome of massive pulmonary emoblization without infarction of the lung may occur with sudden crushing pain, simulating that of acute myocardial infarction. The diagnosis of pulmonary embolism is suggested by intense cyanosis, profound dyspnea, cough with hemoptysis, and tachypnea, whereas referred pain in the arms or jaw ordinarily indicates myocardial infarction.

When pulmonary infarction develops, pleuritis may be identified. The pain is located in the lateral portion of the chest in these patients and is aggravated by breathing.

Chest auscultation reveals a loud P_2 (second component of the second heart sound), decreased breath sounds, and rales or a pleural rub over the region of the involved vessel. The right ventricle may be enlarged, and a gallop (S_3) may be heard or a right ventricular or pulmonary artery impulse palpated. Pulmonic valve murmurs may be heard. If the embolus (emboli) is (are) large enough to compromise the circulation, the patient may be acutely ill, cyanotic, unconscious, and in shock. Another clue to the diagnosis of a pulmonary embolism may be the presence of phlebitis.

Classic ECG findings are present in only a small number of patients and are best observed soon after the embolic event. Sinus tachycardia with S-T segment depression of variable degree is common; in fact, the pulse rate is rarely less than 100 beats per minute following an acute pulmonary embolism.

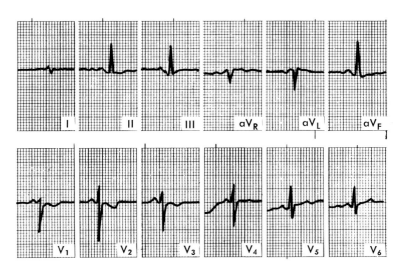

Fig. B-2. Acute pulmonary embolism. This tracing illustrates vertical axis with S wave in leads I and V_6. Inverted T waves in V_1 to V_3 are present. In an earlier tracing, lead III showed upright T waves and no Q waves. This tracing shows a flattening of T waves in lead III, plus a Q wave in leads II, III, and aV_F.

The ECG may reveal right axis deviation and an S wave in leads I and V_6. A terminal R wave in aV_R and V_1 may be seen, plus inverted T waves in V_1 through V_3. In addition, a Q wave in leads II, III, and aV_F may be present, which suggests a diaphragmatic (inferior) myocardial infarction (Fig. B-2).

PULMONARY HYPERTENSION AND NONDISSECTING ATHEROSCLEROTIC ANEURYSMS

Chest pain may occur in patients with pulmonary hypertension. In contrast to angina pectoris, this form of pain is almost invariably associated with dyspnea, which may be the dominant symptom. Severe pulmonary hypertension may occur with recurrent pulmonary emboli or pulmonary disease, with congenital and acquired heart disease, and as a primary idiopathic condition. Chest pain may also be a symptom of nondissecting atherosclerotic aneurysms that are compromising other chest structures.

Pulmonary disorders
SPONTANEOUS PNEUMOTHORAX

Sudden, tearing pleuritic pain located over the lateral thorax and associated with dyspnea suggests a spontaneous pneumothorax. The physical signs include hyperresonance and decreased breath sounds over the involved lung. The trachea may deviate and the mediastinal structures shift toward the side of the collapse in more severe cases. X-ray study shows the collapsed lung. The ECG is usually normal.

PNEUMONIA WITH PLEURISY AND BRONCHITIS

Inflammatory involvement of the pleura, secondary to underlying disease of the adjacent lung, is manifested by chest pain that occurs with respiration. Bronchial infections tend to produce mild substernal pain of a raw or burning quality, often associated with a sensation of pressure and usually accompanied by a significant cough. The ECG is often normal, and x-ray films usually confirm the infectious nature of the illness.

The patient demonstrates typical signs and symptoms of a respiratory illness.

Gastrointestinal disorders

Pain in the lower substernal area may arise as a result of inflammation of the esophageal mucosa or distention or spasm of the muscle layers of the esophagus. It may be gripping, squeezing, or burning in character and at times may be accompanied by regurgitation. Like that of angina pectoris, the discomfort may be precipitated by recumbency or by meals, but not by exercise. Esophageal spasm is often associated with hiatal hernia and may respond to nitroglycerin administration, thereby causing confusion in the diagnosis. Studies such as a cine-esophogram or esophageal pressure dynamics may be necessary to confirm this diagnosis.

Various abdominal disorders may cause chest pain with radiation to the shoulders and back. Cholecystitis can be mistaken for angina pectoris and myocardial infarction. Acute pancreatitis is more likely confused with acute myocardial infarction, except in mild conditions without shock. The hypotension that may occur with acute pancreatitis can produce a reduction of coronary blood flow with the production of angina pectoris.

Gastric or duodenal peptic ulcer may occasionally cause pain in the lower chest rather than in the upper abdomen. Appropriate x-ray and laboratory studies usually provide the necessary information in confirming a diagnosis. Although it is usually normal, the ECG may show nonspecific S-T and T wave changes.

Musculoskeletal disorders

Pain in the chest and arms can be produced by many musculoskeletal disorders. Examples are costochondritis, xyphoiditis, and cervical or thoracic spine diseases. In contrast to angina pectoris, the pain may last for seconds or for hours, and prompt relief is not afforded by nitroglycerin. Clues to a diagnosis may be revealed by x-ray examination or reproduction of the pain by appropriate physical maneuvers. Local infiltration of the involved areas with procaine, or patient response to systemic anti-inflammatory agents may confirm clinical suspicion.

Neurologic disorders

Chest pain can be produced by a variety of processes involving the intercostal nerves. The most commonly recognized of these conditions is herpes zoster (shingles), which usually occurs in older people. Shingles is produced by infection of the dorsal nerve root by a virus and is identified by the appearance of a characteristic vesicular rash in the area of discomfort. Neuritic chest wall conditions are usually dermatomal in distribution. The pain pattern is quite different from coronary pain, usually being unrelated to effort and lasting for prolonged periods of time.

Anxiety states

Anxiety states and other functional disorders producing chest pain are the most common cause of confusion with angina pectoris. The nature of psychogenic chest pain was described in Chapter 8. This presentation emphasizes the recognition of the cardiac neuroses. Clues to the patient's state of mind may come forth during the history recording. For example, the patient may relate the occurrence of chest pain to crowded places (claustrophobia). During conversation the patient may manifest sighing respirations (hyperventilation). Other differential diagnositc features of the patient's description of pain have been discussed previously. Hopefully, emotional states causing chest pain can be recognized and treated. If there is doubt or hesitation, however, on the part of the hospital staff in accepting the patient's complaint, or if the patient is emotionally insecure, the anxiety state may become aggravated, and the patient may be seriously disabled by a disorder that has no organic basis.

Other self-limiting conditions

Chest discomfort is a common accompaniment to acute viral illness such as grippe or influenza. On occasion such pain is quite severe, as in epidemic pleurodynia caused by coxsackievirus infection. The actual mechanism causing this type of pain is obscure and the clinician must rely on clinical judgment and occasionally on a period of observation to differentiate between these patients and those more seriously afflicted.

REFERENCES

Bishop, L. F.: Pericarditis vs. myocardial infarction, Hosp. Med. 3:5, 1967.

Freidberg, C. K.: Diseases of the heart, Philadelphia, 1966, W. B. Saunders Co.

Gefter, W. I., Pastor, B. H., and Meyerson, R. M.: Synopsis of cardiology, St. Louis, 1965, The C. V. Mosby Co.

Hurst, J. W., Logue, R. B., Schlant, R. C., and Wenger, N. K.: The heart: arteries and veins, ed. 4, New York, 1978, McGraw-Hill Book Co.

INDEX